Health Emergency and Disaster Risk Management

Health Emergency and Disaster Risk Management

Editor: Lawanna Boone

AMERICAN
MEDICAL PUBLISHERS
www.americanmedicalpublishers.com

AMERICAN
MEDICAL PUBLISHERS
www.americanmedicalpublishers.com

Cataloging-in-Publication Data

Health emergency and disaster risk management / edited by Lawanna Boone.
p. cm.
Includes bibliographical references and index.
ISBN 979-8-88740-169-0
1. Medical emergencies. 2. Disaster medicine. 3. Hazard mitigation.
4. Emergency medical services--Management. 5. Emergency management.
6. Public health. I. Boone, Lawanna.
RC86.7 .H43 2023
616.025--dc23

American Medical Publishers,
41 Flatbush Avenue,
1st Floor, New York,
NY 11217, USA

ISBN 979-8-88740-169-0 (Hardback)

Contents

Preface

Health emergency and disaster risk management (H-EDRM) is the intersection of health and disaster risk reduction (DRR). In recent years, H-EDRM research has emerged as an important interdisciplinary field. This field involves various aspects including emergency and disaster medicine, DRR, humanitarian response, community health resilience, and health system resilience. The public health prevention hierarchy consists of primary, secondary and tertiary prevention. These are the most essential public health principles which guide policy and program development. The objective of primary prevention is to prevent the onset of disease with strategies including health protection and health promotion. Health protection involves the establishment of policies, regulations and programs such as vaccinations, while health promotion is mainly concerned with health education and information sharing. This book unravels the recent studies in the field of health emergency and disaster risk management. It will serve as an invaluable resource for undergraduate and post graduate students, researchers and scholars.

This book is a result of research of several months to collate the most relevant data in the field.

When I was approached with the idea of this book and the proposal to edit it, I was overwhelmed. It gave me an opportunity to reach out to all those who share a common interest with me in this field. I had 3 main parameters for editing this text:

1. Accuracy - The data and information provided in this book should be up-to-date and valuable to the readers.

2. Structure - The data must be presented in a structured format for easy understanding and better grasping of the readers.

3. niversal Approach - This book not only targets students but also experts and innovators in the field, thus my aim was to present topics which are of use to all.

Thus, it took me a couple of months to finish the editing of this book.

I would like to make a special mention of my publisher who considered me worthy of this opportunity and also supported me throughout the editing process. I would also like to thank the editing team at the back-end who extended their help whenever required.

Editor

1

Sociodemographic Predictors of Health Risk Perception, Attitude and Behavior Practices Associated with Health-Emergency Disaster Risk Management for Biological Hazards: The Case of COVID-19 Pandemic in Hong Kong, SAR China

Emily Ying Yang Chan [1,2,3,*], Zhe Huang [1], Eugene Siu Kai Lo [1], Kevin Kei Ching Hung [1,4], Eliza Lai Yi Wong [3] and Samuel Yeung Shan Wong [3]

1 Collaborating Centre for Oxford University and CUHK for Disaster and Medical Humanitarian Response (CCOUC), The Chinese University of Hong Kong, Hong Kong, China; huangzhe@cuhk.edu.hk (Z.H.); euglsk@cuhk.edu.hk (E.S.K.L.); kevin.hung@cuhk.edu.hk (K.K.C.H.)
2 Nuffield Department of Medicine, University of Oxford, Oxford OX37BN, UK
3 JC School of Public Health and Primary Care, The Chinese University of Hong Kong, Hong Kong, China; lywong@cuhk.edu.hk (E.L.Y.W.); yeungshanwong@cuhk.edu.hk (S.Y.S.W.)
4 Accident & Emergency Medicine Academic Unit, The Chinese University of Hong Kong, Prince of Wales Hospital, Hong Kong, China
* Correspondence: emily.chan@cuhk.edu.hk

Abstract: In addition to top-down Health-Emergency and Disaster Risk Management (Health-EDRM) efforts, bottom-up individual and household measures are crucial for prevention and emergency response of the COVID-19 pandemic, a Public Health Emergency of International Concern (PHEIC). There is limited scientific evidence of the knowledge, perception, attitude and behavior patterns of the urban population. A computerized randomized digital dialing, cross-sectional, population landline-based telephone survey was conducted from 22 March to 1 April 2020 in Hong Kong Special Administrative Region, China. Data were collected for socio-demographic characteristics, knowledge, attitude and risk perception, and various self-reported Health-EDRM behavior patterns associated with COVID-19. The final study sample was 765. Although the respondents thought that individuals (68.6%) had similar responsibilities as government (67.5%) in infection control, less than 50% had sufficient health risk management knowledge to safeguard health and well-being. Among the examined Health-EDRM measures, significant differences were found between attitude and practice in regards to washing hands with soap, ordering takeaways, wearing masks, avoidance of visiting public places or using public transport, and travel avoidance to COVID-19-confirmed regions. Logistic regression indicated that the elderly were less likely to worry about infection with COVID-19. Compared to personal and household hygiene practices, lower compliance was found for public social distancing.

Keywords: COVID-19; urban; health risks; Health-Emergency and Disaster Risk Management; biological hazard; pandemic; PHEIC; Hong Kong

---

1. Introduction

The COVID-19 pandemic was considered a Public Health Emergency of International Concern (PHEIC) by the World Health Organization (WHO) on 30 January 2020 [1]. The SARS-CoV2 belongs to the coronavirus family, which is the same family as the severe acute respiratory syndrome (SARS) and middle east respiratory syndrome (MERS) viruses [2]. It was first reported as a cluster of respiratory illnesses in Wuhan, China, on 30 December 2019. As of 12 April 2020, there were 1,844,863 confirmed cases and 117,021 deaths according to the World Health Organization report [3]. The case-fatality rate resulting from SARS-CoV2 is believed to be around 1%–2% for symptomatic cases [4,5], and the proportion of asymptomatic cases of COVID-19 is much higher [6]. With a higher basic reproductive number than SARS and MERS, and the finding of viral shedding in asymptomatic patients [7], the total number of people infected and killed by COVID-19 exceeds SARS and MERS combined, even though it is less deadly than them [8]. As of April 2020, although more than 200 countries have reported confirmed cases and have implemented travel restrictions [9], social distancing [10] and other response measures to this PHEIC, the global COVID-19 epidemic is yet to end.

The Situation in Hong Kong and Past Experiences of Similar Pandemics

Figure 1 shows that on 23 January 2020, Hong Kong reported its first imported case of COVID-19 [11] and the first local transmission emerged on 31 January 2020 [12]. As of 14 April, there were 1013 confirmed cases [13]. As soon as cases were confirmed in Hong Kong, the Hong Kong government implemented various infection control measures (Figure 1a), including declaring emergency response levels in relation to COVID-19 infection [14], suspending class resumption for all schools and community services [15,16], and prohibiting citizen outdoor activities and gatherings [17–20]. At that time, there were a substantial number of confirmed cases of the epidemic (Figure 1b).

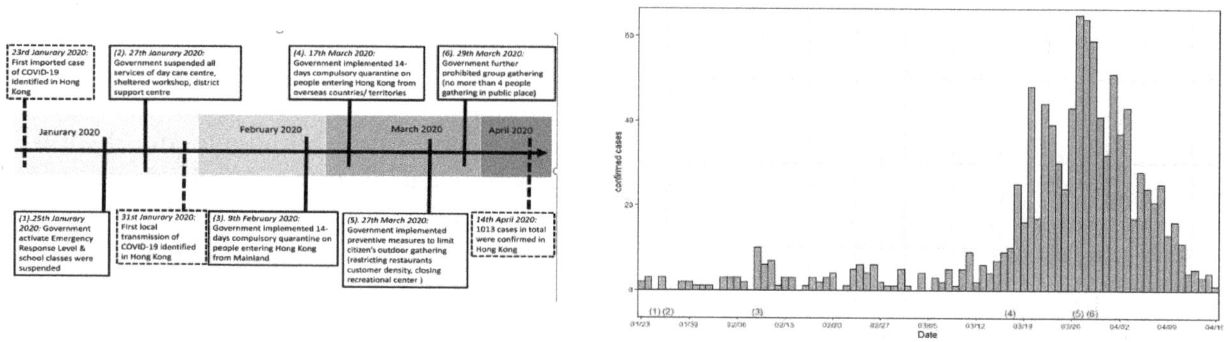

(a) (b)

Figure 1. (**a**) Timeline of the COVID-19 outbreak in Hong Kong and the preventive measures implemented by the Hong Kong government. (**b**) The confirmed cases in Hong Kong from 23 January 2020 to 16 April 2020. Note: (1) to (6) in Figure 1b correspond to (1) to (6) in Figure 1a.

The Health-Emergency and Disaster Risk Management (Health-EDRM) Framework provides a common language and a comprehensive approach for all actors in health and other sectors, to reduce health risks and consequences of emergencies and disasters [21]. Biological hazards, such as infectious disease outbreaks, are considered one of the major health risks for the human population. Besides top-down government efforts in infection control and management, efforts at the individual and household level also have crucial roles in bottom-up resilience of Health-EDRM for biological hazards. Currently, limited scientific evidence is available to understand patterns of knowledge, perception, attitude and behavior undertaken by urban populations for relevant disaster risk reduction programs and policy planning. Hong Kong, as an Asian metropolis in Southern China, has encountered various infectious disease outbreaks, like SARS [22] and avian influenza (e.g., H5N1 and H7N9) [23,24]. Its healthcare system has pre-existing policies and practices against emerging infectious diseases [25]. For example, wearing face masks, washing hands, and disinfecting living quarters for SARS [26], and avoiding contact with birds for the avian influenza [27], are examples of community bottom-up Health-EDRM practices for self-help and contribution to infection control. This study, using a population-based, computerized randomized digital dialing landline telephone survey, intends to examine and explore various primary Health-EDRM prevention efforts in the community through self-reported knowledge, perception and behaviors related to COVID-19 and various droplet borne-transmission control-related Health-EDRM preventive measures among the Hong Kong population [28,29].

2. Materials and Methods

2.1. Study Design and Study Population

A computerized randomized digital dialing (RDD), cross-sectional, population landline-based telephone survey was conducted from 22 March to 1 April 2020. The study population consisted of Hong Kong residents aged 18 years or above, including those holding valid work or study visas. Sample exclusion criteria included (i) non-Cantonese-speaking respondents; (ii) overseas visitors holding tourist visas to Hong Kong or two-way permit holders from mainland China; (iii) those unable to be interviewed due to medical reasons; and iv) non-institutional residents. For the sample size estimation, an assumption was made that 50% of the Hong Kong population were concerned about contracting COVID-19. A sample size of 750 participants was calculated with a 3.6% margin of error and 95% confidence interval.

2.2. Data Collection

The computerized random digit dialing (RDD) method was used for each of Hong Kong's 18 districts to randomly select a representative sample. Stratified random sampling was used to ensure the demographic representation of the general population in Hong Kong in terms of age, gender, and district of residence. This data collection method has been used for other similar local studies on infectious diseases [30,31]. Most of the calls were made during evenings (6:30 pm to 10:00 pm) to avoid an under-representation of the working population. An eligible family member whose birthday was closest to the survey date was invited to participate in the study. If the selected participant was busy at the time, up to four follow-up calls would be made before that number was considered unanswered. All telephone interviews were conducted by trained interviewers in Cantonese. Figure 2 shows that 765 eligible participants were recruited to account for missing values and increase the modelling flexibility.

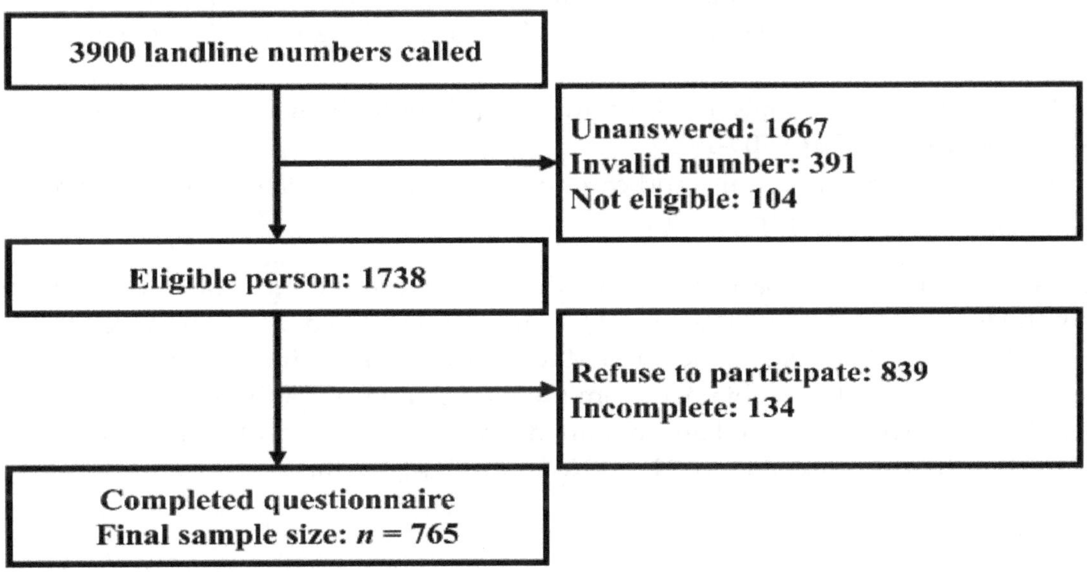

Figure 2. The algorithm of the final data collection.

2.3. Study Instrument

A self-reported structured Chinese questionnaire with 141 questions was designed on the basis of a literature review and previous research experience [27,30–34] on data collection. Information was collected on socio-demographic characteristics, knowledge, attitude and risk perception, and various behavior patterns associated with COVID-19. Sociodemographic information, current and preferred channels of information acquisitions were similar to a number of published study tools of human behavior in extreme events in the same context [30,35,36]. Questions related to "knowledge about COVID-19", "risk perception", "self-reported perception and Health-EDRM practices" and "caregiving", were adopted from previous studies [27,30,31]. A summary of the survey questions can be grouped into six major subgroups as follows.

1. Sociodemographic information was collected for age, gender, district of residence, household income, household size, marital status, education, size of housing, occupation and employment status.
2. Knowledge about COVID-19, including the transmission route, and the comparison between COVID-19 and other respiratory diseases.
3. Risk perception of Health-EDRM behavior associated with COVID-19, including the perceived impacts (e.g., physical, mental, social, financial and the whole impact), perceived sufficient knowledge to manage COVID-19, perceived severity and infectivity. Five-point Likert scales were used to measure the level of agreement or disagreement for the questions (from 1 to 5, 1 = strongly disagree, 2 = disagree, 3 = neutral, 4 = agree, 5 = strongly agree). The 6-item short form of the State-Trait Anxiety Inventory (STAI) was used for measuring their current anxiety level concerning the outbreak [32]. A binary question of whether the respondent was worried about getting infected with COVID-19 was asked.
4. Self-reported perceived usefulness and actual Health-EDRM behavioral practice of nine personal or household health emergency disaster risks management related behaviors and practices of COVID-19 prevention behavior. These include: (1) washing hands before meals and after toileting, (2) washing hands with soaps, (3) avoiding dining or gathering together, (4) using serving utensils, (5) ordering takeaways more often, (6) bringing one's own utensil when dining out, (7) wearing a mask when going out, (8) avoiding going to public places or using public transport, and (9) avoiding going to COVID-19-confirmed regions outside Hong Kong. The four-point Likert scale was used to ascertain the level of the practices (from 1 to 4, 1 = always, 2 = usually, 3 = sometimes, 4 = never).
5. Current and preferred channels of information acquisition, the information they were interested in and the awareness of COVID-19.
6. Questions about home quarantine and caregiving to non-suspected family members during the COVID-19 outbreak were also asked.

We focused on the general patterns of health risk perception, attitude and behavior practices associated with Health-Emergency Disaster Risk Management. Each interview took about 20–40 min. A pilot survey study ($n = 28$) was conducted in March 2020 to ensure interpretability and feasibility of the questions. Verbal consent was obtained from the participants and ethics approval and the consent procedure of the study were reviewed and obtained from the Survey and Behavioral Research Ethics Committee at The Chinese University of Hong Kong (SBRE-19-498).

2.4. Statistical Analysis

Descriptive statistics were reported for the study sample socio-demographic characteristics, awareness, perception and knowledge of COVID-19. Statistical association tests (Pearson's χ^2 test, Fisher's exact test, or McNemar's test) were conducted where appropriate. A binary variable of whether the respondent was worried about getting infected with COVID-19 was used as the dependent variable in logistic regression. Explanatory variables entered into multivariable logistic regression if the p-value < 0.10 in bivariate analysis. Apart from the worry, various community patterns and individual uptake of Health-EDRM behavior associated with COVID-19 as dependent variables were dichotomized for logistic regression ("always" or "usually" versus "sometimes" or "never"). The level of significance of the statistical test was 0.05. All statistical analyses were conducted by using IBM SPSS 21 (IBM Corp., Armonk, NY, USA) for Windows.

3. Results

The final study sample consisted of 765 respondents and a response rate of 44.0% (765/1738) (Table 1). The final study sample was comparable and representative of the population data in the Hong Kong Census 2016 [37] with respect to their age, gender, marital status and residential districts. However, the level of education and household income in our sample were higher than the population census.

Table 1. The respondent's socioeconomic characteristics and comparison with Census population data.

Demographics	2016 Population Census		Study Sample		p-Value [d]
Age	n	%	n	%	0.332
18–24	600,726	9.50%	71	9.30%	
25–44	2,228,566	35.26%	248	32.40%	
45–64	2,328,430	36.84%	303	39.60%	
65 or older	1,163,153	18.40%	143	18.70%	
Gender					0.425 [e]
Male	2,850,731	45.10%	356	46.50%	
Female	3,470,144	54.90%	409	53.50%	
Marital status					0.962 [e]
Non-married	2,523,742	39.93%	304	39.80%	
Married	3,797,133	60.07%	459	60.20%	
Residential district [a,b]					0.334
Hong Kong Island	1,120,143	17.2%	147	19.20	
Kowloon	1,987,380	30.6%	231	30.20	
New Territory	3,397,499	52.2%	387	50.60	
Education [a]					<0.001
Primary level or below	1,673,431	25.7%	61	8.00%	
Secondary	2,841,510	43.7%	330	43.30%	
Tertiary level	1,991,189	30.6%	371	48.70%	
Household Income [c]					<0.001
<2000–7999	378,451	15.1	66	9.3	
8000–19999	649,450	25.9	101	14.1	
20000–39999	699,450	27.8	191	26.6	
40000 or more	782,383	31.2	360	50.2	

[a] The Hong Kong population Census data additionally included age 15 to 17 years old. [b] Marine population was excluded. [c] The analysis was conducted with household data; only 718 households were available in our sample. [d] The χ^2 test was used to measure the overall difference between this survey and the 2016 Hong Kong Population Census data. A p-value < 0.05 indicates a significant difference. [e] The χ^2 test with continuity correction was used.

3.1. Perception of Various Health and Economic Impacts of COVID-19

Figure 3 describes the respondents' perception of various health impacts brought on by COVID-19. Although 94.4% (722/765) of the study respondents believed that COVID-19 had a large impact on their community, social health was reported as the most affected (72.0%). In addition, participants reported the role of government policy (68.6%) would be similar to the effort put in at the household or individual level (67.5%). However, although 63.9% (489/765) believed they had enough knowledge for regular communicable diseases (e.g., influenza), less than half of the participants (47.8%) reported that they had sufficient knowledge to manage the health risk and safety during the outbreak of COVID-19. After adjusting for age, gender, education, household income, and occupation, multiple logistic regression suggested that people aged 65 or above were less likely to be impacted by COVID-19 in terms of their mental, social and financial status, while people with less household income were more likely to be affected financially. In addition, females were more likely to report a large impact on their mental health, but none of the above sociodemographic variables were associated with the reported physical health (Appendix A Table A1).

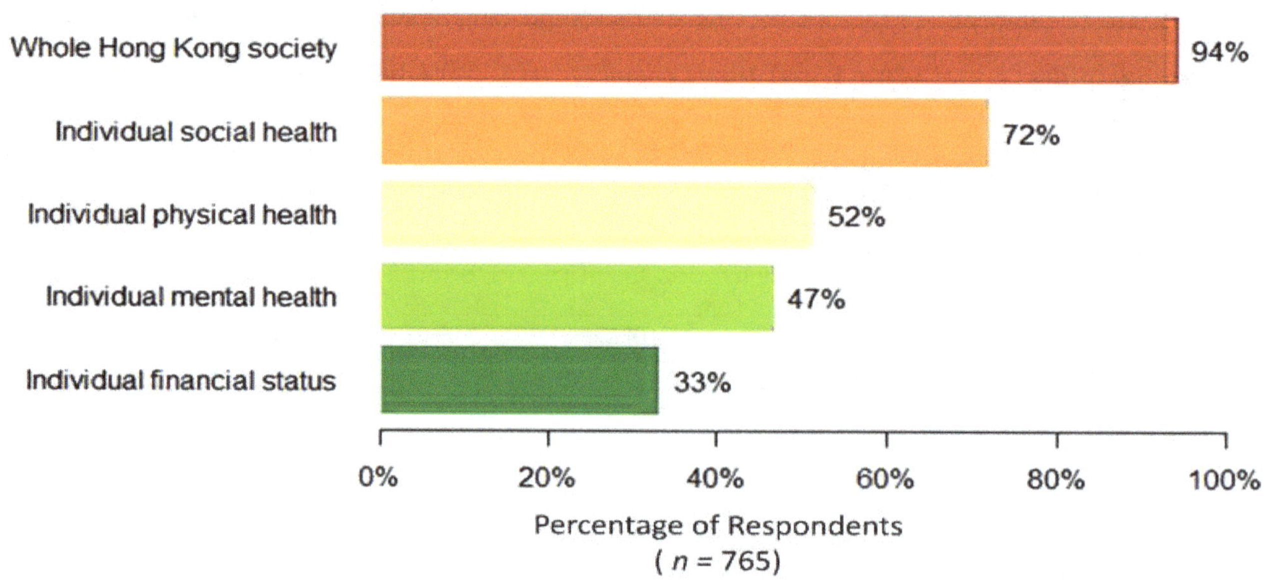

Figure 3. Self-reported large or very large impacts of COVID-19 on various dimensions.

3.2. Knowledge and Risk Perception of COVID-19

Regarding the overall knowledge and understanding of COVID-19, results indicated that most respondents could identify that the disease could be transmitted through droplets, direct or indirect hand contact, fecal contamination, and contact with asymptomatic patients (Figure 4). Yet, confusion was found with some reporting of unconfirmed transmission routes (e.g., insects as vectors) and about 24% (181/764) of the respondents did not believe that asymptomatic patients could transmit the disease, which might affect adoption of appropriate practices. Respondents with a higher level of education were more likely to correctly identify whether insects and asymptomatic patients can transmit the virus (Appendix A Table A1).

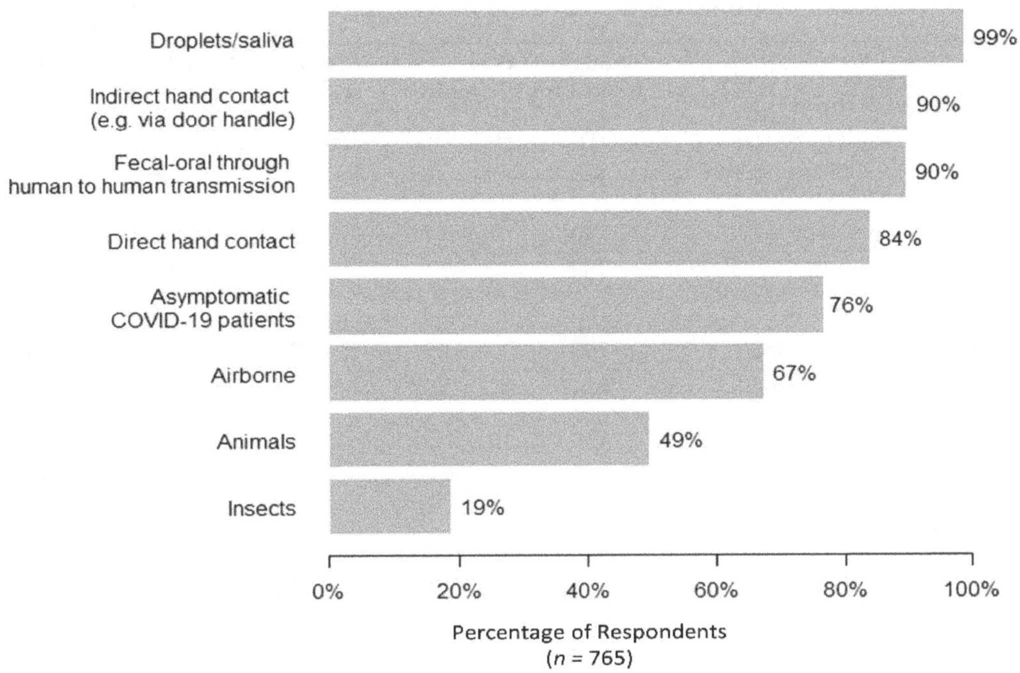

Figure 4. Reported believed transmission mode for COVID-19.

For the perceived infectivity of COVID-19, about 96% (34/765) believed the infectivity was high or very high and that it was much higher than SARS (78.0%) and seasonal influenza (52.5%). For the perceived severity, about 80% (156/765) believed it had a severe or very severe harm to health, which was less than SARS (90.5%) but higher than seasonal influenza (21.6%).

3.3. *Attitude and Uptake of Health-EDRM Behavior Practice towards COVID-19*

Although the uptake of Health-EDRM practice varied, most respondents agreed that personal or household preventive measures could reduce the transmission of COVID-19 (Table 2). Significant statistical differences were found between attitude and practice in regards to washing hands with soap, ordering takeaways more often, wearing masks when going out, avoidance of visiting public places or using public transport, and avoidance of travelling beyond COVID-19-confirmed regions outside Hong Kong. Furthermore, a comparison of the behavior of wearing masks before and after the epidemic found that when going outdoors, mask wearing had increased from 11.3% (86/764) before the epidemic to 97.4% after the disease outbreak (McNemar's test, p-value < 0.001). Compared to personal and household hygiene, compliance of social distancing in public was lower. After adjusting for age, gender, education, household income, and occupation, multiple regression revealed that male gender was significantly negatively associated with the behavior of washing hands with soap and the avoidance of dining and gathering together. Compared to white collar workers, housewives and the unemployed or retired were more likely to avoid going to public places or using public transport (Appendix A Table A2).

Table 2. Perceived usefulness and practice of preventive measures against COVID-19.

Control Measures that Can Protect from COVID-19 Infections	Thought It Was Useful for Prevention		Always or Usually Practicing Currently		Attitude vs. Practice [a]
	n	%	*n*	%	*p*-Value
Wash hands before meals and after toilet	749	97.9	749	97.9	0.555 [b]
Wash hands with soaps	740	96.7	706	92.3	<0.001
Wear mask when going out	753	98.4	745	97.4	<0.001 [b]
Use serving utensil	708	92.5	568	74.2	0.174
Bring own utensils when dining out †	542	81.9	52	7.9	0.199
Order takeaway more often	474	62.0	262	34.4	<0.001
Avoid dining or gathering together	742	97.0	616	85.0	0.178
Avoid going to public place or using public transport	713	93.4	408	53.5	0.002
Avoid going to COVID-19 confirmed regions outside Hong Kong	714	93.3	628	88.0	<0.001

[a] Chi-square or Fisher's exact test was used to test whether the perceived usefulness and practice are dependent. [b] Fisher's exact test was used. † This analysis only included people who will go outdoors for a meal during the epidemic (n = 662).

Around 32.7% (n = 249) of respondents believed in religion. Among them, analysis of mass gathering activity showed that 68.7% (171/249) reported that they reduced their religious gathering behavior during this pandemic. In addition, about a quarter of the study population (n = 181) reported that they had traveled abroad since January 2020. Mainland China (30.6%) and Japan (25.0%) were the most popular travelling areas.

3.4. Sociodemographic Factors Affecting Anxiety around Getting COVID-19

Among all the respondents, 66.7% (252/757) worried that they would become infected with COVID-19 with a mean STAI score of 2.57. Bivariate analyses of different socio-demographics, perception of the effect of COVID-19, and perceived infectivity and severity towards the worry about getting COVID-19 were conducted (Table 3). A multivariable logistic regression (Omnibus tests of model coefficients chi-square: 86.9, df = 10) revealed that young age, respondents who perceived significant COVID-19 impact on their physical, mental health, and/or social life were more likely to express anxiety of being infected. In addition, as the first global metropolis to report house pet SARS-CoV2 infection, our study showed that among the 124 respondents who are house pet owners, 18.5% (23/124) worried that their pets will also be infected with COVID-19.

The multivariable regression revealed that except for age, sociodemographic factors including gender, chronic disease status, education, marital status, household income, household floor area and district of residence were not significantly associated with the concern of becoming infected, which suggested that the worry of COVID-19 was indiscriminate across different sociodemographic factors in Hong Kong. Meanwhile, believing COVID-19 had a large effect on their physical, mental or social health was more likely to cause worry that they will be infected.

Table 3. Factors affecting concern of getting COVID-19.

Characteristics		Not Worry or Don't Know † (n = 252)	Worry (n = 505)	p-Value	AOR (95% CI)	p-Value
Age	18–24	15 (6.0%)	55 (10.9%)	0.037	1	
	25–44	77 (30.6%)	169 (33.5%)		0.567 (0.294–1.095)	0.091
	45–64	103 (40.9%)	198 (39.2%)		0.606 (0.318–1.153)	0.127
	65 or more	57 (22.6%)	83 (16.4%)		0.493 (0.244–0.995)	0.048
Gender	Male	132 (52.4%)	220 (43.6%)	0.022	1	
	Female	120 (47.6%)	285 (56.4%)		1.323 (0.956–1.831)	0.092
Chronic disease	No	206 (81.7%)	412 (81.6%)	0.957		
	Yes	46 (18.3%)	93 (18.3%)			
Education level	Primary level or below	25 (10.0%)	33 (6.6%)	0.249		
	Secondary level	108 (43.0%)	220 (43.7%)			
	Tertiary level	118 (47.0%)	250 (49.7%)			
Marital status	Non-married	99 (39.4%)	201 (39.9%)	0.908		
	Married	152 (60.2%)	303 (60.1%)			
Residential district	Hong Kong Island	52 (21.0%)	93 (18.4%)	0.207		
	Kowloon	83 (32.9%)	145 (28.7%)			
	New Territories	116 (46.0%)	267 (52.9%)			
Families members with chronic disease	No or don't know	209 (82.9%)	393 (77.8%)	0.100		
	Yes	43 (17.1%)	112 (22.2%)			
Household floor area	350 ft or below	53 (21.6%)	100 (21.1%)	0.964		
	351 ft to 800 ft	157 (64.1%)	304 (64.0%)			
	801 ft or above	35 (14.3%)	71 (14.9%)			

Table 3. *Cont.*

Characteristics		Not Worry or Don't Know † (n = 252)	Worry (n = 505)	p-Value	AOR (95% CI)	p-Value
Household income	<2000–7999	29 (12.1%)	36 (7.6%)	0.147		
	8000–19,999	36 (15.0%)	65 (13.8%)			
	20,000–39,999	66 (27.5%)	123 (26.1%)			
	40,000 or more	109 (45.4%)	248 (52.5%)			
Believing COVID-19 had large effect on their physical health	No	158 (62.9%)	206 (40.9%)	<0.001	1	
	Yes	93 (37.1%)	298 (59.1%)		1.583 (1.111–2.256)	0.011
Believing COVID-19 had large effect on their mental health	No	183 (72.6%)	219 (43.4%)	<0.001	1	
	Yes	69 (27.4%)	286 (56.6%)		2.490 (1.719–3.608)	<0.001
Believing COVID-19 had large effect on their financial status	No	181 (71.8%)	324 (64.2%)	0.035	1	
	Yes	71 (28.2%)	181 (35.8%)		0.927 (0.644–1.336)	0.685
Believing COVID-19 had large effect on their social life	No	104 (41.3%)	108 (21.4%)	<0.001	1	
	Yes	148 (58.7%)	397 (78.6%)		1.657 (1.138–2.413)	0.008
Believing COVID-19 had large effect on whole Hong Kong society	No	22 (8.7%)	20 (4.0%)	0.007	1	
	Yes	230 (91.3%)	485 (96.0%)		1.205 (0.608–2.385)	0.593
Perceived sufficient knowledge to manage COVID-19	No	127 (50.4%)	269 (53.3%)	0.456		
	Yes	125 (49.6%)	236 (43.7%)			
Perceived COVID-19 infectivity	Very low to medium or don't know	16 (6.3%)	17 (3.4%)	0.058	1	
	High or very high	236 (93.7%)	488 (96.6%)		1.290 (0.610–2.728)	0.505
Perceived COVID-19 severity	Very low to medium or don't know	58 (23.0%)	63 (19.0%)	0.197		
	High or very high	194 (77.0%)	409 (81.0%)			

† 248 participants reported "not worried" and 4 reported "don't know".

3.5. Other Related Behavioral Experiences: Home Quarantine and Caregiving to Non-Infected Family Members during COVID-19

Of the study respondents, 4.2% (32/765) reported that they practiced home-quarantine for COVID-19, where 71.9% (23/32) were volunteers and 28.1% (9/32) were compulsory quarantined. Most cited reasons for home-quarantine was history of recent travel abroad (13/32 = 40.6%) and close contact with confirmed patients (6/32 = 18.8%). About 83.8% subjects believed that quarantine was effective in infection control. During the COVID-19 epidemic, 25.1% of respondents (n = 192) reported that they engage in regular home and social care responsibilities. Among all the care providers, around 20% reported that they previously used community services and centers (e.g., school and day care centers) before COVID-19. Meanwhile, among these community service users, about 40% had stopped or decreased the use of those services due to closure during the epidemic. Respondents reported the need to take care of one (45.8%) or two family members (35.4%). About 28% and 7.4% of these respondents had been caring for frail older adults and those with disabilities, respectively. More details on caregiving to non-infected family members will be reported separately.

3.6. Information Channel and Type of Information of Health Information Seeking for COVID-19

More than 95% of the respondents reported that they were continuously concerned about the development of the COVID-19 epidemic. The main reported information seeking channels were television (36.1%), internet (28.8%) and smartphone apps (27.6%). When asked what kind of information they wanted to know, 88.3% and 87.7% of respondents wanted to know information about a vaccine and the situation of the epidemic, respectively.

4. Discussion

Using the standard computerized RDD method, this population landline-based study showed the self-reported perceived health impact, and the health emergency and disaster risk management (Health-EDRM) related preventive measures uptake (both individual or household level, and government level) against COVID-19 among the Hong Kong population. Consistent with other telephone survey results at early stages of the pandemic reported in Hong Kong, most respondents continued to report high perceived severity of COVID-19 [38]. In addition, a higher anxiety level during COVID-19 (STAI of 2.57) was seen in this study when compared with previous studies using the comparable scales conducted during SARS (2.24) in 2003 [39], and the H7N9 epidemic (1.85) in 2014 [27].

For various health impacts on demographic subgroups, people aged 65 or above reported that they were less affected by COVID-19 in terms of mental and social health, and these factors were also found to be significantly associated with concern of COVID-19. Findings were consistent with the online survey study results in mainland China [40] that also reported a higher anxiety level among younger respondents. The previous published online survey held in Hong Kong in February 2020 [41] had reported a higher proportion of respondents in distress from COVID-19, which might be explained by the differences in sampling of that study, which had recruited a lower proportion of the elderly. In contrast, the health severity perception of COVID-19 in this telephone survey was lower. This could be due to feeling fatigue with the epidemic news [42] or due to receiving more information about the situation and the virus, as the epidemic had evolved when compared with previous reported findings. Study findings indicated that respondents with chronic disease did not have higher levels of worry of getting COVID-19 when compared with those without chronic disease, even though the literature suggested that having chronic disease was considered as a risk factor for disease severity (complications and mortality) in COVID-19 [43–46]. Strengthening of information about those at higher risk in the community should be provided to raise the awareness of people at risk. Of note, the local population reported their belief that individuals (68.6%) bore comparable responsibility compared to the government (67.5%) to engage in infection control. Less than half of the respondents reported to have sufficient knowledge and accurate concepts to manage the health risk and safety during the outbreak [47]. For example, a quarter of the respondents did not perceive asymptomatic patients as infectious, which was similar to published findings in Egypt [48]. This misconception may affect the effectiveness of COVID-19 prevention efforts because the literature indicates that infected people can transmit the virus regardless of symptoms [7] and a high asymptomatic proportion of all infected patients was reported in Japan and Italy [6,49]. Furthermore, respondents with a misconception of the transmission route were found to be more likely to use television or radio as their main information source. As this misconception may likely be due to the lack of emphasis on asymptomatic patients as a transmission route, additional information related to the transmission route should be tailored to those with a lower education level.

Health-EDRM encompasses a wide range of components, where the component "Community Capacities for Health-EDRM" highlights the importance of the participation of the local population for managing the health risks in an emergency. Among the Health-EDRM behavioral practices [28], which are related to primary disease prevention practices [29], significant differences were found between attitude and practice in regards to washing hands with soap, ordering takeaways more often, wearing masks when going out, and avoiding going to COVID-19-confirmed regions outside Hong Kong. People who regarded these behaviors as useful tended to have a higher uptake rate. Consistent with Kwok et al. and Cowling et al. [38,41], the Hong Kong population showed a high compliance of wearing masks (94.2%), and there was a significant difference before and after the outbreak, which might be due to the high awareness of the outbreak, mass public health information announced through different channels, and the previous experience of SARS. However, more than half of respondents still reported traveling to COVID-19-confirmed regions before and during the study period. In addition, moderate and low uptake rates were found in using serving utensils (74.2%) and bringing their own utensils to meals (7.9%). Uptake patterns were found to be higher when compared with a previous study conducted during the H7N9 pandemic [27], where rates of 45.9% and 1.6%, respectively, were reported.

Meanwhile, no significant differences were found between perceived usefulness and practice of avoidance of dining or gathering together. This might suggest that even though people thought social avoidance might be useful to prevent COVID-19, they were unwilling to practice this socially limiting preventive behavior. As our study findings showed, males were less likely to avoid dining or gathering together, this might also provide the hypothesis that gender behavior might at least be associated with the gender imbalance in confirmed cases (with male predominance) at the beginning of the local outbreak [50]. In addition, "ordering takeaway food" was found to have increased by respondents during the epidemic. This increase may due to the social distancing promotion and regulations by the government (e.g., encouraging restaurants to provide takeaways as an option and avoiding table sharing) [51,52]. To promote better self-protection against infectious diseases, targeted interventions may focus on increasing the awareness towards the outbreak for the behaviors with a significant attitude–practice gap, while for the behaviors without an attitude–practice gap, additional measures to reinforce the practice were suggested. Further studies focusing on the barriers and self-efficacy might also be needed. Appropriate Health-EDRM health education and risk communication might wish to target subgroups who revealed suboptimal behavioral practices to further improve bottom-up response efforts.

Television, internet and smartphone apps were the top three channels for obtaining infectious disease information, covering more than 90% of the population. In Hong Kong, habits of television consumption have developed among the middle-aged and elderly, while the use of internet or smartphone apps were more popular in the younger age group. Consistent with the survey previously held in Hong Kong in February [41], almost all of the respondents would like to know more about the current situation of the outbreak, and how the government and themselves should respond. The availability and safety of COVID-19 vaccine were also of interest to general population.

Study limitations included the methodological limitations of telephone surveys. Firstly, households with no land-based telephone service may be missed. Nonetheless, the penetration rate of residential fixed line services in Hong Kong was 85.5% in December 2019 [53]. In addition, our study was conducted during the peak period of confirmed cases of COVID-19 in Hong Kong. During the data collection period, Hong Kong had 492 confirmed cases, accounting for almost half of the cases as of 14 April. Furthermore, the data collection occurred during the lockdown period in Hong Kong when people were advised to stay at home, and the government prohibited group gatherings of more than four people in public places under the Prohibition on Group Gathering Regulation. In addition, a landline telephone survey allows for more accurate geographic and demographic targeting when compared with mobile and online surveys. In general, specific subgroups, such as the elderly and the poor are more likely to be reached via landline than young adults [54]. Moreover, the landline telephone study methodology might capture populations that might be less technological or digital literate and it also offers the opportunity for researchers to compare with previous study findings with similar study methodology of other extreme events and disaster context. Finally, our sample was collected over a short period and comparable with the population census data in terms of age, gender, district of residence and marital status, which was generalizable to the Hong Kong population.

Secondly, the cross-sectional study design can only demonstrate associations between patterns and social-demographic predictors and causation cannot be attributed to the findings. A further cohort-based study design should be considered to monitor and assess changes in knowledge, attitude and practice patterns. Thirdly, this study might be subject to reporting bias since the information collected was self-reported, and data from non-respondents could not be obtained. In addition, the enquired personal or household health emergency disaster risks management (Health-EDRM) related behaviors and practices of COVID-19 prevention behavior were developed based on previous health and hygiene behavioral practices that might be relevant to contact transmission of the disease [33]. Yet, there are other relevant Health-EDRM behavioral practices in other cultural (non-Asia) and living contexts (e.g., rural community's settings) that are worth exploring to generate evidence and develop health-risk education.

Last but not least, as the survey study was conducted after the implementation of the government preventive social distancing measures (e.g., restricting restaurant's customer density, prohibition of group gathering), behavioral patterns might be subject to further changes if authorities have regulation and policy changes.

5. Conclusions

The Health-EDRM Framework is an integrated approach to manage health risks and build resilience. The COVID-19 pandemic offers an opportunity for the global community to understand how community and individuals might engage in disease prevention and health protection Health-EDRM behaviors that address a major biological hazard. The study findings indicated elderly and people with low education attainment had relatively poor knowledge and were less likely to adopt preventive Health-EDRM practices toward COVID-19. Tailored information with relevant information channels should be considered to reach these at-risk groups. Better understanding of uptake of knowledge, perception, attitude and behavior patterns by urban populations might facilitate better program and policy planning for Health-EDRM.

Author Contributions: Conceptualization, E.Y.Y.C.; methodology, E.Y.Y.C. and E.S.K.L.; validation, Z.H.; formal analysis, E.S.K.L.; investigation, E.S.K.L., E.Y.Y.C., Z.H., E.L.Y.W., S.Y.S.W. and K.K.C.H.; data curation, E.S.K.L. and Z.H.; writing—original draft preparation, E.S.K.L., E.Y.Y.C. and Z.H.; writing—review and editing, E.S.K.L. E.Y.Y.C., Z.H., E.L.Y.W., S.Y.S.W. and K.K.C.H.; visualization, E.S.K.L.; supervision, E.Y.Y.C.; project administration, Z.H. All authors have read and agreed to the published version of the manuscript.

Appendix A

Table A1. Association between demographic variables and risk perception and knowledge about COVID-19.

Demographics	Risk Perception					Knowledge	
	Large Impact on Mental Health	Large Impact on Social Health	Large Impact on Financial Status	Large Impact on Hong Kong	Can be Prevented at Government Level	Can Be Spread by Insect	Can Be Spread by Asymptomatic Patient
Education							
Primary			1.10 (0.51–2.38)	0.15 (0.04–0.51) *		2.89 (1.35–6.18) *	0.45 (0.21–0.96) *
Secondary			1.81 (1.22–2.69) *	0.51 (0.21–1.23)		1.40 (0.87–2.26)	0.50 (0.32–0.78) *
Post-secondary			1	1		1	1
Gender							
Male	1	1					
Female	1.41 (1.02–1.95) *	1.60 (1.10–2.33) *					
Age							
18–24	2.00 (0.77–5.18)	6.12 (1.78–21.54) *	7.93 (2.76–22.76) *		3.06 (0.88–10.61)		
25–44	2.21 (1.19–4.12) *	4.03 (1.99–8.15) *	7.05 (3.35–14.81) *		2.12 (1.10–40.9) *		
45–64	1.26 (0.73–2.19)	2.98 (1.60–5.55) *	4.32 (2.22–8.42) *		0.96 (0.55–1.69)		
65+	1	1	1		1		
Household income							
<2000–7999			1				
8000–19,999			0.43 (0.20–0.92) *				
20,000–39,999			0.33 (0.16–0.72) *				
40,000 or more			0.25 (0.12–0.54) *				
Occupation							
White collar		1					
Blue collar		1.70 (0.99–2.93)					
Housewife		1.95 (0.98–3.90)					
Student		1.35 (0.36–5.05)					
Unemployment or retired		3.41 (1.72–6.76) *					

Note: Multivariable regression was not performed on outcome variables with a small number of cases (probability of that happening <0.05 or >0.95). Only variables with significant odds ratios in the multivariable logistic regression are shown in the table. None of these five demographic variables were significantly associated with believing COVID-19 had a large impact on their physical health, perceived sufficient knowledge of COVID-19, believing COVID-19 can be prevented at the household or individual level, perceived high infectivity and perceived severity of COVID-19. * indicates $p < 0.05$.

Table A2. Association between demographic variables and the practices (always or usually) of preventive measures against COVID-19.

Demographics	Wash Hands with Soaps	Avoid Dining or Gathering Together	Use Serving Utensil	Avoid Going to Public Place or Using Public Transport
Education				
Primary	0.31 (0.12–0.84) *		0.15 (0.04-0.51) *	
Secondary	0.68 (0.33–1.42)		0.51 (0.21–1.23)	
Post-secondary	1		1	
Gender				
Male	1	1		
Female	2.27 (1.17–4.43) *	1.82 (1.21–2.74) *		
Age				
18–24	2.15 (0.39–11.97)			2.48 (0.93–6.65)
25–44	4.62 (1.47–14.52) *			2.08 (1.09–3.98) *
45–64	2.83 (1.15–6.95) *			1.37 (0.77–2.44)
65+	1			1
Household income				
<2000–7999				
8000–19,999				
20,000–39,999				
40,000 or more				
Occupation				
White collar				1
Blue collar				0.70 (0.44–1.23)
Housewife				3.47 (1.87–6.42) *
Student				0.99 (0.37–2.65)
Unemployment or retired				2.29 (1.28–4.07) *

Note: Multivariable regression was not performed on outcome variables with a small number of cases (probability of that happening <0.05 or >0.95). Only variables with significant odds ratio in the multivariable logistic regression are shown in the table. None of these five demographic variables were significantly associated with bringing one's own utensils when dining out, ordering takeaway food more often, and avoiding going to COVID-19-confirmed regions outside Hong Kong. * indicates $p < 0.05$.

References

1. Rolling Updates on Coronavirus Disease (COVID-19). Available online: https://www.who.int/emergencies/diseases/novel-coronavirus-2019/events-as-they-happen (accessed on 23 April 2020).
2. Ye, Z.W.; Yuan, S.; Yuen, K.S.; Fung, S.Y.; Chan, C.P.; Jin, D.Y. Zoonotic origins of human coronaviruses. *Int. J. Biol. Sci.* **2020**, *16*, 1686. [CrossRef]
3. Coronavirus Disease 2019 (COVID-19) Situation Report–85. Available online: https://www.who.int/docs/default-source/coronaviruse/situation-reports/20200414-sitrep-85-covid-19.pdf?sfvrsn=7b8629bb_2 (accessed on 23 April 2020).
4. Rajgor, D.D.; Lee, M.H.; Archuleta, S.; Bagdasarian, N.; Quek, S.C. The many estimates of the COVID-19 case fatality rate. *Lancet Infect. Dis.* **2020**. [CrossRef]
5. Kim, D.D.; Goel, A. Estimating case fatality rates of COVID-19. *Lancet Infect. Dis.* **2020**. [CrossRef]
6. Day, M. Covid-19: Identifying and isolating asymptomatic people helped eliminate virus in Italian village. *BMJ* **2020**, *368*, m1165. [CrossRef] [PubMed]
7. Kimball, A. Asymptomatic and presymptomatic SARS-CoV-2 infections in residents of a long-term care skilled nursing facility—King County, Washington, March 2020. *Morb. Mortal. Wkly. Rep.* **2020**, *69*, 377–381. [CrossRef]
8. Mahase, E. Coronavirus: COVID-19 has killed more people than SARS and MERS combined, despite lower case fatality rate. *BMJ* **2020**, m641. [CrossRef]
9. Wells, C.R.; Sah, P.; Moghadas, S.M.; Pandey, A.; Shoukat, A.; Wang, Y.; Galvani, A.P. Impact of international travel and border control measures on the global spread of the novel 2019 coronavirus outbreak. *Proc. Natl. Acad. Sci. USA* **2020**, *117*, 7504–7509. [CrossRef]
10. Lewnard, J.A.; Lo, N.C. Scientific and ethical basis for social-distancing interventions against COVID-19. *Lancet Infect. Dis.* **2020**. [CrossRef]

11. Novel Coronavirus (2019-nCoV) SITUATION REPORT-3 23 JANUARY 2020. Available online: https://www.who.int/docs/default-source/coronaviruse/situation-reports/20200123-sitrep-3-2019-ncov.pdf?sfvrsn=d6d23643_8 (accessed on 23 April 2020).
12. CHP Investigates Two Additional Cases of Novel Coronavirus Infection. Available online: https://www.info.gov.hk/gia/general/202001/31/P2020013100015.htm?fontSize=1 (accessed on 23 April 2020).
13. Latest Situation of Cases of COVID-19 (as of 14 April, 2020). Available online: https://www.chp.gov.hk/files/pdf/local_situation_covid19_en.pdf (accessed on 15 April 2020).
14. CE Announces Activation of Emergency Response Level in Relation to Novel Coronavirus Infection (with Photo). Available online: https://www.info.gov.hk/gia/general/202001/26/P2020012600087.htm (accessed on 23 April 2020).
15. LNY Welfare Services Set. Available online: https://www.news.gov.hk/eng/2020/01/20200127/20200127_233955_845.html (accessed on 23 April 2020).
16. Deferral of Class Resumption for All Schools Together, We Fight the Virus. Available online: https://www.edb.gov.hk/attachment/en/sch-admin/admin/about-sch/diseases-prevention/edb_20200331_eng.pdf (accessed on 23 April 2020).
17. Compulsory Quarantine Implemented Smoothly. Available online: https://www.info.gov.hk/gia/general/202002/09/P2020020900715.htm?fontSize=1 (accessed on 23 April 2020).
18. Quarantine Measures Enhanced. Available online: https://www.news.gov.hk/eng/2020/03/20200317/20200317_202509_713.html (accessed on 23 April 2020).
19. Prevention and Control of Disease (Requirement and Directions) (Business and Premises) Regulation Gazette. Available online: https://www.info.gov.hk/gia/general/202003/27/P2020032700878.htm?fontSize=1 (accessed on 23 April 2020).
20. Prevention and Control of Disease (Prohibition on Group Gathering) Regulation. Available online: https://www.info.gov.hk/gia/general/202003/28/P2020032800720.htm?fontSize=1 (accessed on 23 April 2020).
21. Health Emergency and Disaster Risk Management Framework. Available online: https://www.who.int/hac/techguidance/preparedness/health-emergency-and-disaster-risk-management-framework-eng.pdf?ua=1 (accessed on 23 April 2020).
22. Wan, Y.K.P. A comparison of the governance of tourism planning in the two Special Administrative Regions (SARs) of China–Hong Kong and Macao. *Tour. Manag.* **2013**, *36*, 164–177.
23. Kung, N.Y.; Morris, R.S.; Perkins, N.R.; Sims, L.D.; Ellis, T.M.; Bissett, L.; Peiris, M.J. Risk for infection with highly pathogenic influenza A virus (H5N1) in chickens, Hong Kong, 2002. *Emerg. Infect. Dis.* **2007**, *13*, 412. [CrossRef]
24. Cheng, V.C.C.; Lee, W.M.; Sridhar, S.; Ho, P.L.; Yuen, K.Y. Prevention of nosocomial transmission of influenza A (H7N9) in Hong Kong. *J. Hosp. Infect.* **2015**, *90*, 355–356. [CrossRef] [PubMed]
25. Wong, A.T.; Chen, H.; Liu, S.H.; Hsu, E.K.; Luk, K.S.; Lai, C.K.; Tong, A.Y. From SARS to avian influenza preparedness in Hong Kong. *Clin. Infect. Dis.* **2017**, *64* (Suppl. S2), S98–S104. [CrossRef] [PubMed]
26. Lau, J.T.; Tsui, H.; Lau, M.; Yang, X. SARS transmission, risk factors, and prevention in Hong Kong. *Emerg. Infect. Dis.* **2004**, *10*, 587. [CrossRef] [PubMed]
27. Chan, E.Y.Y.; Cheng, C.K.; Tam, G.; Huang, Z.; Lee, P. Knowledge, attitudes, and practices of Hong Kong population towards human A/H7N9 influenza pandemic preparedness, China, 2014. *BMC Public Health* **2015**, *15*, 943. [CrossRef] [PubMed]
28. West, R.; Michie, S.; Rubin, G.J.; Amlôt, R. Applying principles of behaviour change to reduce SARS-CoV-2 transmission. *Nat. Hum. Behav.* **2020**, *4*, 1–9. [CrossRef] [PubMed]
29. Chan, E.Y.Y.; Shahzada, T.S.; Sham, T.; Dubois, C.; Huang, Z.; Liu, S.; Shaw, R. Non-Pharmaceutical Behavioural Measures for Droplet-Borne Biological Hazards Prevention: Health-EDRM for COVID-19 (SARS-CoV-2) Pandemic. 2020; Manuscript Submitted for Publication.
30. Chan, E.Y.Y.; Cheng, C.K.Y.; Tam, G.; Huang, Z.; Lee, P. Willingness of future A/H7N9 influenza vaccine uptake: A cross-sectional study of Hong Kong community. *Vaccine* **2015**, *33*, 4737–4740. [CrossRef] [PubMed]
31. Tam, G.; Huang, Z.; Chan, E.Y.Y. Household preparedness and preferred communication channels in public health emergencies: A cross-sectional survey of residents in an Asian developed urban city. *Int. J. Environ. Res. Public Health* **2018**, *15*, 1598. [CrossRef]
32. Marteau, T.M.; Bekker, H. The development of a six-item short-form of the state scale of the Spielberger State-Trait Anxiety Inventory (STAI). *Br. J. Clin. Psychol.* **1992**, *31 Pt 3*, 301–306. [CrossRef]

33. Chan, E.Y.Y.; Wong, C.S. Public health prevention hierarchy in disaster context. In *Public Health and Disasters-Health Emergency and Disaster Risk Management in Asia*; Chan, E.Y.Y., Shaw, R., Eds.; Springer: Tokyo, Japan, 2020; pp. 7–17.

34. Chan, E.Y.Y. *Building Bottom-up Health and Disaster Risk Reduction Programmes*; Oxford University Press: Oxford, UK, 2018.

35. Chan, E.Y.Y.; Huang, Z.; Mark, C.K.M.; Guo, C. Weather information acquisition and health significance during extreme cold weather in a subtropical city: A cross-sectional survey in Hong Kong. *Int. J. Disaster Risk Sci.* **2017**, *8*, 134–144. [CrossRef]

36. Chan, E.Y.Y.; Huang, Z.; Hung, K.K.C.; Chan, G.K.W.; Lam, H.C.Y.; Lo, E.S.K.; Yeung, M.P.S. Health emergency disaster risk management of public transport systems: A population-based study after the 2017 subway fire in Hong Kong, China. *Int. J. Environ. Res. Public Health* **2019**, *16*, 228. [CrossRef]

37. Hong Kong SAR Census and Statistics Department. Available online: https://www.bycensus2016.gov.hk/en/bc-dp.html (accessed on 23 April 2020).

38. Cowling, B.J.; Ali, S.T.; Ng, T.W.; Tsang, T.K.; Li, J.C.; Fong, M.W.; Wu, J.T. Impact assessment of non-pharmaceutical interventions against coronavirus disease 2019 and influenza in Hong Kong: An observational study. *Lancet Public Health* **2020**, *5*, e279–e288. [CrossRef]

39. Leung, G.M.; Lam, T.H.; Ho, L.M.; Ho, S.Y.; Chan, B.H.Y.; Wong, I.O.L.; Hedley, A.J. The impact of community psychological responses on outbreak control for severe acute respiratory syndrome in Hong Kong. *J. Epidemiol. Community Health* **2003**, *57*, 857–863. [CrossRef] [PubMed]

40. Huang, Y.; Zhao, N. Generalized anxiety disorder, depressive symptoms and sleep quality during COVID-19 epidemic in China: A web-based cross-sectional survey. *MedRxiv* **2020**, *288*, 112954.

41. Kwok, K.O.; Li, K.K.; Chan, H.H.; Yi, Y.Y.; Tang, A.; Wei, W.I.; Wong, S.Y. Community Responses during Early Phase of COVID-19 Epidemic, Hong Kong. *Emerg. Infect. Dis.* **2020**, *26*. [CrossRef]

42. Collinson, S.; Khan, K.; Heffernan, J.M. The effects of media reports on disease spread and important public health measurements. *PLoS ONE* **2015**, *10*, e0141423. [CrossRef]

43. Shahid, Z.; Kalayanamitra, R.; McClafferty, B.; Kepko, D.; Ramgobin, D.; Patel, R.; Jain, R. COVID-19 and older adults: What we know. *J. Am. Geriatr. Soc.* **2020**, *68*, 926–929. [CrossRef]

44. Kalligeros, M.; Shehadeh, F.; Mylona, E.K.; Benitez, G.; Beckwith, C.G.; Chan, P.A.; Mylonakis, E. Association of Obesity with Disease Severity among Patients with COVID-19. *Obesity* **2020**. [CrossRef]

45. Hussain, A.; Bhowmik, B.; do Vale Moreira, N.C. COVID-19 and diabetes: Knowledge in progress. *Diabetes Res. Clin. Pract.* **2020**, *162*, 108142. [CrossRef]

46. Cook, T.M. The importance of hypertension as a risk factor for severe illness and mortality in COVID-19. *Anaesthesia* **2020**. [CrossRef]

47. World Health Organization. Modes of Transmission of Virus Causing COVID-19: Implications for IPC Precaution Recommendations: Scientific Brief, 27 March 2020 (No. WHO/2019-nCoV/Sci_Brief/Transmission_modes/2020.1). Available online: https://apps.who.int/iris/bitstream/handle/10665/331601/WHO-2019-nCoV-Sci_Brief-Transmission_modes-2020.1-eng.pdf (accessed on 23 April 2020).

48. Abdelhafiz, A.S.; Mohammed, Z.; Ibrahim, M.E.; Ziady, H.H.; Alorabi, M.; Ayyad, M.; Sultan, E.A. Knowledge, Perceptions, and Attitude of Egyptians Towards the Novel Coronavirus Disease (COVID-19). *J. Community Health* **2020**, 1–10. [CrossRef]

49. Mizumoto, K.; Kagaya, K.; Zarebski, A.; Chowell, G. Estimating the asymptomatic proportion of coronavirus disease 2019 (COVID-19) cases on board the Diamond Princess cruise ship, Yokohama, Japan, 2020. *Eurosurveillance* **2020**, *25*, 2000180. [CrossRef] [PubMed]

50. Coronavirus Disease (COVID-19) in HK. Available online: https://chp-dashboard.geodata.gov.hk/covid-19/en.html (accessed on 23 April 2020).

51. Let's Beat COVID-19 Together. Available online: https://www.cfs.gov.hk/english/whatsnew/whatsnew_fstr/whatsnew_fstr_Beat_COVID-19.html (accessed on 18 May 2020).

52. New Regulations to Fight COVID-19. Available online: https://www.news.gov.hk/eng/2020/03/20200327/20200327_202339_445.html (accessed on 18 May 2020).

53. Office of the Communications Authority Key Communications Statistics. Available online: https://www.ofca.gov.hk/en/data_statistics/data_statistics/key_stat/ (accessed on 23 April 2020).
54. Petrovčič, A.; Vehovar, V.; Dolničar, V. Landline and mobile phone communication in social companionship networks of older adults: An empirical investigation in Slovenia. *Technol. Soc.* **2016**, *45*, 91–102. [CrossRef]

2

Inter-Organisational Exercises in Dry and Wet Context—Why Do Maritime Response Organisations Gain more Knowledge from Exercises at Sea than those on Shore?

Eric Carlström [1,2,*], Leif Inge Magnussen [2], Elsa Kristiansen [2], Johan Berlin [3] and Jarle Løwe Sørensen [2]

1 Institute of Health and Care Sciences, Sahlgrenska Academy, University of Gothenburg, SE-405 30 Goteborg, Sweden

2 USN School of Business, University of South-Eastern Norway, P.O. Box 235, 3603 Kongsberg, Norway; leif.magnussen@usn.no (L.I.M.); elsa.kristiansen@usn.no (E.K.); jarle.sorensen@usn.no (J.L.S.)

3 Department of Social and Behavioural Studies, University West, SE-461 86 Trollhättan, Sweden; johan.berlin@hv.se

* Correspondence: eric.carlstrom@gu.se

Abstract: This is a study of inter-organisational exercises arranged by on-shore organisations (ONSOs) and off-shore organisations (OFFSOs). The aim was to compare findings from trained emergency staffs' perceptions of the impact of exercises. The data were retrieved from surveys conducted by the research team in conjunction with exercises. The surveys included staff from the coast guard, sea rescue, police department, fire department and ambulance services. A total of 94 professional emergency personnel participated in the ONSO exercises and 252 in the OFFSO exercises. The study was based on the suggestion that collaborative elements during an inter-organisational exercise promote learning, and learning is important to make the exercises useful. Collaboration proved to be a predictor for some of the items in learning, and learning was a predictor for some of the items in utility. There was, however, a stronger covariation between collaboration, learning and utility in the OFFSOs exercises than in the ONSOs. One reason might be the different cultures of emergency staff involved in on-shore and off-shore organisations. The OFFSOs' qualifications may be dominated by seamanship, together with professional practice, and all parties are expected to act as first responders. ONSOs, on the other hand, practice exercises from a strict professional and legal perspective.

Keywords: exercises; learning; inter-organisational; off-shore; on-shore; emergencies

---

1. Introduction

Strategic sustainability infers a built-in resistance to the prominence and effects of crisis events. A common way to maximise society sustainability is by maintaining the emergency response via regular exercises. Inter-organisational exercises are supposed to help authorities to become better at handling accidents, crises and disasters. Exercises involving different emergency services are carried out with the purpose of strengthening the inter-organisational ability to deal with difficult events that require extensive resources in a short time. There are, however, few studies of the efficiency of inter-organisational exercises in terms of learning and utility. One exception is Scandinavia, where inter-organisational exercises at sea and ashore have been studied [1–5]. The concept of inter-organisational exercises, as it is used in Scandinavia, describes exercises aiming to prevent organisational fragmentation, and develop integration and distribution of tasks [6,7].

In this article, we compare data from nine exercises (three ONSOs and six OFFSOs) from five published studies in order to find similarities and differences in terms of learning and utility. Comparing inter-organisational exercises arranged by on-shore and off-shore organisations can reveal context specific challenges and differences in learning outcomes. When extrapolated, it can pin-point strengths and weaknesses in different contexts of emergency preparedness. Such knowledge can, in turn, offer suggestions on how to improve the outcome from exercises and emergency response.

During the management of a societal crisis, the need for collaboration between emergency services has been actualised. As a result of criticism towards the management of rescue work during the 2011 attacks on the government blocks in Oslo and the Labour Parties Youth League summer camp on the island of Utoya, Norway in 2012, an extra principle was added to the national emergency preparedness legislation. It was the principle of collaboration, which was supposed to facilitate inter-organisational actions during emergencies [8]. In Sweden, as well as in Norway, where the data for this study were collected, the governments emphasise the importance of exercises to develop collaboration on different societal levels. In particular, inter-organisational collaboration is highlighted as a particularly important task to be practiced, specifically by getting employees to take the initiative to help each other across organisational boundaries [9–12]. This is especially true during time constraining emergencies [13,14].

In several studies, the inclusion of collaborative elements in exercises has proved to contribute to learning, and learning contributes to usefulness in real life situations. However, the studies show that even if there was a significant learning effect because of collaboration, the impact was, in some cases, moderate [13,15,16] and emergency staff have difficulties in learning from past mistakes [17]. Even if emergency response organisations are supposed to collaborate, they tend to prioritise the specific tasks they are trained for, instead of seeing the big picture [18]. Staff may engage in tasks they are accustomed to but are inactive when unaccustomed tasks need to be performed [19]. This is contradictory to collaboration, i.e., only focusing on one's own responsibilities, but being prepared to take initiatives beyond [20].

Here, learning is studied at the collective level [21]. Different patterns of action are built within the organisations, where individuals share experiences, learn from each other, and develop common approaches [22]. Learning occurs from communication across borders, different organisational agendas, the use of common resources and the different skills of collaborating professionals. According to Stein, the knowledge can be shared by permeable boundaries, ensuring multifunctional networks and integration. Demarcated boundaries and hierarchical grouping where activities are distributed into segmented tasks, on the other hand, may prevent knowledge sharing [21]. Institutional learning is accomplished by repeated action patterns, which over time create institutions that are stable in nature [23]. In this study, learning is considered to be the effect of a successful inter-organisational exercise, and learning is assumed to have impact on actual practice. Successful exercises, in terms of learning, may integrate professions at the fictive accident site [24]. Therefore, learning may occur when new patterns of thought are constructed and considered useful [25,26]. During exercises, learning is assumed to stand for change and development [27] and contribute to being open to different options and encourages initiatives to collaborate with others to achieve improved results [28]. According to Stein, inter-organisational learning builds trust, team building and coherence crossing professional borders [21]. Hence, learning can facilitate the development of routines, rules and models that have influence on daily work [29,30]

2. Maritime and Land-Based Collaboration

The collaborative culture seems to be different between emergency staff in maritime versus land-based contexts. Collaboration in the maritime context crosses national and cultural borders and is, in contrast to land-based, regulated by bi- and multi-lateral agreements and treaties. One such example of collaboration is in the high north area, where resources for search and rescue missions are lacking. Even if some areas, such as coastal Norway close to the mainland, are well-developed, distant areas are wastelands that are occasionally trafficked by crowded cruise vessels and oil installations.

The risks related to going aground or collisions with ice, or fire are not in accordance with the number of available rescue services, especially in remote areas. Disasters in wastelands and distant maritime areas put collaboration over organisational and national borders to the test [31]. Rescue missions at sea are, however, performed by all available actors and not just those who are specialised in emergency response. Long distances and severe weather conditions have forced different parties to collaborate, regardless of whether they are publicly financed rescue services, voluntary financed services (e.g., Red Cross and Society for Sea Rescue), fishing fleets or the merchant navy [32].

Several catastrophes have led to updated and sharpened legislations in the maritime context. This was intensified after a series of shipping accidents with grave environmental damages during late 1960s and early 1970s. The subsequent investigations concluded that the main cause of these accidents was human errors, resulting from poor training and lack of inter-organisational competencies [33]. Subsequently, maritime mass-casualty disasters like the Scandinavian Star disaster in 1990 [34], the Estonia disaster in 1994 [35] and the Costa Concordia wreckage in 2012 [36] shed light on the need to put more efforts in inter-organisational education and training. Hence, the maritime domain started harmonising and regulating its educational standards worldwide.

The International Maritime Organisation (IMO)—a technical agency of the United Nations—was introduced in 1959 to harmonise standards of international maritime activities, including training and qualification of mariners who navigate ships. In 1978, the IMO launched its first educational standards—the Standards of Training, Certification and Watch Keeping for Seafarers (STCW). It was considered a breakthrough, as there were practically no international standards in maritime exercises [37]. However, the STCW did not succeed in harmonizing the already established national standards around the world. Several revisions seeking to repair the shortcomings of its predecessors were made, and new conventions were prepared including the recent Manilla amendments, STCW 2010. STCW 2010 highlighted and homogenised concepts of intra-organisational exercises for mariners. The STCW standardised security exercises in different scenarios such as attacks by pirates and operations in polar waters [38].

With regard to collaboration during emergencies in land-based contexts, there are no such standards as those provided by IMO. Some standardisation in crisis organisations and crisis work can be seen within certain covenants like the European Union. Nonetheless, there is still a lack of international as well as national standards in inter-organisational exercises. At the country level, there is some fragmentation. It has been reported about intra-organisational autonomy during emergency response operations from Sweden and Norway. The official evaluation following the 2011 terrorist attacks in Norway found, among other conclusions, that the emergency response had been insufficient, and that inter-organisational collaboration efforts in particular had been inadequate [10]. An article titled "Why is collaboration minimized at the accident scene?" reported on the difference between rhetoric and practice in connection with accident work. Collaboration is seen as a rhetorical ideal rather than something that is carried out in real life accident work. The results from the study showed that police force, fire fighters and prehospital healthcare staff have an intention to develop excellent forms of collaboration at the accident scene but avoid this because of asymmetries in standards and lack of incentives [39]. A study from a tunnel exercise in Norway showed a risk for competition within organisations with unclear hierarchies. A lack of clarity in the distribution of roles and power struggles was identified as potential risks affecting the handling of emergencies [40]. Short distances and high accessibility can also be reasons why land-based emergency staff can uphold a degree of autonomy. In contrast to operations at sea, land-based operations can most often be reached by all the required resources within reasonable time and normally do not need to rely on each other's willingness to cross professional borders [41]. Information exchange during land-based emergency response operations is also known to uphold a certain degree of autonomy. Each organisation in the response network has operational field units at different levels, different functional command structures, separate back offices and intraorganisational radio communications channels [42,43].

Scandinavian countries like Norway and Sweden have a lot of similarities and few differences. Because of a long border between Norway and Sweden, partly in populated areas, they have agreements on sharing resources and coordinating actions during emergencies. The response organisations of the two countries perform common inter-organisational exercises; moreover, the radiocommunication systems, "Nødnett" in Norway and "Rakel" in Sweden, have been connected since 2016 (MSB 2018). The open borders between the countries have a long tradition, based on similar languages, constitutional monarchies, democracy and governments appointed by a parliament in both countries. They share national emergency preparedness principles of responsibility, equality and proximity in their respective legislations [8].

The dependence between organisations at incident locations is well known, which justifies the need for inter-organisational exercises to be conducted regularly [39,44]. Obviously, there are similarities and differences between OFFSOs and ONSOs' collaborative strategies during emergencies. After decades of naval disasters, OFFSOs have developed harmonised standards, while, in the ONSO context, the routines are still fragmented. The ONSO context seems to be more affected by the perception of collaboration as a rhetorical ideal while OFFSOs are characterised by a willingness to cross organisational boarders. We still do not know if collaboration exercises differ in their impact on OFFSOs and ONSOs. Despite a lack of studies [45], inter-organisational exercises arranged by off-shore organisations (OFFSOs) as well as on-shore organisations (ONSOs) are practised at considerable cost, with the supposition that they contribute to learning and utility in real life disasters [3]. We aim to find similarities and differences in the outcome from inter-organisational exercises, in terms of learning and utility, in the maritime versus land-based contexts. The study is supposed to reveal context-specific challenges, weaknesses and differences in traditions of emergency preparedness in order to suggest how to improve the outcome from inter-organisational exercises [46].

3. Methods

Five studies from a Norwegian/Swedish research team was chosen to compare inter-organisational exercises arranged by ONSOs and OFFSOs. One of the studies provided data from three ONSO exercises. Four studies contained data from six OFSO exercises, four of the OFSO exercises were pooled into two datasets. The questionnaire used to collect data during all included exercises was the collaboration, learning and utility instrument (CLU) measuring collaboration, perceived learning and utility from 1 (strongly disagree) to 5 (strongly agree) on a Likert scale [1–5] (see the Supplementary Materials). The CLU scale has been applied in similar studies of crisis exercises [1,4,47,48]. Primarily, it was developed by a team of academic instrument-developers together with emergency practitioners from response organisations. The development was made in different steps based on Stein's [21] learning theories, which have their out spring from Klabber's [49] perspectives on how institutions learn, Meyer and Rowan's 1977 decoupling theory [50], Berlin and Carlström's theories on sequential, parallel and synchronous collaboration [51]. The collaboration dimension encompassed questions about the collaborative characteristics of an exercise. The learning dimension elaborated lessons learnt from collaboration during the exercises. The utility dimension determined if the exercise was perceived to be useful during real emergencies. In addition, questions were elaborated about experience and affiliation.

The CLU surveys were all distributed and collected from emergency personnel in connection with inter-organisational exercises at the included ONSOs exercises. Regarding the OFFSOs exercises, the survey was e-mailed to the participants from an e-mail list. The homogeneity of the 17 items showed a Cronbach's α of between 0.68 and 0.88. Statistical significance was established at $p = 0.05$, and all tests were two-tailed [52]. The analysis stems primarily from descriptive data and regressions (bivariate and multiple). Data were imported and analysed in Statistical Packages for the Social Sciences (SPSS) version 24.0.

3.1. *The Context of the Survey*

The studied inter-organisational exercises were full-scale field exercises. All the organisations that normally participated in the scenario, e.g., coast guard, sea rescue, police department, fire department and ambulance services, were engaged in each exercise. Moreover, the exercises aimed to improve inter-organisational collaboration, crossing organisational boundaries during accidents and disasters. The exercises took place in different parts of Norway and Sweden (Table 1).

Table 1. Distribution of respondents in the on-shore organisation (ONSO) and off-shore organisation (OFFSO) exercises.

Published	Exercise/Scenario	Exercise Arrangement	Number of Organisations Involved in the Exercise	Number of Participants in the Study	Declined to Participate in the Study
[1]	Car ferry accident handled by ONSOS	ONSO	3	39	2
[1]	Fire at school	ONSO	4	28	1
[1]	Fire at work	ONSO	4	27	3
SUBTOTAL ONSOS:			11	94	5
[48]	1. Maritime oil spill 2. Maritime search and rescue	OFFSO	21	79	336
[4]	1. Fire at passenger ferry 2. Maritime search and rescue	OFFSOS	22	53	11
[50]	Maritime search and rescue	OFFSO	8	30	32
[49]	Maritime search and rescue	OFFSO	27	90	472
SUBTOTAL OFFSOS:			78	252	852
TOTAL ALL:			89	346	857

3.2. *Procedures*

The survey included staff in different positions, for example, operational staff in the field, and staff officers from levels of management. Informed consent was obtained from the organisers, and each respondent was provided with written information. They were informed about confidentiality and the opportunity to withdraw from participation in the survey at any time. The data were collected with informed verbal consent.

Self-administered questionnaires collecting data were distributed. The questionnaires were coded for each exercise, and the completed questionnaires were collected anonymously by the authors. The questionnaires from the ONSOs were in paper form, and the later was outlined as web-based documents, while the questionnaires of the OFFSOs were web based.

4. Results

4.1. *Participants*

A total of 94 participants responded to the ONSO paper form survey and 252 to the web-based OFFSO survey.

The response rate was 95% for the ONSO survey and 49% for the OFFSO survey. The participants of the ONSOs and the OFFSOs had previously participated in 1 to 12 exercises (ONSOs $M = 2.87$, $SD = 2.24$; OFFSOs $M = 3.53$, $SD = 1.64$) before the study. Their age ranged from 25 to 49 years for the ONSOs and 18–55 for the OFFSOs. In the ONSO survey, all participants (100%) belonged to the public sector (police personnel, fire fighters and ambulance services). For the OFFSO survey, 86% belonged to the public sector, 10% to private sector and 4% to volunteer sector.

4.2. Collaboration

A majority of the ONSOs (75.6%, M = 4.07, SD = 0.72) and even more of the OFFSOs (88.1%, M = 4.44, SD = 0.87) considered the exercises to be focused on collaboration. Less than half of the ONSOs (41.4%, M = 3.13, SD = 1.11) and 63.5% of the OFFSOs (M = 4.00, SD = 1.19) experienced that the collaboration began without an unnecessary waiting time. Additionally, 42.6% (M = 3.34, SD = 0.98) of the ONSOs and 57.2% (M = 3.97, SD = 1.22) of the OFFSOs considered that the exercises encompassed alternative strategies to collaborate. Moreover, 53.2% (M = 3.70, SD = 1.01) of the ONSOs and 79.7% (M = 4.40, SD = 0.99) of the OFFSOs considered that staff who needed to practice collaboration were engaged in the exercises. Discussions took place after the practical activities in the studied exercises; however, 33% of the ONSOs thought these discussions were insufficient, and they wanted more seminar activities after the practical actions (M = 3.17, SD = 1.00). In contrast, 29.8% of the OFFSOs considered the discussions to be insufficient, while 20.6% remained neutral (M = 3.42, SD = 1.42). Out of all the ONSO respondents, 44.6% did not consider the exercises to be those they usually practiced (M = 2.82, SD = 1.30), while only 5.2% of the OFFSOs considered the same (M = 4.46, SD = 0.93). The mean for all items within the collaboration dimension was 3.52 (SD = 1.01) for the ONSOs and 4.06 (SD = 0.64) for the OFFSOs (Figure 1).

4.3. Learning

The majority of the ONSO and the OFFSO respondents replied that they learnt new things to a certain degree during the exercises (ONSOs M = 3.66, SD = 1.28; OFFSOs M = 4.16, SD = 1.16). Nearly half of the ONSOs (45.7%, M = 3.26, SD = 1.34) and more than half of the OFFSOs (66.6%, M = 3.84, SD = 1.14) considered themselves to have learnt new things about the organisations involved in the exercise. Less than a quarter of the ONSOs (21.4%, M = 2.72, SD = 1.03) and under half of the OFFSOs (42.5%, M = 3.22, SD = 1.30) learnt something about the concepts and acronyms used by the organisations involved as well as their communication patterns (ONSOs 22.4%, M = 2.74, SD = 1.05; OFFSOs 60.3%, M = 3.72, SD = 1.19). Quite a few of the ONSOs (17%, M = 2.79, SD = 0.88) and half of the OFFSOs (47.9%, M = 3.72, SD = 1.19) considered themselves to have learnt about prioritising activities. The mean for all items within the learning dimension was 3.03 (SD = 0.97) for the ONSOs and 3.67 (SD = 0.93) for the OFFSOs (Figure 1).

4.4. Utility

Most of the ONSO and the OFFSO respondents (84.1% and 77.7%) considered the exercises to be useful during actual emergency work (ONSOs M = 4.45, SD = 0.90; OFFSOs M = 4.20, SD = 1.11). Furthermore, they regarded the inter-organisational exercises as having an impact on their everyday work (ONSOs 61.7%, M = 3.69, SD = 1.16; OFFSOs 44.0% M = 3.26, SD = 1.22). It should be noted here that 27.4% of the OFFOS remained neutral. The exercises were considered to be more valuable for the command officers (ONSOs 58.5%, M = 3.54, SD = 1.30; OFFSOs 50.4%, M = 3.68, SD = 1.18) than for the operative staff in the field (ONSOs 30.8%, M = 2.97, SD = 1.22; OFFSOs 29.3%, M = 3.21, SD = 1.23). The mean for all items within the utility dimension was 3.66 (SD = 1.08) for the ONSOs and 3.59 (SD = 0.71) for the OFFSOs (Figure 1).

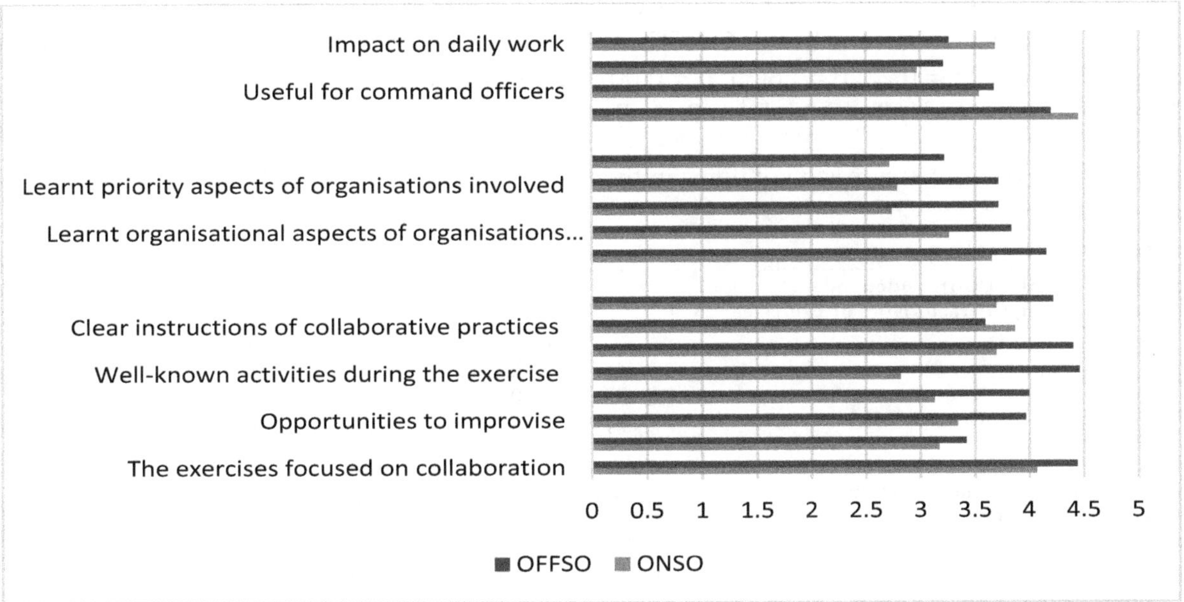

Figure 1. Mean values for the 94 ONSO and 252 OFFSO emergency personnel answering the collaboration, learning and utility instrument (CLU) scale, distributed in the dimensions utility (four items), learning (five items) and collaboration (eight items).

4.5. Bivariate Regressions

The causal effects of collaboration, learning and utility in the ONSO and OFFSO contexts were tested in a number of bivariate regressions. The collaborative dimension of the exercises was significantly correlated to the mean learning score across most of the items associated with the learning measurements in both exercise contexts. The strongest significant correlation on ONSOs was found between the item 'well-known activities during the exercise' and learning (R = 0.48), with this item explaining a significant proportion of variance in the mean learning score ($R^2 = 0.23$, F = 27.67, $p < 0.00$). The strongest significant correlation on OFFSOs was the item 'my point of view was regarded' and learning (R = 0.40), with this item explaining a significant proportion of variance in the mean learning score ($R^2 = 0.16$, F = 48.86, $p < 0.00$) (Table 2).

Table 2. Bivariate regression of items in the collaborative dimension of learning (sig. = $p < 0.05$).

Bivariate Regression ONSO N = 94 OFFSO N = 252						
Dependent Variables: Learning Independent Variables: Collaborative Characteristics of Exercises						
		Pearson R	R-square	F-Value	T-Value	Sig.
1. The exercises focused on collaboration	ONSO	0.27	0.08	7.31	5.03	0.00
	OFFSO	0.33	0.10	30.92	5.56	0.00
2. Discussions immediately after the exercise	ONSO	0.22	0.05	4.55	9.90	0.03
	OFFSO	0.16	0.02	7.08	2.66	0.01
3. Opportunities to improvise	ONSO	0.21	0.04	4.18	9.19	0.04
	OFFSO	0.24	0.05	15.93	3.99	0.00
4. Collaboration was initiated immediately	ONSO	0.39	0.16	16.81	10.19	0.00
	OFFSO	0.18	0.03	8.90	2.98	0.00
5. Well-known activities during the exercise	ONSO	0.48	0.23	27.67	13.73	0.00
	OFFSO	0.11	0.01	3.46	−1.85	0.06
6. Staff that needed to exercise participated	ONSO	0.27	0.07	7.37	7.99	0.00
	OFFSO	0.14	0.01	5.11	2.26	0.02
7. Clear instructions of collaborative practices	ONSO	0.43	0.19	21.33	8.69	0.00
	OFFSO	0.26	0.06	17.47	4.18	0.00
8. My point of view was regarded	ONSO	0.42	0.18	19.85	6.02	0.00
	OFFSO	0.40	0.16	48.86	6.99	0.00

Some of the items in the learning dimension were significantly correlated to the usefulness items. The strongest significant correlation of ONSOs was found between the item 'learnt new things' and usefulness (R = 0.47, R^2 = 0.22, F = 26.35, $p < 0.00$). A somewhat weaker correlation was found for the OFFSOs for the same item (R = 0.35, R^2 = 0.11, F = 31.99, $p < 0.00$) (Table 3).

Table 3. Bivariate regression of items in the learning dimension of utility (sig. = $p < 0.05$).

Bivariate Regression ONSO N = 94 OFFSO N = 252						
Dependent Variable: Utility Independent Variables: Learning Characteristics of Exercises						
		Pearson R	R-Square	F-Value	T-Value	Sig.
1. Learnt new things	ONSO	0.47	0.22	26.35	13.32	0.00
	OFFSO	0.35	0.11	31.99	5.65	0.00
2. Learnt organisational aspects of organisations involved	ONSO	0.30	0.09	8.89	16.58	0.00
	OFFSO	0.32	0.10	27.44	5.23	0.00
3. Learnt communicational aspects of organisations involved	ONSO	0.24	0.06	5.58	15.71	0.02
	OFFSO	0.29	0.08	21.82	4.67	0.00
4. Learnt priority aspects of organisations involved	ONSO	0.15	0.02	2.09	13.48	0.15
	OFFSO	0.31	0.09	25.64	5.06	0.00
5. Learnt new concepts	ONSO	0.14	0.02	1.89	16.04	0.17
	OFFSO	0.25	0.06	16.24	4.03	0.00

4.6. Multiple Regressions

Significant variables from the bivariate regressions were tested separately for the ONSOs and the OFFSOs in multiple regressions. In the case of ONSOs, the collaborative features together predicted 53% (R^2 = 0.53) of learning and for the OFFSOs, they predicted 25% (R^2 = 0.25) of the variance in learning. This meant that 47% and 75% of the predicted variance was non-unaccounted for in the case of ONSOs and OFFSOs, respectively. In the case of ONSOs, four variables were still significant: 'opportunities to improvise', 'well-known activities during the exercise', 'clear instructions for collaborative practices during the exercises' and 'my points of view were regarded'. The OFFSOs showed one still significant variable: 'my points of view were regarded'. The remaining variables displayed somewhat lower t-values and lacked significance on their own (Table 4).

Table 4. Significant variables of a multiple regression of items in the collaboration dimension of learning, (sig. = $p < 0.05$).

Multiple Regression ONSO N = 94 OFFSO N = 252					
Dependent Variable: Learning Independent Variables: Collaborative Characteristics of Exercises					
ONSO R = 0.73 R-SQUARE = 0.53					
	Bivariate St.Beta.	Multi.regr.St.Beta.	Diff.	T-value	Sig.
3. Opportunities to improvise	0.21	0.04	4.18	9.19	0.04
5. Well-known activities during the exercise	0.48	0.23	27.67	13.73	0.00
7. Clear instructions for collaborative practices.	0.43	0.19	21.33	8.69	0.00
8. My point of view was regarded	0.42	0.18	19.85	6.02	0.00
OFFSO R = 0.52 R-SQUARE = 0.25					
8. My point of view was regarded	0.40	0.29	0.11	4.78	0.00

In the next multiple regression, it was found that the items of learning predicted 26% (R^2 = 0.26) of the variance in usefulness in the ONSO and the OFFSO context. This meant that 74% of the predicted variance was still missing in the regressions. One variable was still significant, 'learnt new things' in the ONSO and the OFFSO contexts and 'learnt new concepts' in the OFFSO context. The other variables displayed moderate t-values and lacked significance on their own (Table 5).

Table 5. Significant variables of a multiple regression of items in the learning dimension of usefulness (sig. = $p < 0.05$).

Multiple Regression ONSO N = 94 OFFSO N = 252					
Dependent Variable: Utility. Independent Variable: Learning Characteristics of Exercises					
ONSO R = 0.50 R-SQUARE = 0.26	Bivariate St.Beta.	Multi.regr.St.Beta.	Diff.	T-value	Sig.
1.Learnt new things	0.46	0.46	0.00	4.21	0.00
OFFSO R = 0.52 R-SQUARE = 0.26					
1. Learnt new things	0.47	0.32	0.15	4.71	0.00
5. Learnt new concepts	0.63	0.13	0.50	2.04	0.04

5. Discussion

The OFFSOs considered the exercises to be focused on collaboration to a higher degree (88.1%) than the ONSOs (75.6%). In all items of collaboration, the OFFSOs scored a stronger result except on the item, 'if the actions were those they usually practiced'. Only 5.2% of the OFFSOs did not consider the actions to be those they usually practiced (ONSOs, 44.6%). A similar relation was found within the learning dimension. The majority replied they learnt new things, but the mean for all items within the learning dimension was higher for the OFFSOs (3.67) than for the ONSOs (3.03). The OFFSOs reported they learnt about communication patterns such as concepts and acronyms (60.3%) as well as prioritising (47.9%) to a higher degree than the ONSOs (22.4% and 17%). However, both OFFSOs and ONSOs showed equal results in the utility dimension. A few more participants in the ONSOs dimension perceived the exercises to be more useful during real life events than the OFFSOs (84.1% and 77.1%, respectively).

The multivariate regressions proved that collaboration had a higher degree of explanatory impact on learning for the ONSOs ($R^2 = 0.53$) than the OFFSOs ($R^2 = 0.25$). The impact of learning on the utility dimension was similar at sea and on dry land ($R^2 = 0.26$). The still significant items contributing to learning was 'my point of view was regarded' (OFFSOs and ONSOs). Additionally, 'well-known activities', 'clear instructions' and 'opportunity to improvise' had impact on learning in the ONSOs context.

The results of the study boil down to the finding that communication, learning new things and different points of view are regarded as important to achieve learning and utility from inter-organisational exercises. This calls for communicative and interactive processes during exercises [43]. There are, however, obstacles to achieving such a process. ONSOs repeat well-known activities and are known to be organisationally differentiated. OFFSOs seem to be more integrated than ONSOs, but they are restricted by international regulations. Furthermore, inter-organisational exercises often seem to strictly follow a predetermined manuscript, not allowing much room for improvisation. Consequently, exercises tend to restrict the learning and to be repetitive, drill-like and intra-organisational because of the lack of timeouts, spontaneous assessments and inter-organisational discussions, allowing for reflections on alternative ways to handle tricky situations [24,25,53]. The bivariate regressions, however, display that well-known activities had some impact on learning, especially in the ONSOs context ($R^2 = 0.23$ and OFFSO, $R^2 = 0.03$). A potential explanation can be the use of instrumental learning objectives, leaving little opportunity for improvisation [54]. This means that it is important to exercise well-known and repetitive everyday scenarios, and that new strategies may be developed to improve emergency responses. The result suggests that none of these extremes, (the unknown versus the familiar) can be excluded from inter-organisational exercises [42].

Lessons can be learned from inter-organisational exercises, both on- and offshore if they make room for the participants to talk informally before and after the training. In a recent study, the labelled side effect of the collaborative exercise was highlighted as more important than intra-organisational practices [40]. The opportunity to get to know each other and discuss structures improved collaboration in real life emergencies. This means that even though the inter-organisational exercise per se seems to have poor results, it might lead to the creation of a collaborative culture among the participants. The ability to form and develop relationships might be more valuable than the planned formal learning.

The reason for the surprisingly high degree of learning from OFFSOs exercises, in terms of communication patterns, may be traced to the fact that crisis management in the maritime context is a high-tech sector. Due to several digital and analogous communication and positioning systems as well as international and national regulations, the complexity in training for an accident, or a disaster at sea will be very educational, even if the techniques and scenarios have been practised before. Moreover, if the size of the exercise is too big, it can hamper the possibility for learning, as different actors may focus more on their individual goals and solve discipline-specific tasks rather than on cross-border collaboration and the sharing of resources [40].

Another reason for the stronger learning outcomes in the maritime context may be different cultures at sea and on dry land. ONSOs practise manoeuvres unique to their intra-organisational context, e.g., weapons, advanced medical equipment, fire and rescue equipment from a strict professional and legal perspective. The OFFSOs qualifications, on the other hand, may primarily be dominated by seamanship together with professional practice. The seamanship is a common necessity for all collaborating OFFSOs, whereas the different professions, to some extent, are limited within the physical boundaries of the ship itself. A second factor that is important for the evolvement of cultural bonds is a tradition of spontaneous communication between crews at sea. On dry land, we have bystanders, i.e., the public, and first responders, but in the maritime context all parties are expected to act as first responders, regardless of whether they are publicly financed rescue services. In densely populated areas on land, it is easier to hide behind the crowd during an emergency than it is at sea. Petrenj studied collaboration during accidents on land and highlighted that the main obstacles to collaboration was a lack of incentives and ambiguity in roles and expectations [55]. In the maritime context, actors have proven to be aware of a common and core value of understanding and agreement [56]. Such a value can offer synergies focused on the big picture rather than just prioritising specific tasks they are trained for [19]. In contrast to ONSOs, collaboration at sea seems to be part of the preparedness for everyday work and the ethos of seamanship.

5.1. Practical Implications

This study shows collaboration and learning may be obtained from exercises based on already well-known activities. In this study, well-known activities were combined with opportunities as independent factors for learning. These results can inspire exercise planners to combine the unknown with familiar scenarios. The results may also encourage planners to use timeouts, seminars and repetitions of actions in order to elaborate highly efficient types of inter-organisational collaboration. The use of scripts may hamper learning and utility. This can be addressed by increased the focus on improvisation, together with a new training methodology. Crossing organisational borders during exercises can contribute to a culture that stimulates collaboration, learning and utility in actual emergency work.

5.2. Limitations

There are limited studies on exercises and even fewer conducting meta-analysis of exercises. This study is based on five studies on nine exercises and the ONSOs were collected from only one study. In order to verify the results, several more context specific explorations have to be performed. Furthermore, studies on inter-organisational exercises on land and in the maritime context should be extended to other areas such as the aerospace industry and other security-intensive contexts. Even though Norway and Sweden, where the data for this study were collected, have a lot of similarities, exercises from different cultural contexts can provide important results, contributing to the understanding of how to improve learning and utility from inter-organisational exercises.

The poor participation for the OFFSO survey may be due to a lack of research interest among participants, but also the lack of influence of big scale exercises. It can also be related to intra-organisational focus- and sector-specific objectives. Another reason may be the web-based questionnaires. Compared to paper questionnaires, web-based questionnaires have proven to be less responsive in the Scandinavian context [57].

Author Contributions: Conceptualization, all; methodology, E.C. and J.L.S.; writing—original draft, E.C.; writing—review and editing, all; supervision, E.C. All authors have read and agreed to the published version of the manuscript.

References

1. Berlin, J.; Carlström, E. Collaboration Exercises. What Do They Contribute?: A Study of Learning and Usefulness. *J. Contingencies Crisis Manag.* **2015**, *23*, 11–23. [CrossRef]
2. Berlin, J.; Carlström, E. Learning and usefulness of collaboration exercises: A study of the three level collaboration (3LC) exercises between the police, ambulance, and rescue services. *Int. J. Mass Emergencies Disasters* **2015**, *33*, 428–467.
3. Kristiansen, E.; Löve-Sörensen, J.; Carlström, E.; Magnussen, L.I. Time to rethink Norwegian maritime collaboration exercises. *Int. J. Emerg. Serv.* **2017**, *6*, 14–28. [CrossRef]
4. Magnussen, L.I.; Carlström, E.; Sörensen, J.L.; Torgersen, G.E.; Hagenes, E.F.; Kristiansen, E. Learning and Usefulness stemming from collaboration in a maritime crisis management exercise in Northern Norway. *Disaster Prev. Manag.* **2018**, *27*, 129–140. [CrossRef]
5. Sorensen, J.; Magnussen, L.-I.; Torgersen, G.-E.; Christiansen, A.M.; Carlström, E. Old dogs new tricks? A Norwegian study on whether previous collaboration exercise experience impacted participants' perceived exercise effect. *Int. J. Emerg. Serv.* **2018**, *8*, 122–133. [CrossRef]
6. Axelsson, R.; Bihari-Axelsson, S. Integration and collaboration in public health: A conceptual framework. *Int. J. Health Plan. Manag.* **2006**, *21*, 75–88. [CrossRef]
7. Berlin, J.; Carlström, E. The Dominance of Mechanistic Behaviour: A Critical Study of Emergency Exercises. *Int. J. Emerg. Manag.* **2013**, *9*, 327–350. [CrossRef]
8. Norwegian Ministry of Justice and Public Security. Emergency Preparedness Principles. Available online: https://www.regjeringen.no/no/tema/samfunnssikkerhetog-beredskap/innsikt/hovedprinsipper-i-beredskapsarbeidet/id2339996/ (accessed on 30 April 2020).
9. MSB. *Så Bygger vi Säkerhet i Norden: Ett Svenskt Myndighetsperspektiv*; Myndigheten för Samhällsskydd och Beredskap: Stockholm, Sweden, 2011.
10. Norwegian Official Report. NOU 2012. Report from the July 22 Commission. Available online: https://www.regjeringen.no/contentassets (accessed on 6 June 2020).
11. Skr. *Strengthened Collaboration: Improved Safety, Stated by the Swedish Government*; Regeringskansliet/Försvarsdepartementet: Stockholm, Sweden, 2009.
12. Swedish Civil Contingencies Agency. *Civil Emergency Planning/Crisis Management in Sweden*; Myndigheten för Samhällsskydd och Beredskap: Stockholm, Sweden, 2018.
13. Berlin, J.; Carlström, E. Collaboration Exercises: The Lack of Collaborative Benefits. *Int. J. Disaster Risk Sci.* **2014**, *5*, 192–205. [CrossRef]
14. Van Wart, M.; Kapucu, N. Crisis Management Competencies. The Case of Emergency Managers in the USA. *Public Manag. Rev.* **2011**, *13*, 489–511. [CrossRef]
15. Aedo, I.; Bañuls, V.A.; Canós, J.-H.; Díaz, P.; Hiltz, S.R. Information Technologies for Emergency Planning and Training. In Proceedings of the 8th International ISCRAM International Conference on Information Systems for Crisis Response and Management Conference, Lisbon, Portugal, 8–11 May 2011.
16. Drennan, L.; McConnell, A. *Risk and Crisis Management in the Public Sector*; Routledge: New York, NY, USA, 2007.
17. Deverell, J. *Crisis-Induced Learning in Public Sector Organisations*; Elanders: Stockholm, Sweden, 2012.
18. Christensen, T.; Laegrid, T.; Rykkja, L. After a Terrorist Attack: Challenges for Political and Administrative Leadership in Norway. *J. Contingencies Manag.* **2013** *21*, 167–177. [CrossRef]

19. Scholtens, A. Controlled Collaboration in Disaster and Crisis Management in the Netherlands, History and Practice of an Overestimated and Underestimated Concept. *J. Contingencies Manag.* **2008**, *16*, 195–207. [CrossRef]
20. Groenendaal, J.; Helsloot, I.; Scholtens, A. A Critical Examination of The Assumptions Regarding Centralized Coordination in Large-Scale Emergency Situations. *Homel. Secur. Emerg. Manag.* **2013**, *10*, 113–135. [CrossRef]
21. Stein, J. How Institutions Learn: A Socio-Cognitive Perspective. *J. Econ. Issues* **1997**, *3*, 729–740. [CrossRef]
22. Corbacioglu, S.; Kapucu, N. Organisational learning and selfadaption in dynamic disaster environment. *Disasters* **2011**, *30*, 212–233. [CrossRef]
23. Bush, P.D. The Theory of Institutional Change. *J. Econ. Issues* **1987**, *21*, 1075–1116. [CrossRef]
24. Moynihan, D.P. From intercrisis to intracrisis learning. *J. Contingencies Crisis Manag.* **2009**, *17*, 189–198. [CrossRef]
25. Gredler, M. *Evaluating Games and Simulations, a Process Approach*; Kogan Page: London, UK, 1992.
26. Moynihan, D.P. Learning under Uncertainty: Networks in Crisis Management. *Public Adm. Rev.* **2008**, *68*, 350–361. [CrossRef]
27. Sommer, M.; Braut, G.S.; Njå, O. A Model for Learning in Emergency Response Work. *Int. J. Emerg. Manag.* **2013**, *9*, 151–169. [CrossRef]
28. Nemeth, C.; Wears, R.L.; Patel, S.; Rosen, G.; Cook, R. Resilience is not control: Healthcare, crisis management, and ICT', Cognition. *Technol. Work* **2011**, *13*, 189–202. [CrossRef]
29. Sullivan, H.; Williams, P.; Jeffares, S. Leadership for Collaboration. *Public Manag. Rev.* **2012**, *14*, 41–66. [CrossRef]
30. Torres, R.T.; Preskill, H. Evaluation and organisational learning: Past, present, and future. *Am. J. Eval.* **2001**, *22*, 387–395. [CrossRef]
31. Marchenko, N.A.; Borch, O.J.; Markov, S.V.; Andreassen, N. Maritime Safety in the High North:Risk and Preparedness. In Proceedings of the Twenty-Sixth International Offshore and Polar Engineering Conference, Rhodes, Greece, 26–27 July 2016.
32. Carlström, E.; Sörensen, J. Forberedt pa krise. In *Samvirke: En Larebok i Beredskap*; Kristiansson, E., Magnussen, L.I., Carlström, E., Eds.; Universitetsforlaget: Oslo, Norway, 2017; pp. 45–58.
33. Emad, G.; Roth, W. Policy as Boundary Object: A New Way to Look at Educational Policy Design and Implementation. *Vocat. Learn.* **2008**, *2*, 19–35. [CrossRef]
34. Almersjö, O.; Ask, E.; Brokopp, T.; Brandsjö, K.; Hedelin, A.; Jaldung, H.; Lundin, T. Branden på Scandinavian Star den 7 April 1990. In *SOS-Rapport 1993:3*; Socialstyrelsen: Stockholm, Sweden, 1993.
35. Cornwell, B.; Harmon, W.; Mason, M.; Merz, B.; Lampe, M. Panic or Situational Constraints? The Case of the M/V Estonia. *Int. J. Mass Emergencies Disasters* **2001**, *19*, 5–26.
36. Alexander, D.E. The 'Titanic Syndrome': Risk and Crisis Management on the Costa Concordia. *J. Homel. Secur. Emerg. Manag.* **2011**, 9. [CrossRef]
37. Zec, D.; Komadina, P.; Pritchard, B. Toward a global standard MET system: An analysis of the strengths and weaknesses of present MET systems. In Proceedings of the 1st International Association of Maritime Universities, Inaugural General Assembly & Congress, Istanbul, Turkey, 26–29 June 2000.
38. IMO. The STCW Convention & Code 2010 Manila Amendments. 2019. Available online: http://www.imo.org/en/OurWork/HumanElement/TrainingCertification/Pages/STCW-Convention.aspx (accessed on 1 August 2019).
39. Berlin, J.; Carlström, E. Why is collaboration minimised at the accident scene? A critical study of a hidden phenomenon. *Disaster Prev. Manag.* **2011**, *20*, 159–171. [CrossRef]
40. Kristiansen, E.; Håland Johansen, F.; Carlström, E. When it matters most. Collaboration between first responders in incidents and exercises. *J. Contingencies Crisis Manag.* **2018**, *27*, 72–78. [CrossRef]
41. Carlström, E.; Fredén, L. The First Single Responders in Sweden: Evaluation of a pre-hospital single staffed unit. *Int. Emerg. Nurs.* **2017**, *32*, 15–19. [CrossRef]
42. Comfort, L.K.; Kapucu, N. Inter-Organisational Coordination in Extreme Events: The World Trade Center Attacks, September 11, 2001. *Natl. Hazards* **2006**, *39*, 309–327. [CrossRef]
43. Wolbers, J.; Groenewegen, P.; Mollee, J.; Bím, J. Incorporating Time Dynamics in the Analysis of Social Networks in Emergency Management. *Homel. Secur. Emerg. Manag.* **2013**, *10*, 1–31. [CrossRef]

44. Borodzicz, E.P.; Van Haperen, K. Individual and group learning in crisis situations. *J. Contingencies Crisis Manag.* **2002**, *10*, 139–147. [CrossRef]
45. Sinclair, H.; Doyle, E.E.; Johnston, D.M.; Patton, D. Assessing Emergency Management Training and Exercises. *Disaster Prev. Manag.* **2012**, *21*, 507–521. [CrossRef]
46. McConnell, A.; Drennan, L. Mission Impossible? Planning and Preparing for Crisis. *J. Contingencies Crisis Manag.* **2006**, *14*, 59–70. [CrossRef]
47. Sorensen, J.L.; Magnussen, L.-I.; Torgersen, G.-E.; Christiansen, A.; Carlström, E. Perceived Usefulness of Maritime Cross-Border Collaboration Exercises. *Arts Soc. Sci. J.* **2019**, 9. [CrossRef]
48. Sorensen, J.L. Norwegian Maritime Crisis Collaboration Exercises: Are they Useful? Ph.D. Thesis, Graduate Faculty of the School of Business and Technology Management, Northcentral University, San Diego, CA, USA, 2017.
49. Klabbers, J. *The Exercises Planners Guide*; HMSO: London, UK, 1999.
50. Meyer, J.W.; Rowan, B. Institutionalized organizations: Formal structure as myth and ceremony. *Am. J. Sociol.* **1977**, *83*, 340–363. [CrossRef]
51. Berlin, J.; Carlström, E. *Samverkan på Olycksplatsen: Om Organisatoriska Barriäreffekter*; University West: Trollhättan, Sweden, 2009.
52. Altman, D.G. *Practical Statistics for Medical Research*; Chapman and Hall: New York, NY, USA, 1991.
53. Landgren, J. Spontant organiserad samverkan kompenserar för de centrala aktörernas misslyckande. In *Samverkan för Säkerhets Skull, Myndigheten för Samhällsskydd och Beredskap*; Nilsson, N.-O., Ed.; Myndigheten för Samhällsskydd och Beredskap: Stockholm, Sweden, 2011.
54. Magnussen, L. Didactics and Innovation in Collaboration for the Unforeseen in Training Practice Preparation. In *Interaction: 'Samhandling' Under Risk: A Step Ahead of the Unforeseen*; Torgersen, G.-E., Ed.; Cappelen Damm Akademisk: Oslo, Norway, 2018; pp. 339–353.
55. Petrenj, B.; Letterie, E.; Trucco, P. Towards enhanced collaboration and information sharing towards Critical Infrastructure resilience: Current barriers and emerging capabilities. In Proceedings of the 4th Annual International Conference on Next Generation Infrastructures, Washington, DC, USA, 16–19 November 2011.
56. Rykkja, L.H. Övelser i sammfunnsikkerhet som styrnings-och samordningsverktöy. *Nord. Organ.* **2011**, *12*, 2–25.
57. Ebert, J.F.; Huibers, L.; Christensen, B.; Christensen, M.B. Paper- or Web-Based Questionnaire Invitations as a Method for Data Collection: Cross-Sectional Comparative Study of Differences in Response Rate, Completeness of Data, and Financial Cost. *J. Med. Internet Res.* **2018**, *20*, e24. [CrossRef] [PubMed]

3

Acute Mental Health Needs Duration During Major Disasters: A Phenomenological Experience of Disaster Psychiatric Assistance Teams (DPATs) in Japan

Sho Takahashi [1,2,*], Yoshifumi Takagi [3], Yasuhisa Fukuo [4,5], Tetsuaki Arai [6], Michiko Watari [4] and Hirokazu Tachikawa [1,2]

1 Department of Disaster and Community Psychiatry, Faculty of Medicine, University of Tsukuba; Tsukuba, Ibaraki 305-8577, Japan; tachikawa@md.tsukuba.ac.jp
2 Department of Community and Disaster Assistance, Ibaraki Prefectural Medical Center of Psychiatry, Asahi-machi, Kasama, Ibaraki 309-1717, Japan
3 Nihon Fukushi University, Okuda, Mihama-cho, Chita-gun, Aichi 470-3295, Japan; cch61030@gmail.com
4 DPAT secretariat, commissioned by the Ministry of Health, Labor and Welfare, Kasumigaseki Chiyoda-ku, Tokyo 100-8916, Japan; josukef3@gmail.com (Y.F.); watari@dpat.jp (M.W.)
5 Kanagawa Psychiatric Center, Serigaya, Konan Ward, Yokohama, Kanagawa 233-0006, Japan
6 Department of Psychiatry, Division of Clinical Medicine, Faculty of Medicine, University of Tsukuba, Tsukuba, Ibaraki 305-8577, Japan; 4632tetsu@md.tsukuba.ac.jp
* Correspondence: takahashi.sho.fn@u.tsukuba.ac.jp

Abstract: Background: How long acute mental health needs continue after the disaster are problems which must be addressed in the treatment of victims. The aim of this study is to determine victims' needs by examining activity data from Disaster Psychiatric Assistance Teams (DPATs) in Japan. Methods: Data from four disasters were extracted from the disaster mental health information support system (DMHISS) database, and the transition of the number of consultations and the activity period were examined. Results: Common to all four disasters, the number of consultations increased rapidly from 0–2 days, reaching a peak within about a week. The partial correlation coefficient between the number of days of activity and the maximum number of victims showed significance. The number of victims and days of activity can be used to obtain a regression curve. Conclusions: This is the first report to reveal that mental health needs are the greatest in the hyper-acute stage, and the need for consultation and the duration of needs depends on the number of victims.

Keywords: disaster; Kumamoto earthquake; DMHISS; disaster psychiatry; Japan; acute mental health needs; duration of activity; DPAT (Disaster Psychiatric Assistance Team)

1. Introduction

In recent years, the question of how to respond to psychiatric disorders, as well as psychological problems, that arise among disaster victims has become a significant challenge. Many investigative studies have shown that the incidence of disorders such as post-traumatic stress disorder (PTSD) and depression increase markedly after disasters [1]. The criteria for PTSD require that the person was exposed to actual or threatened death, serious injury, or sexual violence [2]. There is a relationship between PTSD and disaster response. It is also known that psychosocial problems that accompany disasters, such as poverty, community breakdown, and the exacerbation of pre-existing psychiatric disorders, have long-term effects on the well-being of victims. Furthermore, existing psychiatric hospitals and health centers in disaster areas lose functionality during disasters and become unable to adequately undertake their consultations and diagnostic functions.

Following recent disasters around the world, such as Hurricane Katrina, the 9/11 terrorist attacks, and major earthquakes, postdisaster mental health services (MHS) have been organized and various kinds of mental health support have been provided [3]. The Inter-Agency Standing Committee (IASC), a nongovernmental organization (NGO), established a set of guidelines in 2007 on how mental health support should be conducted during disasters. These guidelines position mental health support for disaster areas within the broader context of psychosocial support, to create a system of combined mental health services and psychosocial support services (MHPSS), with interventions divided into four levels of specialized services, namely, focused specialized services, nonspecialized support, community and family support, and basic services and security [4]. Concerning specialized services, the guidelines state that interventions by specialists in psychiatry or psychology are necessary, but that due to the diverse social and cultural backgrounds of people in disaster areas, it is not possible to provide guidelines with regard to the specific services to be offered or the types of organized activities to be carried out.

Japan has been significantly affected by disasters, with one quarter of global disasters having occurred there in recent decades [5]. In the Hanshin-Awaji Earthquake of 1995, many people suffered from PTSD, and a psychiatric aid station was established to provide assistance. This led to a broader awareness of the need for psychological support for disaster victims. The 2011 East Japan Earthquake caused many people to suffer from PTSD due to the tsunami, along with the considerable stress suffered by those living in evacuation shelters. In response, several organizations and institutions, such as universities with psychiatry departments, academic associations, and NGOs organized disaster medical services [6], involving the creation of mental health care (*kokoro no care* in Japanese) teams, which carried out support work in the disaster areas. However, a lack of coordination among the teams, as well as their varied composition, led to confusion when providing assistance. There were also tragic cases in which patients in psychiatric hospitals were left behind during evacuation procedures immediately after the disaster, and who died because they could not be brought to the evacuation sites.

Drawing on these experiences, the DMAT system was modified to take into account specific psychiatric needs, and officially approved disaster psychiatric assistance teams (DPATs), which are dispatched to provide mental health support services to people in disaster areas, were established in 2013. The Ministry of Health, Labor, and Welfare (MHLW) determined the definition and role of a DPAT, set up a DPAT head office in Tokyo, and established DPATs in each prefecture and in designated cities in Japan. Since then, the number of teams across the country has gradually increased to 374 in 2017. Meanwhile, the support activities of DPATs have expanded as various disasters have occurred, such as volcanic eruptions, landslides, floods, and earthquakes. We found no other reports of such teams that have been organized to respond to mental health needs in acute phases of disasters in such a specialized and sophisticated manner.

However, clear guidelines have still not been determined for DPATs concerning the scale of activities to be carried out and at what point the work should be concluded. Because *kokoro no care* team that was active before the creation of DPATs focused primarily on mid- to long-term psychological support, data cannot be obtained that would contribute to the development of practical guidelines for acute phase activities. In relation to DPATs, a disaster mental health information support system (DMHISS) and an online database where all teams document their consultation activities have been established and are used in support activities, and it is now possible to do comparative studies using shared disaster support activity data. Therefore, we have examined data on support activities from multiple disasters that have occurred since the creation of DPATs. The aims of this study were to consider: (1) the scope of mental health needs in the acute phase of disasters, (2) whether organized MHS composed of specialists is necessary, and (3) the scale and time period necessary for the activities of acute-phase MHS.

2. Materials and Methods

2.1. *Subject of Investigation*

The period of investigation extended from 2013, when the DPAT system was first created, until 2016. The subject of investigation concerned the activity reports of DPATs, as well as daily reports from the DMHISS database, in relation to four disasters where support activities were conducted during that period, namely, the eruption of Mount Ontake (2014), the Hiroshima landslides (2014), the Kanto-Tohoku torrential rains (2015), and the Kumamoto earthquake (2016).

In the 2012fiscal year, the Toshiba Solutions Corporation was commissioned by the MHLW to develop a disaster mental health information support center. This resulted in the creation of the DMHISS, an online information system that aims to consolidate the activity logs of MHS and contribute to support that is appropriate for the needs of specific disaster areas. It came into nationwide operation in March 2013.

The functions of the DMHISS are divided to cover: (1) a normal period (prior registration of support teams), (2) an initial response period (coordination of support teams to be dispatched), (3) an activity period (collection of activity logs), and (4) a postactivity period (processing and analysis of activity logs). To facilitate these functions, an activity log collection tool allows data to be divided into microdata to record individual consultation trends and to record the daily activity logs of each DPAT team.

Items to be entered into the activity logs include team information (for example, team name, affiliation, and dispatch period) and type of support (for example, the results of processed data). Before and after its period of activity, each DPAT team enters its activity records into the DMHISS microdata sheet and the daily activity log. As a result, information concerning the people receiving consultations and details about the support activities of that day can be shared in real time between the disaster area itself, the base headquarters, the coordination headquarters, and the DPAT head office, thus making it possible to acquire detailed information about the activities of each DPAT [7].

2.2. *Methods of Investigation*

The definition of a DPAT, the structure of the organization, and an overview of its activities are first set out, followed with an explanation of the methods of investigation.

2.2.1. The Definition of a DPAT, the Structure of the Organization, and an Overview of Its Activities

A DPAT is a psychiatric team that has received specialized training for disaster management, which enables it to be dispatched to disaster areas. Additionally, DPATs are organized according to the administrative districts responsible for responding to disasters.

The main activities of a DPAT are: (1) responding directly or indirectly to the psychological problems experienced by residents in a disaster area at evacuation shelters, (2) coordination of the transport of patients from psychiatric hospitals whose functionality has been affected by the disaster, and (3) support for disaster relief workers. When DPATs are called into action, they move quickly to the disaster area or accident site, i.e., within 48 h, and in coordination with government agencies, fire departments, police departments, and defense forces, they conduct support activities for up to several months until there is no further need (Figure 1). A DPAT team consists of five people (composed of one psychiatrist, two nurses, and two logistics personnel for administrative work). Each team is dispatched to a site to conduct support activities for approximately one week. A reconnaissance team arrives in the disaster area within 48 h, sets up a DPAT coordination headquarters, coordinates with DMATs, coordinates the dispatched teams, and provides initial services at evacuation shelters. After that, the regional DPATs that follow continue the support activities in one-week rotations (Figure 2). The DPATs engage with the disaster countermeasure headquarters operating at the prefectural level, as well as with appropriate authorities at the health center and evacuation shelter levels, and at the level of each team, and coordinate with the DMATs to determine a plan for conducting support activities.

Under the direction of each DPAT headquarters, each DPAT can carry out its support activities at evacuation shelters and elsewhere in a coordinated and integrated fashion (Figure 3). Under the instructions of the disaster coordinator, DPATs also coordinate with medical teams such as DMATs, while medical teams coordinate with police, fire departments, and defense forces; health workers coordinate with health care centers.

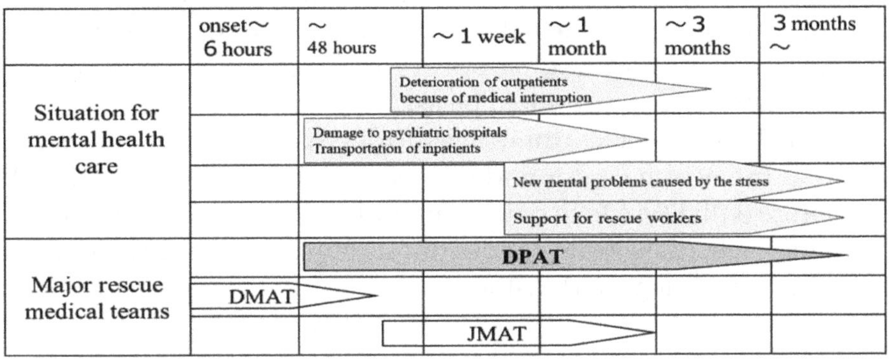

Figure 1. Postdisaster mental health care needs and DPAT dispatch periods. JMAT: Japan medical association team, DMAT; Disaster medical assistance team, DPAT; Disaster psychiatric assistance team.

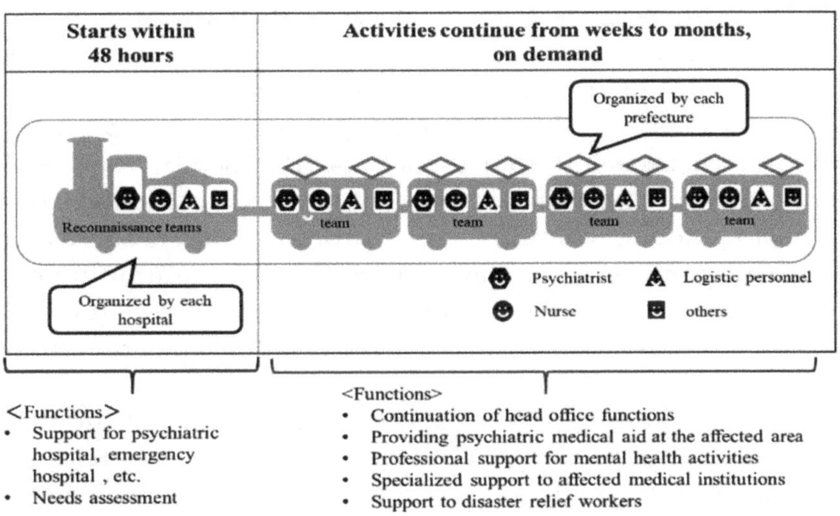

Figure 2. The roles of the reconnaissance Disaster Psychiatric Assistance Team (DPAT) and subsequent DPAT teams.

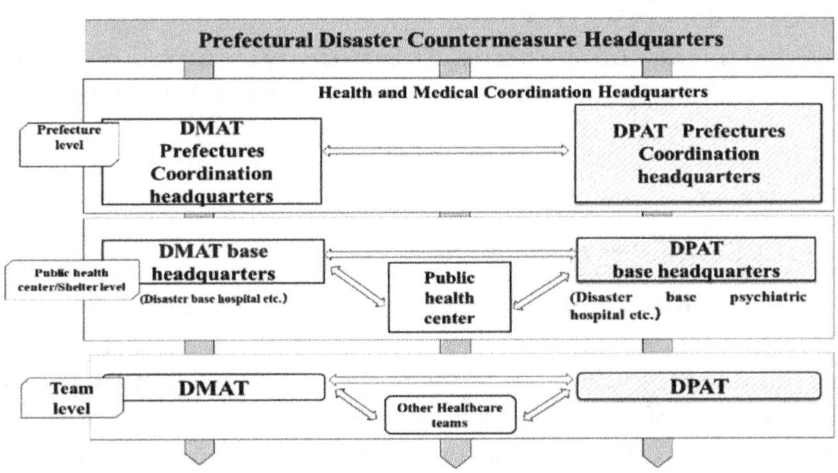

Figure 3. The Disaster Medical Assistance Team (DMAT) operational system.

DPATs arrive slightly later than DMATs, entering the disaster area within 48 h, and continue their activities for longer than DMATs, depending on the scale of the disaster. The timeline of their activities remains unspecified. DPAT: Disaster Psychiatric Assistance Team; DMAT: Disaster Medical Assistance Team; JMAT: Japanese Medical Association Team.

The reconnaissance team enters the disaster area within 48 h, establishes a headquarters, provides support for affected psychiatric hospitals and other health care institutions as required, and conducts need assessments for the disaster area. The subsequent teams provide services such as mental health care assistance, psychological support, and support for disaster relief workers in the affected area. These subsequent teams operate on a rotational basis.

DPATs engage with the disaster countermeasure headquarters at the prefectural level, with appropriate authorities at the health center and evacuation shelter levels, and at the team level with other teams, and collaborate with DMATs to determine a plan for support activities. Under the direction of the DPAT headquarters, each DPAT team carries out its support activities at evacuation shelters and elsewhere in a coordinated and integrated fashion.

2.2.2. Methods of Investigation

First, we summarized the damage situation and DPAT activities in relation to the four aforementioned disasters based on activity reports.

Next, we extracted data from the DMHISS database for these disasters, and created a data set for the daily reports. Following this, we aggregated the information on the dispatch and support structures for each disaster area, changes over time in the number of consultations provided, the number of teams engaged in support activities, and the duration of the period of activity. Furthermore, we divided the dispatch and support structures into four models as proposed by Katō et al. [8]: (a) an outside support model, wherein multiple support workers come from outside the disaster area to provide assistance; (b) a supervision model, wherein outside support workers serve as supervisors, but the support activities are carried out by local staff; (c) a local collaboration model within the region, wherein local organizations such as mental health and welfare centers take the lead in providing support, and; (d) a general support model, wherein mental health is incorporated into ordinary health care services.

We also estimated the duration period of activity for DPATs. At the time of estimation, we supplemented our data with data concerning the support provided by mental health care (*kokoro no kea*) teams before the creation of the DPAT system in relation to the Sayō-chō floods, the Niigata Chūetsu earthquake, the Hanshin-Awaji earthquake, and the East Japan earthquake, as derived from studies published in various documents such as the Cabinet Office's White Papers on Disaster Management and interviews conducted in each disaster area.

Concerning ethical considerations, we used only anonymous aggregated data from the DMHISS and publicly available documents for this study. This study was carried out with the approval of the Japan Psychiatric Hospitals Association Ethics Committee (approval number 161110-01).

3. Results

3.1. Comparison of Dispatch Systems for the Four Disasters

We compared the characteristics of the four disasters and the DPAT dispatch systems (Table 1). The disasters were of diverse types, comprising a volcanic eruption, flood disasters, and an earthquake. Although the number of casualties varied, in terms of damage conditions in relation to the number of people evacuated, the numbers of casualties steadily increased, from low numbers with the volcanic eruption, then rising for the flood disasters, and peaking with the earthquake.

Table 1. Aggregated data on damage situations and DPAT activities for the four disasters.

	Mt. Ontake Eruption	Hiroshima Landslides	Jōsō Floods	Kumamoto Earthquake
Onset date	2014/9/27	2014/8/20	2015/9/9	2016/4/14
Type of disaster	Eruption	Flood	Flood	Earthquake
Maximum evacuees	-	2354	6223	183,882
The number of dead	58	74	2	267
Model (early phase)	c	b	b	a
Model (middle and long term)	-	c	c	b
DPATs dispatch period (days)	6	23	27	90
Total number of DPATs	3	43	28	1242
Total number of consulting cases	12	106	139	2125
Sex (male/female/unknown)	5/7/0	43/63/0	58/70/11	717/1357/51

a–d: due to Models of disaster assistance [8]. Models of disaster assistance. (a) Outside support model: in which many support personnel come from outside the disaster area and provide support. (b) Supervision model: in which external support personnel act as supervisors, with support activities undertaken by regional staff. (c) Local collaboration model: in which the staff of mental health welfare centers mainly comprise locals. (d) General support model: in which mental health support is incorporated into ordinary health care services.

In the acute phase, DPAT dispatch and support operated in accordance with the local collaboration model within the region for the Mount Ontake disaster, the supervision model for the Hiroshima and Kanto-Tohoku disasters, and the outside support model for Kumamoto disaster; that is, the greater the scale of the disaster, the more outside support it required. In the mid- to long-term period, Hiroshima and Jōsō moved to a local collaboration model within the region, while Kumamoto transitioned to a supervision model. The period for which teams were dispatched varied a great deal, from 6 days to 3 months. In terms of the total number of teams dispatched, Mount Ontake had the smallest number of teams dispatched, i.e., three teams, while Kumamoto had the highest number, with 1242 teams taking part in support activities. In terms of the number of consultations, there were a total of only 12 for Mount Ontake, but over 100 each for Hiroshima and Jōsō, and 2125 for Kumamoto. In other words, the greater the scale of the disaster and the greater the number of evacuees, the greater the number of teams that were dispatched, and the longer the period of support activity.

3.2. Changes over Time in the Number of Consultations in the Four Disaster Areas

Next, we compared changes over time for the number of support consultations in each of the four disasters.

Figure 4 shows the changes in the number of consultations over time for three localized disasters, i.e., Mount Ontake, Hiroshima, and Jōsō. In the case of the eruption of Mount Ontake, the period of assistance lasted only four days, since many of the victims were people who had come from other prefectures for sightseeing and who were sent back to their home regions after four days of assistance. For the Hiroshima landslides, the number of consultations per day peaked on the 4th day, and on the 12th day after the flooding. After these days, the number of consultations gradually decreased, reaching 0 after approximately 1 month. For the Jōsō floods, the highest number of consultations occurred on the 1st day, at 27, then hovered in the 10–20 range for the next 3 days, after which it decreased to 7 consultations on the 16th and 20th days, before converging to 0 after approximately 1 month.

The vertical axis shows the number of consultations per day, while the horizontal axis shows the number of days following the disaster. The lines of the graph represent the changes in the number of consultations over time for each disaster.

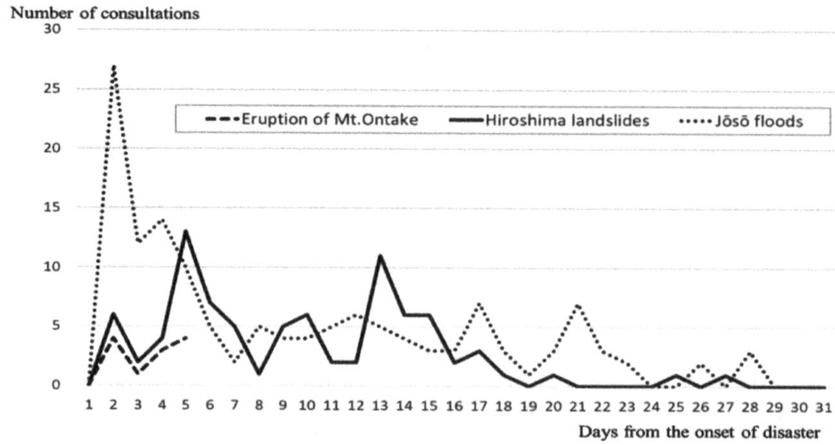

Figure 4. Changes over time in the number of consultations per day for the Mount Ontake eruption, the Hiroshima landslides, and the Jōsō floods.

Figure 5 shows the changes in the number of consultations over time for the Kumamoto earthquake. Immediately after the earthquake, patients were moved out of psychiatric hospitals that were at risk of collapsing, so support consultations at evacuation shelters essentially started on the 5th day. There were 66 consultations on the 6th day after the earthquake, with the number peaking on the 8th day, with 101 consultations. After that, the number of consultations decreased with fluctuations, but there were still more than 20 consultations on the 45th day. Two months after the earthquake, the number finally decreased to 15, and assistance continued with fluctuations before concluding after a total of 2–3 months.

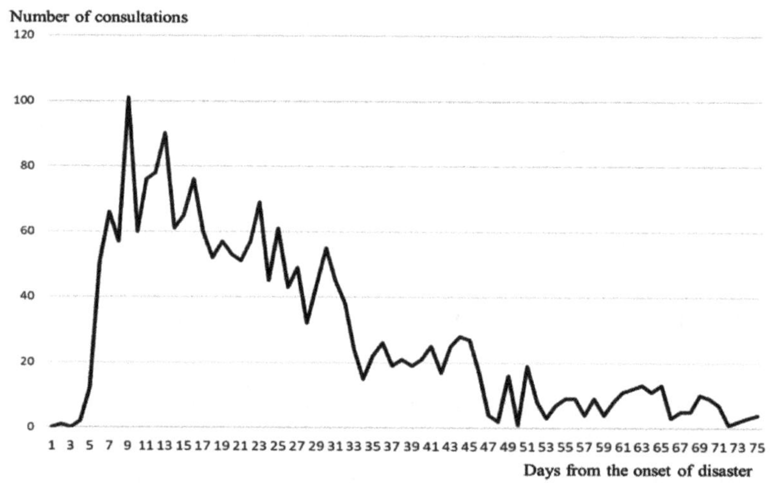

Figure 5. Change over time in the correspondence count per day for the Kumamoto earthquake.

The vertical axis shows the number of consultations per day, while the horizontal axis shows the number of days following the disaster.

For all four disasters, the number of consultations started to increase substantially on days 0–2, and reached a peak within approximately 1 week (1–8 days); the larger the scale of the disaster, the longer it took for the number of consultations to converge to 0. Especially in Kumamoto, the scale of the disaster was significantly greater than for the other three disasters, and the number of consultations also showed greater multimodal variation.

3.3. Estimation of the Period of DPAT Support from the Scale of the Disaster

In order to quantitatively consider the relationship between the scale of the disaster and the duration period of support, we also investigated the duration of the support period, the maximum number of evacuees, the number of dead, and the number of buildings damaged for other large-scale disasters in Japan, and compared the results (Table 2). An investigation of the partial correlation for each index showed that the partial correlation coefficient between the number of days of assistance and the maximum number of evacuees was significantly high, at 0.97 ($p < 0.001$).

Table 2. The number of DMS activity days and major indicators of damages in large-scale disasters.

Name of Disaster	Team Activity Days	Maximum Number of Evacuees	The Number of Dead	Number of Houses Damage
Sayō-chō Floods	22	2219	20	1790
Hiroshima landslides	27	2257	58	4559
Jōsō Floods	32	10,390	2	8327
Niigata Prefecture Chuetsu Earthquake	60	76,615	68	123,664
Kumamoto Earthquake	75	183,882	50	206,148
Great Hanshin-Awaji Earthquake	120	307,022	6400	256,312
Great East Japan Earthquake	120	409,146	15,735	1,137,785
Partial correlation coefficient (R2) with team activity days	-	0.97	−0.01	−0.57

A scatter plot detailing the number of evacuees and the number of days of assistance, where the number of evacuees is x and the number of days of assistance is y, yielded a regressive curve of $y = 0.0002x + 29.797$ (R2 = 0.95) (Figure 6).

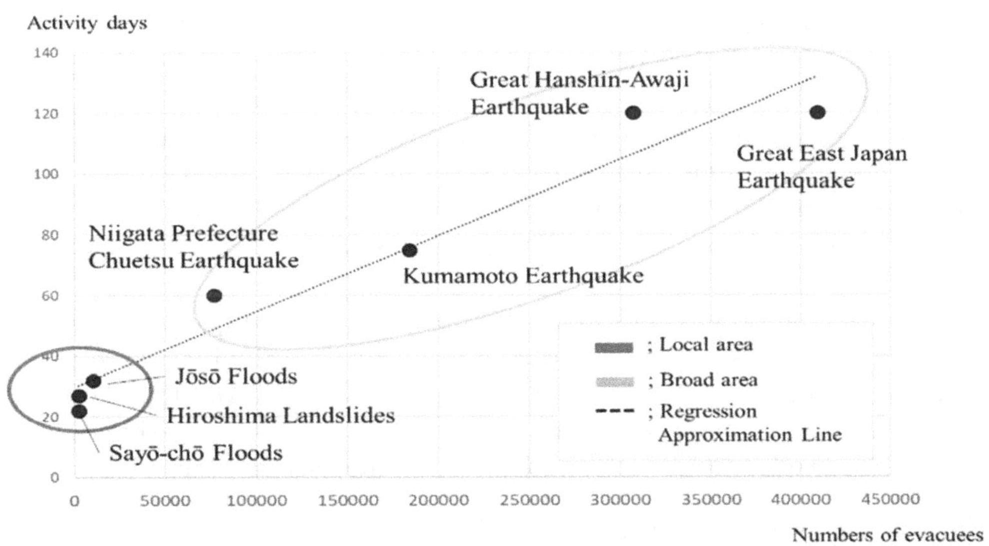

Figure 6. Plot of the team activity days and the maximum number of evacuees.

Figure 6 plots the disasters on a scatter diagram, where the vertical axis represents the team activity period (number of days) and the horizontal axis represents the maximum number of evacuees (number of people). The dotted line represents the regression line, the numerical formula represents the regression line formula and the regression coefficient, and the ellipses show the concentrations of localized disasters (Sayō-chō, Hiroshima, and Jōsō) and large-scale disasters (Niigata, Kumamoto, Hanshin-Awaji, and East Japan).

4. Discussion

Using mainly DPAT activity data, this study elucidated the need for mental health care in the acute phase of a disaster, the systems necessary to provide it, and criteria for determining the duration of team activity. This study is novel, not only because it provides an outline of the assistance activities of DPATs for the first time using real-time and objective data, but also in the sense that it has determined indices not seen in reports thus far to relate mental health needs in the acute phase of a disaster, the duration period of activities typically carried out in MHS in the acute phase, and the scale of the disaster.

In the section below, we provide a summary and interpretation of the results of the investigation.

4.1. *The Role of DPATs Nationally and Internationally*

In the MHPSS teams that existed prior to the DPAT system, mental health needs in the acute phase were not gauged, there was not a clear chain of command, and there was no training for support workers, so various problems tended to arise and were less effectively addressed in disaster areas. It would appear, when considering that in the Jōsō floods the DPATs successfully conducted assistance activities in coordination with the Japan Red Cross, and that in the Kumamoto earthquake, patients were successfully transported in a safe and organized manner, that the DPAT system has proved itself, in comparison to the MHPSS, to be a useful disaster mental health service in Japan, especially in the acute phase.

In the United States, under the assistance of the Federal Emergency Management Agency (FEMA) [9], the administrative agencies of each state have jurisdiction over various disaster support activities. However, although various psychological first aid (PFA) guidelines have been established, there are no specialized and standardized teams for disaster psychiatry. For example, mass shooting episodes have increased in recent decades with crisis response teams, which is not for disasters [10]. In Thailand, the Department of Mental Health established a mental health crisis assessment and treatment team (MCATT) system in 2012 [11]. A MCATT comprises a team of specialists including psychiatrists, doctors, psychiatric nurses, nurses, psychologists, and social workers, to provide assistance to disaster victims; it works in coordination with medical emergency response teams, disaster medical assistance teams, and surveillance rapid response teams. According to official requirements, ministries must configure subdistrict or state-level MCATTs with at least one team in each regional hospital (HEALTH, 2018). In South Korea, Korean disaster psychiatric assistance teams (K-DPATs) have begun activities [12] based on the DPAT system in Japan. However, any results concerning the activities of these teams remain unreported.

Compared with these other international MHPSS systems, a unique characteristic of the DPAT system is that standardized teams, centered around a psychiatrist and which have received specialized training, carry out organized mental health care activities starting from the ultra-acute phase after a disaster. Through sharing the results of DPAT activities both in- and out- side of Japan, this system has the potential to become a leading model in disaster mental health care.

4.2. *Mental Health Care Needs in the Acute Phase of a Disaster*

The number of consultations increased immediately after the disaster, reaching a peak in the ultra-acute to acute phase (ranging from 2 to 7 days), regardless of the disaster. Since psychological reactions result from the physical danger experienced immediately following a disaster, and since the most common conditions that arise in a disaster such as PTSD and depression are diagnosed after a certain period of observation, there has been a conventional general belief that mental health support may best be carried out after the acute phase. However, the results of this study have shown that mental health care needs are highest in the ultra-acute phase, so it is necessary for DPATs to do everything they can during this period. Based on the results of the responses to the four disasters, we also noted that consultation needs depended heavily on factors related to the scale of the disaster, such as the number of evacuees. For DPAT activities henceforth, it would be advisable to conduct overall preparation and training to provide swift and large-scale assistance starting from the ultra-acute phase and proportionate to the number of evacuees.

4.3. *The Duration Period of DPAT Activities*

The required duration period of DPAT activities can be determined by the time it takes for a local area's mental health and welfare system to recover. However, opinions vary as to what constitutes "recovery", and DPATs have struggled from their inception with the question of when to conclude their activities. Based on the regression equation for the two-dimensional scatter plot, $y = 0.0002x + 29.797$, with approximately one month as the y-intercept, we estimate that the recovery period increased by two days for each 10.000-maximum number of evacuees. Further, the same formula suggested that disasters should be considered separately, as both localized disasters, wherein assistance activities may last no more than one month, and disasters that occurred over a wide area, wherein assistance activities may last more than two months, had recovery times which were substantially influenced by the number of evacuees. The use of this kind of predictive formula for determining the duration period of activity has not been reported by DMSs working elsewhere. Furthermore, considering that in the mid- to long-term effects, the support model tended to change to a close collaboration model within the affected region, the basic period of DPAT support should perhaps be set at 1 month as a standard, and a method for smoothly transferring responsibilities back to the local mental health and welfare system should be considered. Furthermore, the periods of time following a disaster are usually divided into the immediate aftermath (ultra-acute phase), the acute phase, the middle phase, and the recovery phase (the long-term), but the number of days comprising each period has not been clearly defined. Considering our results, we suggest that, to facilitate recovery management, the time periods may be defined as an ultra-acute phase lasting 1–2 weeks, an acute phase lasting 1 month, and a mid- to long-term phase for subsequent engagement. As acute-phase mental health care assistance activities by DPATs and other forms of assistance continue to expand in the future, the predictive formula and its interpretation developed in this study should provide practical guidance for recovery interventions.

4.4. Limitations of this Study

This study had various limitations. Only a limited amount of data could be obtained concerning disasters, and there was a lack of prior relevant research. We searched the literature for intervention and comparative studies, but could not find any matches. Also, there was no study like this, so comparisons could not be made. There are only 12 literature publications, but there are few comparable studies, which was a difficult point. A search of past disaster dispatched psychiatric teams for all years showed no results. Few countries have done this, and few have reported on their activities; that is why there are few cited references. Therefore, we think that this paper has novel points.

More data on disasters should be accumulated. Also, the analysis concerning the duration period of activity included recent major disasters, but the MHPSS system was responsible for the mid- to long-term recovery period in relation to support activities conducted following the Hanshin-Awaji Earthquake and the East Japan Earthquake; hence, strictly speaking, its activities cannot be compared with those of the DPATs. In future, further data should be accumulated to aid in the undertaking of more precise analyses.

5. Conclusions

1. We compared activity data from four disasters where DPATs had provided support.
2. We discovered that mental health care needs were greatest in the ultra-acute phase following a disaster.
3. We discovered that the duration of the activity period was 1 month for localized disasters, or longer for disasters covering a wide area, depending on the number of evacuees.
4. It is necessary to accumulate more cases and examples to ensure more precise analyses.

Author Contributions: Conceptualization, S.T. and H.T.; Methodology, S.T. and H.T.; Software, S.T. and Y.F.; Validation, T.A. and H.T.; Formal analysis, S.T. and H.T.; Investigation, S.T., Y.T. and H.T.; Resources, M.W.; Data curation, S.T., Y.T. and Y.F.; Writing—original draft preparation, S.T.; Writing—review and editing, S.T. and H.T.; Visualization, Y.F.; Supervision, T.A. and H.T.; Project administration, S.T., H.T. and M.W.; Funding acquisition, M.W. All authors have read and agree to the published version of the manuscript.

Acknowledgments: We would like to express our sincerest sympathy to those struck by disaster, and once again to express our gratitude to everyone on the DPAT teams who have taken part in support activities from the acute phase to the mid- to long-term phase after a disaster.

References

1. Weisaeth, L. Disaster, Risk and preventive intervention. In *Handbook of Studies on Preventive Psychiatry*; Raphael, B., Burrows, G., Eds.; Elsevier: Amsterdam, The Netherlands, 1995; pp. 301–332.
2. American Psychiatric Association. *Diagnostic and Statistical Manual of Mental Disorders*, 5th ed.; American Psychiatric Publishing: Arlington, VA, USA, 2013; pp. 271–280.
3. Rodriguez, J.J.; Kohn, R. Use of mental health services among disaster survivors. *Curr. Opin. Psychiatry* **2008**, *21*, 370–378. [CrossRef]
4. Iasc Guidelines on Mental Health and Psychosocial Support in Emergency Settings: Inter-Agency Standing Committee. Available online: Https://www.who.int/mental_health/emergencies/guidelines_iasc_mental_health_psychosocial_june_2007.pdf (accessed on 23 December 2019).
5. Cabinet Office, Goverment of Japan. Disaster management in Japan. Available online: http://www.bousai.go.jp/kaigirep/hakusho/h22/bousai2010/html/honbun/2b_1s_1_01.htm (accessed on 23 December 2019).
6. Knouss, R.F. National disaster medical system. *Public Health Rep.* **2001**, *116*, 49–52. [CrossRef]
7. Fukuo, Y.; Tachikawa, H.; Takahashi, S.; Takagi, Y.; Yoshida, W.; Komi, M.; Arai, T.; Watari, M. An activity report of Disaster Psychiatric Assistant Team (DPAT) in the 2016 Kumamoto Earthquake: Special reference to the statistical data from Disaster Mental Health Information Support System (DMHISS). *J. Jpn. Emerg. Psychiatry* **2018**, *21*, 86–94.
8. Kato, H. Progress of Disaster Psychiatry in Japan. *Clin. Psychiatry* **2006**, *48*, 231–239.
9. Federal Emergency Management Agency (FEMA). National Incident Management System. Available online: http://www.fema.gov/national-incident-management-system (accessed on 23 December 2019).
10. Lowe, S.R.; Galea, S. The Mental Health Consequences of Mass Shootings. *Trauma Violence Abuse* **2017**, *18*, 62–82. [CrossRef] [PubMed]
11. Department of Mental Health MoPH, Thailand. Mental Health Crisis Assessment and Treatment Team: MCATT. Available online: http://www.skph.go.th/newskph/Doc_file/ManualMCATT2018.pdf (accessed on 23 December 2019).
12. Jo, S.J.; Na, K.S.; Park, J.E.; Lee, M.S. Decision Making Regarding Key Elements of Korean Disaster Psychiatric Assistance Teams Using the Analytic Hierarchy Process. *Psychiatry Investig.* **2018**, *15*, 663–669. [CrossRef] [PubMed]

4

Health Data Collection Before, During and After Emergencies and Disasters—The Result of the Kobe Expert Meeting

Tatsuhiko Kubo [1,*], Alisa Yanasan [2], Teodoro Herbosa [3], Nilesh Buddh [4], Ferdinal Fernando [5] and Ryoma Kayano [6]

1 Department of Environmental Epidemiology, Institute of Industrial Ecological Sciences, University of Occupational and Environmental Health, Kitakyushu 807-8555, Japan
2 Ministry of Public Health, Nonthaburi 11000, Thailand; yanasan.a@gmail.com
3 UP College of Medicine, University of the Philippines Manila, Manila 1000, Philippines; tjherbosa@up.edu.ph
4 WHO Regional Office for South-East Asia, New Delhi 110002, India; buddhan@who.int
5 The ASEAN Secretariat, Jakarta 12110, Indonesia; ferdinal.fernando@asean.org
6 World Health Organization Centre for Health Development, Kobe 651-0073, Japan; kayanor@who.int
* Correspondence: kubo@med.uoeh-u.ac.jp

Abstract: In October 2018, the World Health Organization (WHO) convened a meeting to identify key research needs, bringing together leading experts from WHO, WHO Thematic Platform for Health Emergency and Disaster Risk Management (Health-EDRM) Research Network (TPRN), World Association for Disaster and Emergency Medicine (WADEM), the Japan International Cooperation Agency (JICA), and delegates to the Asia Pacific Conference for Disaster Medicine (APCDM) 2018. The meeting identified key research needs in five major research areas for Health-EDRM. One of the five major research areas was "Health data collection during emergency and disaster". Experts for this research area highlighted WHO Emergency Medical Team Minimum Data Set (EMT MDS), a standardized medical data collection method during and after disasters, as an example of substantial progress, with knowledge gaps and challenges in implementation in some regions and countries (i.e., information collection methodology in medical facilities of affected local areas, seamless and practical connection between acute phase data collection and post-acute phase local surveillance). The discussion on this research area also identified key research needs in standardization of broader health-related data to inform effective Health EDRM (i.e., community vulnerabilities, hospital functional status, infrastructure, lifelines and health workforce).

Keywords: health emergency and disaster risk management (H-EDRM); Sendai Framework for Disaster Risk Reduction; WHO Thematic Platform for H-EDRM; Emergency Medical Team; Emergency Medical Team Minimum Data Set; epidemiology; Public Health Surveillance

---

1. Introduction

In October 2018 at the Asia Pacific Conference for Disaster Medicine (APCDM) 2018 [1], an expert meeting to identify key research needs in major research areas was organized by the World Health Organization (WHO) Centre for Health Development (WHO Kobe Centre (WKC)), convening the leading experts from the Asia Pacific region, WHO, WHO Thematic Platform for Health Emergency and Disaster Risk Management (Health-EDRM) Research Network (TPRN), World Association for Disaster and Emergency Medicine (WADEM). The expert meeting was conducted, along with progress in the scientific aspect of the implementation of the Sendai Framework on Disaster Risk Reduction 2015–2030 [2], the resulting document of the 3rd UN World Conference on Disaster Risk Reduction

(WCDRR), including establishment of TPRN, and following journal papers on recommended H-EDRM research activities [3–6]. Through the expert meeting and related review of literature and existing projects and activities, key research gaps in five major H-EDRM research areas were identified.

"Health Data collection before, during and after emergencies and disasters" is one of the five proposed major H-EDRM research areas. To conduct effective and timely health support in disaster relief and recovery activities, accurate and comprehensive health-related data is essential. Relief activities not based on relevant and accurate data could lead to negative impacts on recovery, related to the "do no harm" principle of Mary B. Anderson [7]. There have been a number of challenges in data collection in affected areas such as safe access to affected areas, preparing resources for data collection, obtaining informed consent from disaster victims, and fragmentation in data collecting and reporting methodology among different relief teams. All of these challenges cause a significant lack of scientific evidence in Health EDRM, especially the research with quantitative health data. For example, a MEDLINE search with MESH term "Disaster Medicine/statistics and numerical data" hit only 14 articles [8], which indicates a strong requirement of improvement in research and development of related methodology and tools for health data collection during and after disasters.

2. Material and Methods

The expert discussion of this research theme primarily aimed to identify recommended contents and source of health data to be collected, with reviewing the current available tools, methods and background systems and regulations in disaster relief activities. For the follow up of the expert meeting, a supplementary literature review and online discussion among the experts were conducted.

3. Results

Through the expert meeting based on a preliminary literature review, follow up online discussion, and a supplementary literature review, the experts developed the two research questions to be addressed, below. The greater details of the background of the proposed questions are described below.

(a) What are the national and regional challenges inhibiting implementation of the WHO standardized medical data collection systems during and after emergencies and disasters?
(b) What is the broader health-related data needed to inform effective Health-EDRM, i.e., community vulnerabilities, hospital functional status, infrastructure, lifelines and health workforce?

Firstly, the experts highlighted some key points for effective and practical data collection and utilization, including the "keep it simple" concept, which recommends simple and concise data, timely data collection for basic statistics in the manner to support operation, effective connection between collected data and ongoing response activities (i.e., recommendation to include geographical information).

Secondly, the current tools, methods and background systems and regulations in disaster relief were reviewed. A disaster is defined as a situation or event which overwhelms local capacity, necessitating a request for national or international level of assistance [9]. Although local health facilities are expected to function as a fundamental resource for disaster response, previous events revealed that local facilities often lose their functionally in major disasters. In a major disaster, a surge of affected patients further overwhelmed the damaged local capacities. To support local capacities by fulfilling the supply gaps, Emergency Medical Teams (EMTs), defined as a "groups of health professionals and supporting staff providing health care specifically to disaster- and health emergency-affected populations" are deployed to affected area [10]. To register as an EMT, verified by WHO, the team needs to meet EMT minimum standards, prepare resources for their activities by themselves, and regularly report their activities and status during their relief activities [11]. This nature of EMT supports the rationale for EMT to take a fundamental role for health data collection during and after disasters in collaboration with local capacities and under the agreement of affected countries. As EMTs can be deployed from different countries and organizations, the standardization of the data collection and reporting system has been a great challenge. Responding to this challenge, in 2017 EMT Minimum Data Set (MDS), a standardized medical data set to be collected and reported by EMT, was developed [12]. The fact that MDS became available was evaluated as an example of significant progress in health data collection by all of the experts who participated in the meeting.

Following the consensus on the improvement in health data collection by the development of MDS, the experts focused on the gaps and research needs for further comprehensive data collection to inform timely and effective disaster response and recovery. The expert meeting, and a following supplementary literature review, concluded that there is no internationally agreed or standardized methodology for public health data collection during and after a disaster, which indicates the substantial quality gaps between countries in post-acute phase health data collection and following response. The source and available tools and methods for health data collection are listed in Table 1.

Table 1. Source and available tools or methods for health data collection during and after emergencies and disasters.

Source of Data (Reporter)	Acute Phase	Post-Acute Phase
Emergency Medical Team (EMT)	WHO EMT Minimum Data Set (MDS)	(Demobilization)
Local Facilities (i.e., Hospitals)	(Often difficult to function to collect data)	Local surveillance
Public Health Sector	(No international consensus)	Local surveillance

Based on the proposed list of sources and tools for health data collection, several research priorities were identified. First, regarding the acute phase data collection, although WHO EMT MDS is available, some countries are not ready to implement it and need capacity-building and training to adapt their national system to meet international reporting standards. Experts supported research to analyze the best practices of and lessons from the implementation of MDS, for future effective capacity development in different countries.

Second, regarding data collection by and from local facilities, given the damaged capacity of local facilities during the acute phase, research on effective information collection and sharing systems through the collaboration between local facilities and EMTs is worth conducting. To address this research priority, including broader public health and environmental concerns (i.e., infrastructure, lifelines, hospital functional status, and health workforce available in communities) should be considered.

Third, in connection with the above-mentioned broader data collection, because there is no internationally agreed or standardized tool or method, research on setting up essential public health data for disaster response is expected to be conducted. The development process of WHO EMT MDS would inform the establishment of the broader data set.

Fourth, the experts also emphasized the critical knowledge gaps in an effective and harmonized transition from the acute phase, often relying on EMT activities to the post-acute phase relying on local capacities. Research on the seamless and effective connection of activities in those two phases is required.

4. Discussion

This expert discussion highlighted the needs and priorities in health data collection with a focus on on-site relief activities and medical support. To address the identified research needs for more comprehensive data for disaster response and recovery, inclusion of experts from other sectors such as United Nations International Strategy for Disaster Reduction, the World Bank and United Nations Development Programme will be the key. While the focus of this expert meeting was on post-disaster health data collection, understandably proper collection of baseline data before the disaster is essential to conduct efficient health emergency management.

In the Asia Pacific Region there are ongoing efforts to implement MDS, including the establishment and implementation of Surveillance in Post Extreme Emergencies and Disasters (SPEED) in the

Philippines, and the Japanese version of SPEED (J-SPEED). Those two data collection systems have already been used for large scale data collection. For example, in Japan, the health data of 8089 patients in the Kumamoto Earthquake in 2016, 3620 patients in the West Japan Heavy Rain in 2018 and 591 patients in the Hokkaido Earthquake in 2018 were collected through the J-SPEED system, and are being analyzed quantitatively. This experience supports the practical utility of WHO EMT MDS. To maximize the impact of the data collection during and after a disaster, usually health data registration is required as the preparedness before disasters. Strengthening the health system, including capacity building for disaster response, is also the key for successful data collection. More implementation research on practical adaptation of international standards is also required, as countries which still need support for capacity building face the requirement of partial implementation of the MDS to address their ongoing health challenges in disasters.

5. Conclusions

The expert meeting on "Health data collection before, during and after emergencies and disasters" provided a clear view on the sources and currently available tools for health data collection during and after emergencies and disasters, and therefore required research activities for further improvement for comprehensive health data collection for effective, timely and seamless interventions in disaster response and recovery. More implementation research should be conducted.

Author Contributions: Conceptualization, T.K., R.K.; Methodology, T.K., A.Y.; Writing—Original Draft Preparation, T.K.; Writing—Review & Editing, A.Y., T.H., N.B., F.F., R.K.; Project Administration, T.K.

Acknowledgments: The opinions contained in the paper are those of its authors and, except where specifically stated, are not intended to represent the official policies or positions of the WHO. The authors thank all the meeting participants who contributed to achieving the results: Paul Farrell (WADEM), Shuichi Ikeda (Project for Strengthening the ASEAN Regional Capacity on Disaster Health Management (ARCH Project), JICA), Tatruro Kai (Saiseikai Senri Hospital, Japan), Yasushi Nakajima (ARCH Project, JICA), Yosuke Takada (Okayama University, Japan), Nobuyo Tsuboyama-Kasaoka (National Institute of Health and Nutrition, Japan).

References

1. Asian Pacific Conference for Disaster Medicine 2018. Available online: http://www.apcdm2018.org/index.html (accessed on 15 January 2019).
2. Sendai Framework for Disaster Risk Reduction 2015–2030. Available online: https://www.unisdr.org/we/inform/publications/43291 (accessed on 15 January 2019).
3. WHO Thematic Platform for Health Emergency and Disaster Risk Management. Available online: http://www.who.int/hac/techguidance/preparedness/WHO-Thematic-Platform-Health-EDRM-Terms-Reference-2018.pdf?ua=1 (accessed on 15 January 2019).
4. WHO Thematic Platform for Health Emergency and Disaster Risk Management Research Network. Available online: http://www.who.int/hac/techguidance/preparedness/WHO-Thematic-Platform-Health-EDRM-Research-Network-2018.pdf?ua=1 (accessed on 15 January 2019).
5. Chan, E.Y.Y.; Murray, V. What are the health research needs for the Sendai Framework. *Lancet* **2017**, *390*, e35–e36. [CrossRef]
6. Lo, S.T.T.; Chan, E.Y.Y.; Chan, G.K.W.; Murray, V.; Abrahams, J.; Ardalan, A.; Kayano, R.; Yau, J.C.W. Health Emergency and Disaster Risk Management (Health-EDRM): Developing the Research Field within the Sendai Framework Paradigm. *Int. J. Disaster Risk Sci.* **2017**, *8*, 145–149. [CrossRef]
7. Anderson, M.B. *Do No Harm: How aid Can Support Peace or War*; Lynne Rienner Publishers: Boulder, CO, USA, 1999; p. 161.
8. Kubo, T. Disaster Medical Record/J-SPEED—Towards national implementation and international sharing of lessons learned from the Great East Japan Earthquake and the Kumamoto earthquake. *Prehosp. Care* **2018**, *31*, 64–68.

9. World Health Organization. *Definitions: Emergencies. Humanitarian Health Action*; World Health Organization: Geneva, Switzerland, 2018; Available online: http://www.who.int/hac/about/definitions/en/ (accessed on 17 April 2016).
10. World Health Organization. Emergency Medical Team. Available online: http://www.who.int/hac/techguidance/preparedness/emergency_medical_teams/en/ (accessed on 15 January 2019).
11. World Health Organization. *Classification and Minimum Standards for Foreign Medical Teams in Sudden Onset of Disasters*; World Health Organization: Geneva, Switzerland, 2013.
12. Emergency Medical Team Minimum Data Set Working Group. *Minimum Data Set for Reporting by Emergency Medical Teams*; World Health Organization: Geneva, Switzerland, 2017.

5

A Prognostic View on the Ideological Determinants of Violence in the Radical Ecological Movement

Elżbieta Posłuszna

Faculty of Aviation Safety, Military University of Aviation, 08-521 Dęblin, Poland; e.posluszna@law.mil.pl

Abstract: Ecologically motivated violence that manifests itself in the animal-rights and environmental forms is not a declining phenomenon. The fluctuating increase of the number of ecologically motivated crimes during the last 50 years, the multiplicity of the methods used (arson, food poisoning in supermarkets, destruction of equipment, attacks with the use of incentivized devices) should make us look at eco-extremism as a dynamic and difficult to grasp phenomenon. The paper is of both explanatory and prognostic nature; its goal is to present the genesis and essence of ecological radicalism, as well as to formulate the predictions for the future. In these forecasts, I wish to depart from the frequent, albeit somewhat simplistic, argument that, since the environmental extremist groups have not yet resorted to direct violence (targeting humans), and the animal-rights groups have reached for it very rarely, this state of affairs will continue in the future. This claim does not necessarily have to be true. I argue that some aspects of ideology can induce, in certain circumstances (a growing ecological catastrophe, further departure from the anthropocentric perspective), a change of the potential of radicalism within the environmental and animal-rights movements. In the case of animal-rights groups, the principle of not causing harm to people may be openly rejected, and in the case of environmental groups, the actions aimed at the annihilation of the whole human species may be undertaken.

Keywords: ecoterrorism; environmental extremism; animal-rights extremism; deep ecology; ecologically motivated violence

---

1. Introduction

We live in the shadow of the coming crisis. However, this crisis will be different from all the previous ones, for it will cover all spheres of life and will be total in its nature. It is a crisis of paradigms; the paradigms, like anthropocentrism or dichotomism, that for centuries, brought forth achievements of our civilization. These paradigms, however, have eventually led to the threat of self-destruction.

In 1962, Rachel Carson emphasized the need for attention to the emerging ecological crisis, by describing the impact of insecticides (such as DDT or aldrin) on the natural environment and the life support system over the longer term [1]. According to Carson, the greed and egoism of the lethal pesticide industry cannot be easily stopped, just as it is the case with the pursuit of technological progress that has become a permanent element of the post-war world. Therefore, the natural world, and consequently, human beings, are in mortal danger, and this cannot be easily reversed. Many ecological thinkers, such as Clarence Morris, Lynna White, and Christopher Stone followed this way of thinking, as well as numerous radical environmental and animal-rights organizations (Earth First!, Earth Liberation Front, and Animal Liberation Front).

British scientist James Lovelock presented a slightly different vision of the catastrophe (disaster) in his Gaia hypothesis in the early 1970s [2]. According to this hypothesis, the Earth is not merely a collection of living and inanimate entities, but a living superorganism that manipulates the Earth's atmosphere for its benefit, and strives for optimal harmony that promotes the development of life [2].

It is in Gaia's interest to keep all life on Earth in the state of dynamic balance (homeostasis). When this balance is disturbed, e.g., due to pollution or collision with a meteorite, it usually leads to the extinction of species, but not necessarily to the disappearance of life on Earth. The reason might be the fact that the earth will be able to adapt to new conditions and will survive; however, this adaptability may not necessarily be applied to its individual parts that have not developed such capabilities.

Although both concepts differ in the way that they see the future of the ecological system (according to the first, it will degrade, while the second states that it will cope), there is something that undoubtedly links them together, namely the belief that a catastrophe caused by humanity will destroy the foundations of its existence, and thus the whole species. Indeed, the changes that have been taking place in the world do not engender optimism. The surface temperature of our planet has risen by 1 °C over the past 150 years [3]. The effects of global warming include climatic anomalies such as floods, drought, desertification, cyclones, and hurricanes. In many regions of the world, progressive soil degradation occurs, which is manifested by erosion, loss of organic components, desertification, acidification, salinity or alkalization (excessive accumulation of sodium compounds). The increased emission of sulfur oxide (SO_2) contributes to the formation of acid rain, which then cause the degradation of forests, vegetation, and diseases of animals and people [4]. As many as 50% of the animals that once shared the Earth with us have already disappeared. A significant population decrease has been observed in another 30% of species. In recent years, most of them have lost over 40% of their natural habitat area, and almost half of them have lost more than 80% of their areas of occurrence in 1900–2015 [3]. Modern meat production, mass-scale fishing, and modern chemistry-based agriculture destroy the natural environment, and in moral terms, they bring forth the death and suffering of millions of animals. All these changes are brought forth because of human activity. Unfortunately, that is not all. Mass deforestation and the destruction of meadows destroy habitats of wild animals that massively move near human homes. This, in turn, results in the occurrence of numerous zoonoses, such as Spanish flu, AIDS, measles, Nipah disease, Ebola hemorrhagic fever, swine flu, SARS, MERS or COVID-19 [5].

Radical ecologists believe that humans are destructive beings, who use and misuse nature in the process of satisfying their non-vital needs. Being part of nature, they, of course, are entitled to protection, but as misusers, they deserve condemnation, and perhaps even exclusion from the biological community. The aim of this paper is to discuss the risks posed by eco-terrorism, and to investigate which branch of the ecological movement will radicalize and hence create new threats.

It should be noted that many researchers have doubts regarding the usage of the term "terrorism" concerning radical animal rights and environmental groups. Among such scholars, there is, for example, Christopher C. Harmon, according to whom activists whose actions are motivated by the will to protect animals and natural environment do not usually have an inclination towards acts that could be described as "terrorist." This means that they do not seek to destroy the social order, and are usually opposed to all forms of bodily integrity violations. Their goal is not to generate a sense of threat, but to stop the activities of certain classes of people (vivisectors, entrepreneurs, foresters). It is in this narrow-range mode of operation that they try to influence the policy of a given country or region [6]. A similar opinion is expressed by Leonard Weinberg and Paul Davis [7] or Bron Taylor, according to whom "despite the frequent use of revolutionary and martial rhetoric by participants in these movements, they have not, as yet, intended to inflict great bodily harm or death" [8].

Of course, environmental activists, who construct their conceptual framework on a different philosophical basis than their opponents, do not accept the term "terrorism" to be used to describe their actions. They argue, taking a completely "non-anthropocentric" position (egalitarian in relation to sentient beings or holistic in relation to the natural world), that the use of the term "terrorism" to denote activities that do not target natural (the environmentalist perspective) or sentient beings (the animal-rights perspective) is an abuse originating from the traditional (anthropocentric) moral perspective. This perspective leads to the erroneous perception of violence and terrorism as something that can occur only in relation to human beings and their property, and not in relation to other non-human beings. If we abandon this erroneous factor, which is based on our harmful habits of thought and perspective, we will have to recognize that the "real terrorists" are not those who fight for "oppressed beings" (animal and natural), but rather those "that promote or defend the exploitation of the natural world" [9].

The term "terrorism" is not neutral. This word has strong negative connotations and is associated with the need to take decisive defense measures to combat it. Therefore, even if we do not revise our conceptual framework and do not take the non-anthropocentric position, we will have to recognize that using this term to refer to groups that operate according to the non-violence principle must give rise to a feeling of inadequacy, or even injustice. It is especially so when we compare their "violent" actions with the activities of such groups as the Islamist Al-Qaeda or the anti-abortion Army of God, which are undoubtedly much more brutal. Moreover, the radicalism of the animal-rights and natural environment defenders is not particularly "impressive" when compared to other types of radicalism born in Western civilization (e.g., religious, nationalist, single issue, far right, and far left), both in terms of the numbers and violent nature of attacks [10].

At this point, it should be noted that the environmental activists are often the target of "terrorist" attacks. According to David Helvarg, the author of *The War Against the Greens*, some of these attacks in the US are organized by the robust Wise Use movement, that gathers farmers, property developers, hunters, SUV users, miners, free-market advocates, and religious fundamentalists. This movement, in Helvarg's opinion, is, in fact, not a grassroots campaign, but a kind of "astroturf", behind which big business hides [11], as well as those who are responsible for a series of acts of violence, such as intimidation, arson, assault, rape, and even murder towards people involved in the environmental movement [11]. Carl Deal, in his book *The Greenpeace Guide to Anti-Environmental Organizations*, expresses a similar opinion [12]. Public Employees for Environmental Responsibility (PEER) that studies and analyzes the actions of Wise Use, lists on its websites a number of acts of violence perpetrated by supporters of the Wise Use ideology, among which there are shooting at buildings, beating and intimidating, and planting bombs [13–15].

2. Methodology

The goal of the paper is to provide a narrative, based on interdisciplinary research, review on the topic of eco-terrorism. The study was carried out on the philosophical, political, sociological, and historical level. The basis of the entire research process was, of course, analysis and synthesis. The analytical method was deployed to examine original source texts, and all types of other studies (scientific and non-scientific). The purpose of the analysis of the source texts was to extract the truth about a given document, and to ascertain on its basis, as well as on the previously acquired knowledge, what the actual facts were. The goal of the analysis of the secondary literature was to, apart from expanding knowledge about the phenomenon, extract "alternative truths" and confront them with the author's own research intuitions. With the use of synthesis in the research process, the author intends to go beyond the mere merging of reconstructed fragments of the studied phenomenon, and to create a complete, and most importantly, meaningful and rich picture of the whole.

The paper is based on many sources that can be classified into a few groups. The first one are scientific works. Some concern the phenomenon of eco-extremism, others broadly understood security. The second group of sources includes reports of analytical centers and statistical materials. Some reports come from government agencies, some from private agencies. The third group of sources consists of propaganda materials of the discussed groups and the so-called narrative sources, namely "testimonies" (i.e., confessions of environmental radicals). These materials are posted on websites or published in a traditional form. The fourth group consists of documentary sources (official documents, court records, trial transcripts, official letters). The fifth group of sources includes press releases and news agencies reports. There are difficulties related to all those sources because, as it happens, various sources often give contradictory information (sometimes it is due to the imperfection of human memory, and sometimes it stems from a deliberate bending of facts in the sake of one's own, usually ideological, interests). It also happens that the authors are not neutral in their approach, which often leads to a distortion of the image of a given phenomenon. Therefore, in my research, I had to place great emphasis on identifying the most reliable data and distinguishing between facts and ideological propaganda, which I did by relying on my knowledge about the authors, the source of materials, and socio-political context.

3. Results

3.1. The Characteristics of Ecoterrorism

The belief of human superiority over all other beings [16] was rarely negated within the European culture. However, everything changed in the 1970s, when, within the framework of the culture, an extremist trend appeared that changed gentle activism into unprecedented committed radicalism. Today, ecologically motivated violence is no longer a marginal phenomenon. The data published by the FBI shows that among 112 attacks carried out between 1986 and 2005 in the United States, classified as terrorism, 57 were organized by groups or individuals motivated by environmental or animal-rights ideologies, such as Animal Liberation Front, Earth Liberation Front, Stop Huntingdon Animal Cruelty, Arissa, Animal Rights Militia, Band of Mercy, Justice Department, Animal Liberation Brigade, Vegan Dumpster Militia, Sea Shepherd Conservation Society, Direct Action Front.

Although, in the United States, there were only nine attacks in 1986–1997, the number grew to 48 in 1998–2005 [17]. The total number of incidents in the USA between 1979 and 2008 committed by ecological extremists was around 2000, and their total cost was estimated at $110 million [18]. These statistics do not include minor vandalism attacks, or small acts of violence against people, or, finally, botnet swarm attacks [19]. R. L. Young's doctoral dissertation examined the period, 1993–2003, and identified over 1400 incidents of terrorism committed by environmental and animal rights extremists [20], while Varriale-Carson, LaFree, and Dugan documented 1069 criminal incidents committed by these groups between 1970 and 2007 [21].

According to the data of the Foundation for Biomedical Research, in 1981–2005, there were 529 ecology-related crimes committed in the United States, including 53 arson attacks, 123 thefts, 36 bombings, 238 acts of vandalism, and 79 cases of harassment. A particular increase in crimes occurred after 1999. In 1998, there were only seven registered incidents of that kind, but in 1999, the number grew to 27, and the trend continued—in 2000 there were 28 of them, in 2001—42, 2002—17, 2003—101, 2004—99, 2005—82, and so on [22]. According to the data presented by the National Consortium for the Study of Terrorism and Responses to Terrorism, in the United States alone, there were 239 attacks between 1995 and 2010—arson (38%) and bombing attacks (62%), perpetrated by environmental (54.8%) and animal-rights extremists (45.2%)—mainly the ALF (Animal Liberation Front) and the ELF (Earth Liberation Front). More than 42% of these attacks resulted in severe financial losses [23,24]. These data indicate an increase in the number of incidents in 1995 through 2001, a variation in the number of incidents until 2010, and a relatively stable level after 2010 [24].

According to the data gathered by AnimalRighstsExtremism.info, there were 27 serious incidents worldwide between April 2012 and 5 September 2016 [25]. In 2010–2019, animal rights organizations carried out approximately 2521 prohibited acts, including sabotage, arson, "liberation" actions (in 2019—264, in 2018—306, in 2017—225, in 2016—124, in 2015—139, in 2014—214, in 2013—241, in 2012—251, in 2011—387, in 2010—370) [26]. The Global Terrorism Index states that attacks on facilities and infrastructure were the most common form of terrorist attacks in the US between 2002 and 2018, with a total number of 239 attacks. The majority of attacks were carried out by animal rights and environmentalist groups. It should be stressed, however, that these types of attacks result in very low casualties and rarely have loss of life as the main goal [27]. According to William Braniff, the Director of National Consortium for the Study of Terrorism and Responses to Terrorism, between 2000–2009, animal rights and environmentally motivated terrorist attacks were carried out by Animal Liberation Front (Coalition to Save the Preserves, Earth Liberation Front, Environmentalists, Revenge of the Threes,

Revolutionary Cells, Animal Liberation Brigade). In 2010—2019, in the US, there were six terrorist attacks that can be attributed to Animal Liberation Front, one attributed to the Justice Department, and three to environmentalist groups. One deadly attack was carried out by an anonymous person driven by broadly conceived ecological ideology [10]. Of course, these statistics are highly selective and do not take into account the attacks carried out in Europe and other various parts of the world.

3.2. Reasons for the Emergence of Ecological Extremism

The reasons for the emergence of environmental and animal-rights extremisms seem to be different. The sources of the former could be found in the early 1960s, when the correlation between the increase of exploitation of natural resources and the growth of prosperity started to be questioned for the very first time. Moreover, more and more people (mainly in the U.S.) began to realize that the possibility of an ecological crisis is real, and when it occurs, it will threaten all the species living on the earth. This emerging environmental awareness quickly resulted in protective activities. As early as in the second half of the 1960s, the consumer movements in the United States started to demand the right for "the natural environment that would correspond to the needs of the human body and high quality of life." More and more organizations were established to lobby for the natural environment. Despite the high activity of these movements, their actions did not bring forth expected results, or the results did not satisfy all of the members, who increasingly demanded more radical forms of fighting for the conservation of the natural environment. The 1979 decision of the U.S. Forest Service to use 36 million acres of forest areas for commercial purposes; the so-called RARE II ("Roadless Area Review and Evaluation II") was, as it seems, a turning point in the formation of green extremism. The decision was a great shock for some environmental activists. It not only showed the lack of ecological awareness of the agency, but also demonstrated the weakness of the traditional environmental organizations that were not able to oppose it, or did not want to, due to e.g., their relationship with large corporations and government agencies, as well as large internal bureaucracy. Because of general dissatisfaction caused by this decision and the unfavorable climate around the "legal environmental organizations", several groups were established, the sole purpose of which was to decisively (and not necessarily lawfully) combat the growing indifference towards the natural environment [28].

The emergence of the animal rights extremism is more difficult to picture, since it is problematic to point out a turning point that could be considered to be an "ideological trigger" of the animal-rights radicalism. It is so probably because the process of becoming radical was evolutionary, not revolutionary; it was a consequence of ever stronger and courageous demands regarding broadening moral horizons, so they included all previously discriminated groups of beings, including those who are unable to articulate the liberation postulates themselves. The animal rights movement was born in the 19th century in England, and although initially, the source of its motivation were not animals but human beings, more precisely, their spiritual and moral development; the movement relatively quickly tried to reject this "narrow anthropocentric perspective" in order to entirely equalize the respect of the interests of all sentient beings. This was the path that facilitated a formulation; in the 1970s, the most radical (and yet very catchy) claim of the modern "liberation movement" so far, namely that the discrimination of a creature only because of its belonging to a particular species is a superstition as immoral as racism or sexism. In contrast to the environmental extremism, which constituted to the influence of an eco-systemic threat, the radical movement of animal protection came into being, because of an altruistic development of moral awareness.

In the second half of the 20th century, this development brought about a real abundance of radical animal-rights groups fighting for a total ban on exploitation and killing of animals. The activities of radical groups defending the rights of animals, as well as those fighting for protection and conservation of the natural environment, are often analyzed together under the umbrella terms "ecological terrorism" or [29–31]. Such an approach is justified by the fact that many organizations belonging to the two movements closely cooperate, because their objectives, in many respects, confluence. Despite the convergence of the goals and quite similar intra-organizational structure (leaderless resistance model), there are some ideological differences between the radical environment activists and animal rights defenders that prevent them from a complete organizational convergence. Such differences also mean that some researchers (such as Wayman Mullins, Kenneth Dudonis, David Schulz, Sean Eagan) distinguish between ecoterrorism or environmental terrorism, understood as violence in defense of nature, and animal rights terrorism, understood as violence in the defense of animals [32–34]. The Earth Liberation Front and the Animal Liberation Front are, respectively, the most prominent representatives of those two types.

The Earth Liberation Front (ELF) was founded in England in 1992, by former members of Earth First!. The group's aim is to restore the original ecosystems, which in the opinion of the group's members, have been destroyed as a result of immoral and selfish human activities. According to Earth First!, adopting an uncompromising view, based on the philosophy of deep ecology attitude towards the natural environment, is a necessary condition to achieve this goal. Moreover, such an attitude should be expressed by direct actions. The ELF's attacks are aimed primarily at timber companies, institutions promoting genetic engineering, construction companies, car sellers, and power generating and distribution businesses, as well as, it is worth emphasizing, all structures that embody the "greed and injustice of the capitalist state" [35]. This last point requires a short elucidation, for the ELF does not only want to destroy the capitalist system, but also to remove profit as a motive for action from all spheres of social life [36].

The Animal Liberation Front (ALF), the largest extremist animal-rights group, was founded in 1976 by Ronnie Lee. The main goal of the group is to fight all forms of human exploitation of animals. Their attacks are aimed primarily at the meat production, food, pharmaceutical, fur, zoological industries, as well as research institutions. In the first period of its activity, the most frequent method used by the group was sabotage: freeing animals, inserting sticky substances into holes in locks, destroying equipment, painting on windows or breaking them. This relatively mild period of the ALF's activity ended in the 1980s, when the group began to organize acts of economic sabotage, like arson, planting explosive and incendiary devices, devastating laboratory equipment, or bricking up windows in butcher shops. The radicalism of the ALF grew in the mid-1980s, when the group started attacking people. The attacks most often consisted of threats, intimidation, and relatively minor cases of assault and battery, although sometimes, more drastic acts of violence also occurred (planting explosive devices in the homes of people working in companies exploiting animals) [37].

3.3. *Ideological Basis as a Source of Radicalism*

The ideological foundation of the radical environmental and animal rights movements is undoubtedly anti-anthropocentrism that manifests itself in the belief that the human being is not a unique and superior element of the world. Human beings, therefore, should not occupy a privileged place among other beings. However, the category of "other beings" is not shared by the two ecological radical movements. According to the animal rights activists, it is limited to sentient beings (who possess the so-called interests), and according to environmentalists, it includes all-natural creatures (including those inanimate as well).

Another difference is the placement of moral value. In the case of environmental radicals, this placement is of holistic nature, i.e., it is based on the belief that nature is not a mere collection of living and inanimate beings, but a biogenic whole that is infinitely more perfect than its individual human or non-human forms of existence [38]. This whole is not an aggregate—it possesses peculiar characteristics that cannot be reduced to the characteristics of its constituents (i.e., it is not merely a sum of the properties of its individual parts). Analyzing this claim from an ethical perspective, may lead to the conclusion that nature as a whole has a higher moral value than the individuals that constitute it. It is well reflected by the words of Aldo Leopold from his *A Sand County Almanac:* "A thing is right when it tends to preserve the integrity, stability, and beauty of the biotic community. It is wrong when it tends otherwise" [39]. Hence, nature is, primarily, entitled to respect and protection, and its less perfect parts should be considered in the second place. The practical dimension of this claim refers to the threat posed by environmental extremists, which may be the gradation of beings (certain parts of the whole that belong to the lower levels of the food chain have higher moral value than the ones that are on the top, e.g., the existence of oceanic plankton or soil bacteria is essential for the functioning of the ecosystem, while the existence of humans or tigers is not necessary). Secondly, due to the integrity of the ecosystem, the life of the representative of the endangered species should be given a higher value than the life of the human being, whose species is not threatened with extinction. Thirdly, since the human being threatens the entire ecosystem and does not seem to be necessary for its functioning, it can be stated that it would be better for the ecosystem if the human species disappeared entirely from the surface of the planet.

From the perspective of prognostic considerations, it should be acknowledged that the above claim may also lead to a hypothesis that, as long as human activities do not directly threaten nature as a whole, but merely harm certain parts of it that do not possess a full autonomous moral value, it can be expected that the environmental organizations will use non-threatening forms of persuasion. It is especially so because of their strong conviction of the sanctity of all life, including human life precluding such attacks. Still, for many radical environmentalists, the human beings are "problematic"—they are, indeed, a part of nature, but, at the same time, go beyond it through their hostile actions towards nature. As part of nature, they are obviously entitled to protection; as the beings that destroy nature—condemnation, or perhaps even exclusion from the biological community. These two perspectives of looking at the human being overlap and intersect. However, this standoff does not have to be permanent. It may change as soon as a severe ecological crisis occurs; one that will not pose a threat to some parts of the ecosystem, but to nature as a whole, which is given almost divine status by environmentalists. Then, one can expect a significant radicalization of their actions, that might target not only individual people, but all humankind.

Of course, the belief that human activity threatens the ecosystem as a whole is always a subjective, to a certain degree, conviction. Moreover, apparently, such a subjective conviction guided the actions of the R.I.S.E group [40], which, in 1972, hoping for the annihilation of the human species [32], decided to reach for, in their opinion the most reliable remedy—pathogens (corynebacterium diphtheria, neisseria meningitides, salmonella typhi, shigella sonnei) [40]. The pathogens were to be sprayed in supermarkets and large buildings using special aerosols, and for contamination of the water supply system of Chicago. It was not the only case of using a biological weapon by an environmental group. In 1981, a not well-known group called Dark Harvest Commando in protest against anthrax contamination, during World War II, of a small Gruinard Island located close to the Scottish mainland, placed a package containing the soil taken from the island in front of the Chemical Defense Establishment in Porton Down in Wiltshire. A few days later, a similar package was dropped off at the conference of the ruling Conservative Party in Blackpool [41].

The animal rights movements place moral value in individuals. A distinctive feature of their ideology is what could be called an "individual approach", which is manifested in the belief that the life and well-being of the individual has the priority. A person has the right to defend them even if, in consequence, it will necessarily lead to an infringement of the well-being of the ecological community they are a part of. Moral value is attributed here, above all, to individuals [42]. The latter category, according to the defenders of animal rights, includes all living beings capable of feeling pleasure and suffering, and thus has interests [43]. Among such beings, there are, of course, human beings and animals. Killing morally significant individuals (the one possessing moral value) is treated as the greatest crime that has to be firmly fought against. The consequences stemming from the adopted by the animal activists' assumptions are unequivocal. If we accept that animals, as well as people, have the same capacity for suffering and the right to equal treatment, then we must also recognize that their often cruel exploitation is evil and comparable to what slaves experienced at plantations or prisoners in concentration camps [44]. If it is additionally accepted that this evil must be necessarily opposed with the use of all possible and adequate means, then using violence against humans begins to appear as the supreme moral obligation [37].

Still, the evil that the animal rights activists fight against is rather individual, not collective in nature. In their writings, there are not many references to the collective responsibility or catastrophic visions of the end of the world. "Animal executioners" have names and addresses; they are concrete people who must be stopped or even "neutralized" at any cost. There have been several attempts of such "neutralization." One dramatic attempt of resorting to violence in the United States was an incident involving an activist, who in November 1988, was apprehended at the premises of the United States Surgical Corporation (a company that used dogs for testing surgical staples), while she was planting a high-class explosive device equipped with a radio igniter at the parking spot of the head of the facility. In February 1990, the Dean of the Veterinary School of the University of Tennessee was shot to death on his private farm. A month earlier, local police received a warning from the FBI National Crime Information Center that animal rights extremists threatened to murder the Dean in the next 12 months. On 6 May 2002, another activist committed a murder, which was intended to protect the "weakest part of society", in which, as it seems, he included animals [45]. In spite of the attacks of that type, humanity, according to animal-rights extremists, is not an impediment to the liberation of animals. People and animals can live in peace and harmony. Therefore, it seems impossible that the radical animal-rights activists would be willing to target humans. On the other hand, it is plausible and should be assumed that violence against individuals blamed for the oppression of animals is unlikely to diminish. On the contrary, it can even, given the growing willingness to challenge anthropocentrism, significantly escalate and radicalize.

4. Tactics

However, the differences between the two types of groups are not limited merely to ideology. They also manifest themselves in relation to violence and the tactics derived from it. In its struggle for "restoring ecological balance", the environmental movement employs, almost exclusively, indirect violence that is based on acts of ecological sabotage, whereas animal-rights groups, apart from indirect violence, use also, although in a limited scope, direct violence targeting human beings.

a. **Sabotage:** Sabotage, also known as ecotage (ecological sabotage) or "monkeywrenching" (from a monkey wrench, the most popular tool of saboteurs), is a common tactic to both types of groups, and involves a variety of methods, among which the most commonly used are: setting fire to tourist centers in construction, "tree spiking" (inserting long metal rods into the trunks of trees that are to be cut down. When the saw chain hits such a spike, it is torn, and its pieces often hurt the loggers). Destruction of machines and equipment, knocking down billboards, removing signs from the ski trails, dismantling power lines (environmental groups), releasing animals, destruction and setting fire to laboratories, walling up windows in butcher stores, destroying equipment used for transport or the slaughter of animals (animal-rights groups). "Monkeywrenching is believed to be more than just sabotage. It is revolutionary, Jihad, which even affects innocent bystanders, because in these desperate hours, bystanders are not innocent" [8].

b. **Arson**: The most spectacular method of ecotage has always been arson. This method was used in a famous attack on the Vail Ski Resort in Colorado on 19 October 1998. Its purpose was to protect the land inhabited by lynxes, and resulted in the destruction of the restaurant, four hotel buildings, and three chairlifts. Monkeywrenchers caused damage assessed at $12 million. Burning down the Vail Ski Resort is no longer the most costly act of environmental sabotage. Another arson attack that caused a total burn down of a residential complex and a crane in San Diego on 1 August 2003, resulted in losses at around $50 million. The most costly case of sabotage motivated by animal-rights ideology in the United States was undoubtedly the arson attack on the University of California Veterinary Diagnostic Center in Davis on 16 April 1987, in which several buildings and 18 vehicles were destroyed, with a cost of about $3.5 million [46]. This attack was the first classified as "domestic terrorism" by the FBI [47]. In June 2006, ALF members claimed responsibility for a firebomb attack on a UCLA researcher. A firebomb was planted on the doorstep of a house occupied by a 70-year-old tenant. However, it failed to ignite. The attack was used by the acting Chancellor of UCLA, to constitute the Animal Enterprise Terrorism Act. In December 2015, the ALF admitted that they had organized an arson attack on a clubhouse operated by the Fox Terrier Association in Germany, in consequence of which, the building burned down. This attack came after an incident in June of the same year, when the ALF released several foxes from an enclosure on the club's plot [48]. In June 2015, another arson attack took place—fire was set to two trucks belonging to Harlan Laboratory in Mississauga, Canada. The activists accused Harlan of supplying research animals and animal feed for vivisectionists [49].

c. **Direct attacks on humans**: Sabotage actions are not the only ones that radical environmentalists carry out. Some of them who belong to a not a very numerous group fighting for animal rights reach for more violent forms of persuasion, namely, the attacks directly targeting humans. There are two groups that should be mentioned here—the Animal Rights Militia (ARM) and the Justice Department (JD). The ARM's actions have always been organized as single, isolated attacks, and their primal aim was to intimidate "animal enemies." The first action carried out by the ARM probably took place in England on 30 November 1982. Explosives were sent to the offices of the leaders of four major political parties. Three of them were disabled, but the fourth one exploded in the hands of an official, and caused minor injuries [50]. Another ARM's action consisted of poisoning of Mars candy bars on 18 November 1984, which forced the company to withdraw the "suspicious" batch of products from the stores, and a loss of £3 million. A similar action was carried out by the Canadian ARM in 1992 [51]. At the beginning of the 1990s, the ARM's attacks became more violent. The most common practice was planting incendiary bombs in stores. Other attacks reported are; threats to kill (1998), poisoning (2006), contamination (2007) [48,52]. The ARM also took responsibility for attacks in Sweden, mainly against vivisection personnel and fur farm owners. The actions involved planting firebombs at a McDonald's restaurant in Gothenburg in 2011, bomb threats, letter bombs, and vandalism, targeting fur companies and vivisection personnel. According to the Animal Liberation Press Office, in 2011–2012, there was a wave of ARM-claimed attacks in Sweden, which occurred after the arrest of a young animal rights activist, who was sentenced to prison in 2011 [48].

d. **Other methods:** The methods used by the animal-rights group Justice Department were in many respects similar to those employed by the ARM, i.e., beatings, blackmail, and relatively harmless bomb attacks. The first action of the JD consisted of sending several package bombs to people who practiced "bloody" off-road sports, such as hunting or fishing. The packages did not reach the recipients—the explosion occurred at the sorting office in Watford. In 1996, the JD attacked representatives of the leather industry with the allegedly soaked in HIV infected blood razor blades. In 1999, yet again, the Justice Department Anti-Fur Task Force sent a letter containing razor blades to the representatives of the American fur industry. In February 2009, two scientists from Wake Forest University in North Carolina experimenting on animals received letters with razor blades covered in rat poison [53]. A similar action took place on 22 November 2010, when the Justice Department at UCLA sent bloody AIDS tainted razor blades to a neuroscientist and animal researcher. The North American Animal Liberation Press Office posted an anonymous communiqué from the group, who claimed that they had carried out the action because the scientist used primates for government-funded testing of drug addiction [54].

5. Discussion

It is undoubtedly the fact that the sensitivity of society to environmental problems has considerably increased over the past few decades. Nobody now negates the need to care for the welfare of our planet and its inhabitants. Despite sustained development and the increasing popularity of the environmentalist movement, as well as eco-friendly legislation adopted by many governments, the destruction of the natural environment progresses rapidly. Oil stains, clusters of trash in the oceans, the mass felling of Siberian and Amazon forests, air pollution, water poisoning, soil degradation, not to mention the greenhouse effect, are the facts to which, despite the declared indignation, one gets no real widespread and spirited reaction. Environmental and animal-rights activists often see this incapacity for self-restraint as a manifestation of destructive property intrinsic to human nature, which leads to a global ecological disaster/catastrophe. The catastrophe could be avoided not only by rejecting the anthropocentric culture, but also everything that it has created (modern medicine and agriculture, technology, industrialism). There is much skepticism regarding human nature and the possibility of the voluntary abandonment of anthropocentrism, which could foster the occurrence of a hostile attitude towards the human species and the readiness to eliminate it, at least partially [55].

Moreover, the times when animals were considered to be only tools whose sole purpose was to serve humans have already happened. More and more people are willing to see in animals the beings that, due to their ability to experience suffering, must be respected and protected, and even have the right to life and unfettered development. Ninety years ago, when industrial production changed farming into agribusiness, the living conditions of breeding animals have dramatically deteriorated. In those who are sensitive to the suffering of animals, such a state of affairs must necessarily cause frustration and outrage, which can easily lead to a desire to punish those who are responsible for that suffering. Here, as well, it is anthropocentrism (speciesism) that is blamed for that situation, but because of a strong individualistic attitude and a lack of a holistic approach, this "placing blame" is never of a total nature, i.e., it does not encompass the whole species. This is why the response to the evil that is experienced by sentient beings (animals) has to be individual (attacks on particular human individuals).

Can ecological radicalism change its nature or intensity? As it seems, the number of sabotage actions have not significantly changed. Due to a slow overcoming of anthropocentrism, one should instead expect the opposite trend. However, one thing should be noticed—over the past twenty years, radical ecological organizations have constantly broadened the scope of their goals. Nowadays, these organizations do not limit themselves to attacking forest-felling companies, ski resorts, high-voltage power lines, or laboratories where experiments on animals are carried out. More and more often, large corporations, private houses, SUVs, as well as various symbols of capitalism, become the subject of attacks [46]. The anti-capitalist attitude is obviously nothing new among the radical environmentalists and animal-rights activists. It was there before, but open criticism of capitalism and globalization occurred in the late 1990s, especially after the protests in Seattle in the fall of 1999, when people closely associated with anarchism and alter globalism started to have more influence on these movements. For them, the liberation of the earth has become closely linked to the abolition of capitalism and social liberation. The way to achieve that was not a slow reform, but a revolutionary spurt, preceded by mass attacks on the elements of the capitalist system [56]. The actions of the ELF can be comprehended as acts of revolution, not reform. The liberation of the Earth equals the liberation of every one of us [28,57]. Paradoxically, the broadening of the scope of objectives by incorporating the social ones that are specifically human (and hence pro-anthropocentric) can in fact, lead to the intensification of actions, but rather not to their brutalization. Such a situation in the case of environmental groups can even become an ideological safeguard against anti-human activities, which, in the era of the ecological catastrophe and relatively easy access to means of mass destruction, will become more than probable.

The word "jihad" used by many activists should be understood as the "jihad of the sword" but also, and perhaps even above all, as the "jihad of the heart", which is a profound transformation in the way of thinking and feeling, and which must arise in the minds of all monkeywrenchers. It seems that although many interpretations of Islam propagate the intrinsic value of animals [58] and there are even calls for Islamic eco-jihad [59], the above mentioned activists had in mind rather a common perception of the word as a wide-raging fight against the enemy. The actions of destroying machinery and objects that pose a threat to nature are such a fight. It is, however, not only a strategy, but an attempt to reorganize the world; an attempt of introducing an order that initially existed in the world, and which was lost by the people at some moment in time. The destruction of machinery is not violence but the only appropriate and necessary way of restoring these machines to their original form, their true unadulterated nature, which has been brutally taken away from them. Animal-rights radicals speak in a similar vein. In April 1989, the Animal Liberation Front organized a raid on the University of Arizona in Tucson, in the result of which, 1200 animals were liberated, and material losses stemming from the destruction of several buildings that were set on fire amounted to $250,000. After the action, the activists released a statement in which they claimed that the Arizona raid was conducted as "an act of mercy and compassion for the individual animal victims and also as part of a larger international campaign against the scientific/medical industry's misguided, anti-human, anti-earth, profit-oriented practices of vivisection, bio-technology, and synthetic pharmaceutical research" [60]. It is worth noting that the ALF always considered its sabotage activities to be completely violence-free [61]; violence can occur only in actions involving attacks on living beings capable of feeling joy and sadness. Military-type actions targeting objects used for inflicting suffering to animals are, in their opinion, purely defensive, and cannot be compared to bloody acts of terror.

As we observe emerging risk factors that may affect the future occurrence of public health emergencies, we may not forget the impact of eco-terrorism on the future development of the world. The actions conducted by eco-activists may be isolated but may also extend to a larger magnitude than we may be able to handle, resulting in major incidents and disasters. These actions should be taken into serious considerations, and contingency plans should also include suggestions to mitigate the impact of these actions. Whatever the causes, sabotage, arsons, direct violence, threats, bombs, etc. are all methods used in eco-terrorism. As we label these acts as instruments for terrorists, we may also consider that eco-terrorism might be easier to perform and the enemy may not be as visible as we believe.

6. Limitation

There are a few limitations to this study. This narrative review is an evidence-round up, on eco-terrorism, and not a systematic evidence-based investigation. Although this review may not have the same value as a systematic review, given the fact that the topic is seldom discussed, it still gathers enough information for further studies or a systematic review. Having this in mind, the selection of the literature used might be biased and based on the author's preferences.

7. Conclusions

Although the environmental extremist groups have not yet resorted to direct violence (targeting humans), and the animal rights groups have reached for it very rarely, the phenomenon itself and some aspects of ideology can induce, in certain circumstances, such as a growing ecological catastrophe, further departure from the anthropocentric perspective, a change of the potential of radicalism within the environmental and animal-rights movements. In the case of animal-rights groups, the principle of not causing harm to people may be openly rejected, and in the case of environmental groups, the actions aimed at the annihilation of the whole human species may be undertaken. This change may result in more extensive actions, and eventually major incidents and disasters. The will and threats from all radical organizations should be taken into serious considerations, and preventive measures should be established to prevent a future catastrophe.

References

1. Macnagten, P.; Urry, J. *Alternatywne Przyrody. Nowe Myślenie o Przyrodzie i Społeczeństwie*; Scholar: Warszawa, Poland, 2005; p. 67.
2. Lovelock, J. *Gaia: A New Look at Life on Earth*; Oxford University Press: Oxford, UK, 2000; p. 9.
3. Globalne i Regionalne Problemy Środowiskowe. Available online: https://geografia.na6.pl/globalne-i-regionalne-problemy-srodowiskowe (accessed on 1 July 2020).

4. Sustainable Development Goals "UN Report: Nature's Dangerous Decline 'Unprecedented'; Species Extinction Rates 'Accelerating'". Available online: https://www.un.org/sustainabledevelopment/blog/2019/05/nature-decline-unprecedented-report/ (accessed on 1 July 2020).
5. The Environmental Justice Foundation. Lynn Dicks, "Viral Diseases from Wildlife in China. Could SARS Happen Again?". 2020. Available online: https://ejfoundation.org/resources/downloads/EJF_Viral-diseases-from-wildife-in-China-2003-final.pdf (accessed on 1 July 2020).
6. Harmon, C.C. *Terrorism Today*; Frank Cass Publishers: London, UK, 2000; p. 8.
7. Weinberg, L.B.; Davis, P.B. *Introduction to Political Terrorism*; McGraw-Hill: New York, NY, USA, 1989; p. 7.
8. Taylor, B. Religion, violence and radical environmentalism: From earth first! to the Unabomber to the Earth Liberation Front. *Terror. Political Violence* **1998**, *10*, 1. [CrossRef]
9. Best, S. Behind the Mask: Uncovering the Animal Liberation Front. In *Terrorist or Freedom Fighters? Reflections on the Liberation of Animals*; Best, S., Nocella, A.J., II, Eds.; Lantern Books: New York, NY, USA, 2004; p. 31.
10. National Consortium for the Study of Terrorism and Responses to Terrorism (START); Homeland Security and Governmental Affairs Committee. Countering Domestic Terrorism: Examining the Evolving Threat. *Testimony of William Branif*, 25 September 2019, pp. 31–32. Available online: https://www.start.umd.edu/sites/default/files/publications/local_attachments/START_HSGACTestimony_CounteringDomesticTerrorism_Braniff_09252019.pdf (accessed on 14 March 2020).
11. Helvarg, D. *The War Against the Green. The 'Wise Use' Movement, the New Right, and Anti-Environmental Violence*; Sierra Club Books: San Francisco, CA, USA, 1994; pp. 120–122, 374–375, 385–389.
12. Deal, C. *The Greenpeace Guide to Anti-Environmental Organization*; Odonian Press: Berkley, CA, USA, 1993; p. 1.
13. Profile in Courage. Available online: http://www.peer.org/watch/wiseuse/profileincourage.php (accessed on 13 December 2008).
14. Employee Violence Report Covering 2004 Incidents. Available online: http://www.peer.org/watch/wiseuse/employee_violence_report_upto2004.pdf (accessed on 13 December 2008).
15. Vohryzek-Bolden, M.; Olson-Raymer, G.; Whamond, J.O. *Domestic Terrorism and Incident Management. Issue and Tactics*; Charles C Thomas Publisher: Springfield, IL, USA, 2001; p. 151.
16. Gen. 1:26. In *The Holy Bible: New Revised Standard Version*; Cambridge University Press: Cambridge, UK, 2005; p. 1.
17. U.S. Department of Justice, Federal Bureau of Investigation, "Terrorism 2002–2005". Available online: https://www.fbi.gov/stats-services/publications/terrorism-2002--2005 (accessed on 1 September 2019).
18. FBI. Putting Intel to Work: Against ELF and ALF Terrorists. 30 June 2008. Available online: https://archives.fbi.gov/archives/news/stories/2008/june/ecoterror_063008 (accessed on 1 September 2019).
19. Arquilla, J.; Ronfeld, D. Networks and Netwar. Available online: http://radio-weblogs.com/0107127/stories/2002/09/10/networksAndNetwar.html (accessed on 2 September 2019).
20. Young, R.L. A Time Series Analysis of ECO Terrorist Violence in the United States: 1993–2003. Ph.D. Thesis, Sam Houston State University, Huntsville, TX, USA, 2004.
21. Varriale-Carson, J.; LaFree, G.; Dugan, L. Terrorist and non-terrorist criminal attacks by radical environmental and animal rights groups in the United States, 1970–2007. *Terror. Political Violence* **2012**, *24*, 298–319.
22. *Illegal Incidents Report: A 25 Year History of Illegal Activities by Eco and Animal Extremists*; Foundation for Biomedical Research: Washington, DC, USA, 2006.
23. U.S. Department of Homeland Security. An Overview of Bombing and Arson Attacks by Environmental and Animal Rights Extremists in the United States, 1995–2010: Final Report to the Resilient Systems Division, Science and Technology Directorate. May 2013. National Consortium for the Study of Terrorism and Responses to Terrorism A Department of Homeland Security Science and Technology Center of Excellence. Available online: https://www.dhs.gov/sites/default/files/publications/OPSR_TP_TEVUS_Bombing-Arson-Attacks_Environmental-Animal%20Rights-Extremists_1309-508.pdf (accessed on 23 July 2019).
24. START, National Consortium for the Study of Terrorism and Responses to Terrorism. Ideological Motivations of Terrorism in the United States, 1970–2016. Available online: https://www.start.umd.edu/pubs/START_IdeologicalMotivationsOfTerrorismInUS_Nov2017.pdf (accessed on 23 July 2019).
25. AnimalRighstsExtremism.info, ARE INCIDENT MAP. Available online: http://www.animalrightsextremism.info/are-incident-map/ (accessed on 14 March 2020).

26. Bite Back Direct Action Info. Available online: http://www.directaction.info/news.htm (accessed on 14 March 2020).
27. Institute for Economics and Peace. Global Terrorism Index 2019. Measuring the Impact of Terrorism, Sydney, November 2019. Available online: http://visionofhumanity.org/app/uploads/2019/11/GTI-2019web.pdf (accessed on 14 March 2020).
28. Posłuszna, E. *Environmental and Animal Rights: Extremism, Terrorism, And National Security*; Elsevier: Amsterdam, The Netherlands, 2015.
29. Statement of James, F.; Jarboe, Domestic Terrorism Section Chief. Counterterrorism Division Federal Bureau of Investigation Before the House Resources Committee. Subcommittee on Forest and Forest Health. 12 February 2002. Available online: http://www.cdfearchives.org/jarboe.htm (accessed on 1 February 2009).
30. Laqueur, W. *The New Terrorism. Fanaticism and the Arms of Mass Destruction*; Oxford University Press: Oxford, UK; New York, NY, USA, 1999; pp. 199–204.
31. Liddick, D.R. *Eco-Terrorism. Radical Environmental and Animal Liberation Movement*; Praeger, Westport: London, UK, 2006.
32. Mullins, W.C. *A Sourcebook on Domestic and International Terrorism. An Analysis of Issues, Organizations, Tactics and Responses*; Charles C. Thomas Publisher: Springfield, IL, USA, 1997; pp. 229, 232.
33. Kushner, H.W. *Encyclopedia of Terrorism*; Sage Publications: Thousand Oaks, CA, USA; London, UK; New Delhi, India, 2003; pp. 32–35, 116–118.
34. Bolz, F.; Dudonis, K.J.; Schulz, D.P. *The Counterterrorism Handbook. Tactics, Procedures, and Techniques*; Taylor & Francis: Boca Raton, FL, USA; London, UK; New York, NY, USA; Singapore, 2005; pp. 157, 164.
35. U.S. Department of Justice. Federal Bureau of Investigation. Terrorism 2002/2003. Available online: http://www.fbi.gov/publications/terror/terrorism2002_2005.htm#page_21a (accessed on 8 October 2008).
36. Pickering, L.J. *The Earth Liberation Front 1997–2002*; Arissa Media Group: Portland, OR, USA, 2007; p. 47.
37. Henshaw, D. *Animal Warfare, The Story of the Animal Liberation Front*; Fontana Press: London, UK, 1989.
38. Callicott, J.B. Elements of an Environmental Ethics: Moral Considerability and the Biothic Community. *Environ. Ethics* **1979**, *1*, 71–81. [CrossRef]
39. Leopold, A. *A Sand County Almanac*; Oxford University Press: New York, NY, USA, 1991; p. 262.
40. Carus, S. R.I.S.E. In *Toxic Terror*; Tucker, J.B., Ed.; MIT Press: Cambridge, CA, USA; London, UK, 2001.
41. Eagan, S.P. From Spikes to Bombs: The Rise of Eco-Terrorism. *Stud. Confl. Terror.* **1996**, *19*, 7–8. [CrossRef]
42. Singer, P. *Animal Liberation*; Thorsons: New York, NY, USA, 1991.
43. Regan, T. *All that Dwell Therein. Animal Rights and Environmental Ethics*; University of California Press: Berkeley, CA, USA; Los Angeles, CA, USA; London, UK, 1982.
44. Jensen, D.; Opening the cages with the ALF. An Interview with David Barbarash. DerricJensen.org (17 December 2001). Available online: https://www.derrickjensen.org/2001/12/opening-the-cages-with-the-theALF/ (accessed on 1 September 2019).
45. Carnell, B. Volkert van der Graaf in Court, Brian.Carnell.Com. 14 April 2003. Available online: https://brian.carnell.com/articles/2003/volkert-van-der-graaf-in-court/ (accessed on 30 September 2019).
46. ADL. Ecoterrorism: Extremism in the Animal Rights and Environmentalist Movements. Available online: https://www.adl.org/education/resources/reports/ecoterrorism (accessed on 12 September 2019).
47. U.S. Department of Justice, U.S. Department of Agriculture, Report to Congress on the Extent and Effects of Domestic and International Terrorism on Animal Enterprises. 2 September 1993. Available online: http://www.rpoatexasoutreach.org/Brochurs_Flyers/Flyer%20-%20FBI_Report.pdf (accessed on 12 September 2019).
48. START—National Consortium for the Study of Terrorism and Responses to Terrorism. Available online: https://www.start.umd.edu/gtd/search/IncidentSummary.aspx?gtdid=201512020058 (accessed on 15 March 2020).
49. UPDATED: Animal Rights Group Claims Responsibility for Blaze that Destroyed Two Trucks in West Mississauga. Mississauga News. 8 June 2015. Available online: https://www.mississauga.com/news-story/5666768-updated-animal-rights-group-claims-responsibility-for-blaze-that-destroyed-two-trucks-in-west-mississauga/ (accessed on 16 March 2020).
50. Ezard, J. Animal Group says it sent bomb to PM. Guardian.co.uk, 1 December 1982. Available online: http://www.guardian.co.uk/fromthearchive/story/0,,1362801,00.html (accessed on 22 June 2019).
51. Smith, G.D. (Tim), Commentary No. 21: Militant Activism and the Issue of Animal Rights. April 1992. A Canadian Security Intelligence Service Publication. Available online: http://www.datapacrat.com/True/INTEL/CSIS/COM21E.HTM (accessed on 27 June 2019).

52. Facebook. Animal Liberation Press Office. 7 May 2019. Available online: https://www.facebook.com/AnimalLiberationPressOffic/posts/animal-rights-militiathe-animal-rights-militia-arm-is-a-banner-used-by-animal-ri/2278788152207848/ (accessed on 16 March 2020).
53. Bite Back Direct-Action Info. News from the Frontlines. Available online: http://www.directaction.info/news_aug28_07.htm (accessed on 16 March 2020).
54. North American Animal Liberation Press Office. Justice Department at UCLA sent bloody AIDS tainted razor blades to David Jentsch. Available online: https://animalliberationpressoffice.org/NAALPO/2010/11/22/justice-department-at-ucla-sent-bloody-aids-tainted-razor-blades-to-david-jentsch/ (accessed on 17 March 2020).
55. Aiken, W. Ethical Issues in Agriculture. In *Earthbound. New Introductory Essays in Environmental Ethics*; Tom, R., Ed.; Random House: New York, NY, USA, 1984; p. 269.
56. Leslie, J.P. ELF Communique. In *The Earth Liberation Front 1997–2002*; Arissa Media Group: Portland, OR, USA, 2007; p. 29.
57. Pickering, L.J. Final Statement of Leslie James Pickering as Spokesperson of the North American Earth Liberation Front Press Office. In *The Earth Liberation Front 1997–2002*; Arissa Media Group: Portland, OR, USA, 2007; p. 234.
58. Bernat, P. Sustainable development and the values we share—Sustainability as the confluence if islamic and western frameworks. *Probl. Sustain. Dev.* **2012**, *7*, 33–41.
59. Zbidi, M. The Call to Eco-Jihad, Environment and Ecology. 2013. Available online: http://environment-ecology.com/religion-and-ecology/738-the-call-to-eco-jihad.html (accessed on 28 July 2020).
60. Strand, R.; Strand, P. *The Hijacking of the Humane Movement*; Doral Publishing: Wilsonville, OR, USA, 1993; p. 121.
61. Stallwood, K. A Personal Overview of Direct Action in the United Kingdom and the United States. In *Terrorist or Freedom Fighters? Reflections on the Liberation of Animals*; Best, S., Nocella, A., II, Eds.; Lantern Books: New York, NY, USA, 2004; p. 83.

6

Disaster Preparedness and Professional Competence Among Healthcare Providers

Krzysztof Goniewicz [1,*] and Mariusz Goniewicz [2]

1 Department of Aviation Security, Military University of Aviation, 08-521 Dęblin, Poland
2 Department of Emergency Medicine, Medical University of Lublin, 20-059 Lublin, Poland; mariusz.goniewicz@umlub.pl
* Correspondence: k.goniewicz@law.mil.pl

Abstract: The preparedness of a hospital for mass-casualty incident and disaster response includes activities, programs and systems developed and implemented before the event. These measures are designed to provide the necessary medical care to victims of disasters, and to minimize the negative impact of individual events on medical services. Up until now, there has been no systematic survey in Poland concerning the readiness of hospitals, as well as medical personnel, to deal with mass-casualty incidents. Consequently, little is known about the knowledge, skills, and professional competences of healthcare workers. The objective of this pilot study was to start an exploration and to collect data on the competences of healthcare workers, in addition to assessing the preparedness of hospitals for mass-casualty incidents. Utilizing an anonymous survey of a random sample, 134 healthcare providers were asked to respond to questions about the competencies they needed, and hospital preparedness during disaster response. It turned out that the test subjects evaluate their own preparedness for mass-casualty incidents and disasters better than the preparedness of their current place of work. The pilot study demonstrated that a properly designed questionnaire can be used to assess the relationship between hospital and staff preparedness and disaster response efficiency. Evaluation of the preparedness and effectiveness of disaster response is a means of finding and removing possible gaps and weaknesses in the functioning and effective management of a hospital during mass-casualty incidents.

Keywords: disasters; healthcare workers; hospital preparedness; hospitals

---

1. Introduction

In a globalized world, in which crisis incidents are becoming more frequent, more devastating and have a significant impact on the health and lives of societies, the quality of healthcare services, including in particular the operational capacity of hospitals, is crucial for health security. A well-established preparedness program is a prerequisite for the effective response to emergencies of healthcare systems, including hospitals.

The preparedness of a hospital for mass-casualty incident and disaster response includes activities, programs and systems developed and implemented before the event. These measures are designed to provide the necessary medical care to victims of disasters, and to minimize the negative impact of individual events on medical services. These undertakings include, in particular, the appropriate training of medical personnel, appropriate safeguarding of logistics, and having validated emergency response procedures in place in the hospital. Evaluation of preparedness for incidents and disasters, as well as the effectiveness of response, is one way in which to locate and remove possible gaps and weaknesses in the functioning and effective management of the hospital during mass-casualty incidents (events that overwhelm the local healthcare system, where the number of casualties vastly exceeds the local resources and capabilities in a short period of time) [1–3].

Even in a well-prepared hospital, responding effectively to a disaster is a complex challenge. In the literature, there are many methods and evaluations [4–10] of the level of hospital emergency preparedness, but there is no consensus on correct and standardized methods and tools that would clearly define how individual institutions should prepare for crisis incidents [11–14]. This is largely due to the allocation of individual hospitals as well as, among others, geographical, demographic, climatic, social and economic factors, which may impact upon or be associated with the occurrence of particular events in a given region, or the response to them. It is also unclear whether individual procedures can reliably predict, in real time, the effectiveness of hospital functions [15–17]. Although many studies [18–27] have assessed the correlation between the level of hospital preparedness and disaster response, only a few functional elements have actually been assessed.

Although the World Health Organization (WHO) has developed the Hospital Safety Index (HSI) [28], a checklist of all hazards, which is a standardized, globally accepted method for assessing hospital preparedness, to date there have been no legally regulated international standards for hospital preparedness and response to crisis incidents [29–32].

Up until now, there has been no systematic survey in Poland concerning the readiness of hospitals, as well as medical personnel, to deal with mass-casualty incidents. Consequently, little is known about the knowledge, skills, and professional competences of healthcare workers [33–35]. This information is crucial for the development of effective response plans for individual hospitals, as well as for the preparation of training tailored to the needs of medical personnel [36,37]. The above-mentioned factors prompted the authors to undertake this study.

2. Aim

The main aim of the study is to investigate and to collect data on the competences of healthcare workers, in addition to assessing the preparedness of hospitals for mass-casualty incidents. An additional aim is to use the data from this initial survey to design a more comprehensive analysis of disaster preparedness (preparedness is defined by the United Nations International Strategy for Disaster Reduction as knowledge, capabilities and actions of governments, organizations, community groups and individuals "to effectively anticipate, respond to, and recover from, the impacts of likely, imminent or current hazard events or conditions), as well as new training and exercise models, which could improve the preparedness of health services for mass-casualty incidents and disasters.

3. Materials and Methods

3.1. Test Site

The study was conducted between 10 and 21 February 2020 at Public University Hospital No. 1 (polish SPSK No. 1) in Lublin. This hospital was selected as one of the largest hospitals in the Lublin region, and for this reason, it was chosen for the pilot study. SPSK No. 1 has a total of about 550 beds (including chemotherapy beds). It employs about 1600 people (including doctors, nurses and other medical personnel, as well as administration, technical, cleaning and service personnel). According to the latest data provided by the hospital, the number of hospitalizations for the academic year of 2017–2018 was about 40,000 cases, and the number of surgical procedures performed was about 19,000. The average time of hospitalization was 4.4 days.

3.2. Population Studied

The quantitative pilot study was conducted in the form of an anonymous questionnaire on a random sample of 134 healthcare workers, which account for 11.1% of the total number of employed healthcare workers at SPSK 1. More than half of them were women (56%). Men, on the other hand, constituted 44% of the research group. The respondents were mostly people with over 20 years of service (41.8%), while less frequently they had 6–10 years of service (19.4%), 0–5 years (16.4%),

11–15 years (12.7%) or 16–20 years (9.7%). Doctors (41.8%) and nurses (46.3%) represented the highest proportion of the study group, whereas 11.9% of respondents were paramedics.

3.3. Study Design

An extensive analysis of literature, and then the arrangement of the acquired knowledge through categorization and knowledge mapping, led to the development of a research tool in the form of a close-ended questions questionnaire. A qualitative method was used to verify the research tool and the questionnaire was tested on a sample of 10 people in order to check whether the respondents understood the questions it contained and whether the respondents reacted to some questions. This group was then excluded from the pilot study and their answers were not included in the final analysis. The questionnaire was designed in such a way that the time required to complete it did not exceed 15 min.

3.4. Type of Study

In the pilot study, an original questionnaire was available in both paper and online versions, and contained 18 closed questions and two additional descriptive questions. The respondents were asked about their own competences, experience, courses, and training completed, as well as knowledge about preparedness of the workplace for mass-casualty incidents. Respondents were also asked to rate their own preparedness on a scale from 1 to 10, as well as the preparedness of the hospital in which they worked, for mass-casualty incidents.

3.5. Data Analysis

Statistical analyses were conducted using IBM SPSS Statistics version 26. Frequency analyses, analysis of basic descriptive statistics, correlation analysis using Spearman's rho coefficient, the chi square test of independence, the Student's t-test for dependent samples, a one-way analysis of variance, and a Student's t-test for independent samples in addition to Mann Whitney's test were performed. The level of statistical significance was set at the classic level of $\alpha = 0.05$.

3.6. Ethical Considerations

The study is not a medical experiment and legally does not require the approval of the Bioethics Committee.

4. Results

4.1. Frequency Analysis

In response to the question about participation in a mass-casualty incident or disaster as a healthcare worker, the majority of respondents (74.6%) declared that they had not participated in such an event. More than a quarter of the respondents (25.4%) answered in the affirmative to the analyzed question.

The respondents were asked whether the facility where they currently worked has a plan for dealing with mass-casualty incidents and disasters. Most of the respondents (71.6%) answered "yes" to this question. Only 3% of the respondents answered "no" to this question. More than a quarter of the respondents (25.4%) felt they did not know the answer to this question (Table 3).

The respondents most frequently (77.6%) reported that they were familiar with the procedure for dealing with mass-casualty incidents and disasters. Only 22.4% of the research group was not acquainted with the procedure for handling such situations.

Most of the respondents (79.1%) knew who was responsible for managing mass-casualty incidents and disasters in the facility of their current workplace. On the other hand, 20.9% answered in negatively to this question.

In response to the question concerning the knowledge of the procedures to be followed in the event of evacuation during a mass-casualty incident at their workplace, the majority of respondents (87.3%) answered affirmatively. Only 12.7% of respondents did not know the procedures to be followed in this situation.

The respondents were asked whether their workplace had adequate logistical infrastructure for mass-casualty incidents. Most often (41.8%) respondents did not know whether their workplace had such a logistical infrastructure. On the other hand, 39.6% of the respondents believed their workplace to be prepared logistically for mass-casualty incidents. On the other hand, 18.7% of respondents answered negatively to this question.

More than half of the respondents (54.5%) reported a lack of organization with drills regarding disaster management at their workplace. In turn, 45.5% of the respondents stated that such activities had been organized at their workplace.

As far as the frequency of organizing drills is concerned, respondents most frequently reported that such drills were organized less frequently than once every 3 years (91.8%). Individual respondents provided the following answers: once every 3 years (3%), once every 2 years (3%) and annually (2.2%). More than half of the respondents (53.7%) had not received training related to disaster preparedness at their current workplace. However, 46.3% of respondents reported that they had received such training.

In response to the question concerning knowledge of triage, almost all respondents (99.3%) answered yes. Only one person answered negatively to this question.

4.2. Relationship between Sociodemographic Variables and Evaluation of Preparedness for Mass-Casualty Incidents and Disasters

The statistical analyses carried out checked the relationship between sociodemographic variables and the evaluation of preparedness for mass-casualty incidents and disasters. To this end, a correlation analysis using Spearman's rho coefficient and a one-way analysis of variance were performed.

Initially, the relationship between the seniority of the respondents and the evaluation of preparedness for mass-casualty incidents and disasters was tested. For this purpose, correlation analyses using Spearman's rho coefficient were performed. The results of this analysis are presented in Table 1.

Table 1. Results of the analysis of correlation between the length of service of the respondents and the evaluation of preparedness for mass-casualty incidents and disasters.

		Length of Service
Evaluation of the preparedness of the current workplace for a mass-casualty incident or disaster	Spearman's *rho*	0.19
	significance	0.033
Evaluation of one's own preparedness for mass-casualty incidents or disasters	Spearman's *rho*	0.14
	significance	0.108

According to the analyses carried out, seniority is positively linked to the evaluation of the preparedness of the current workplace for a mass-casualty incident or disaster (weak link). This shows that the longer the respondents have been working, the better do they evaluate the preparedness of the institution where they work for a mass-casualty incident or disaster.

A one-way analysis of variance was then carried out to see if occupation differentiates the evaluation of preparedness for mass-casualty incidents or disasters. The results of this analysis are presented in Figure 1.

The results indicate a statistically significant effect for assessing the preparedness of the current workplace for a mass-casualty incident or disaster. In order to investigate the exact differences, Sidak post hoc tests were performed. The test results show no statistically significant difference.

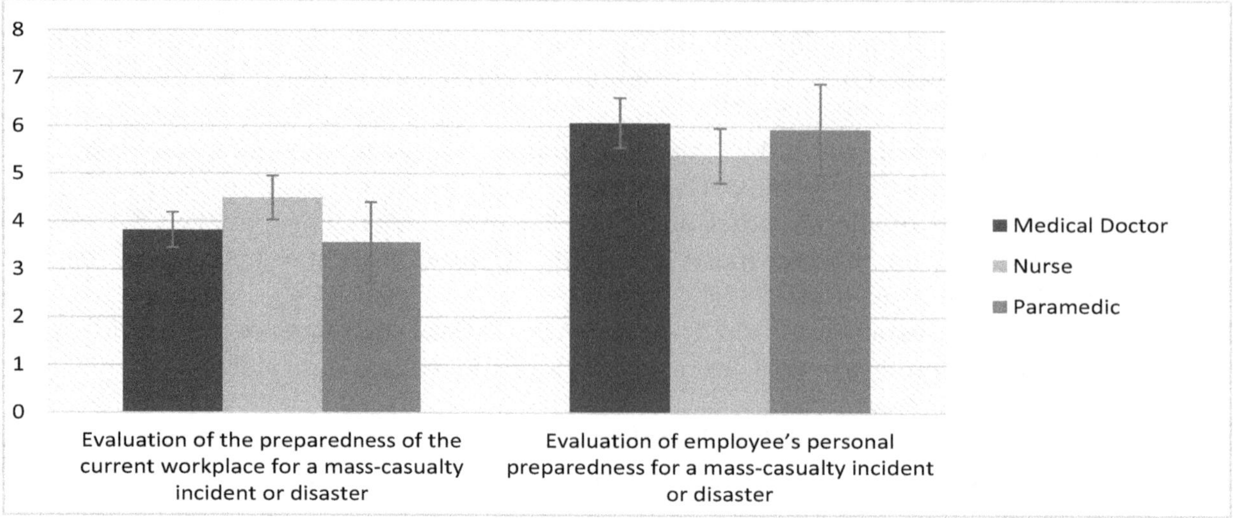

Figure 1. Average with a confidence interval of 95% for the evaluation of preparedness for mass-casualty incidents and disasters by occupation.

4.3. *Differences between the Evaluation of Preparedness for a Mass-Casualty Incident or Disaster in the Current Place of Work and the Evaluation of One's Own Preparedness*

In the next stage of the analyses, it was assessed whether there are differences between the evaluation of one's own preparedness and the evaluation of the current workplace's preparedness for a mass-casualty incident and disaster. For this purpose, Student's t-test was performed for dependent samples. The results of this test are presented in Table 2 and in Figure 2.

Table 2. Differences between the evaluation of preparedness for a mass-casualty incident or disaster in the current place of work, and the evaluation of one's own preparedness.

	Current Place of Work		Own		*t*	*p*	95% *CI*	
	M	*SD*	*M*	*SD*			*LL*	*UL*
Evaluation of preparedness for a mass-casualty incident or disaster	4.10	1.68	5.71	2.14	−9.28	<0.001	−1.95	−1.27

M—mean; *Me*—median; *SD*—standard deviation; *Bias.*—bias; *Kurt.*—kurtosis; *Min & Max.*—the lowest and highest value of distribution; *D*—Kolmogorov–Smirnov test result; *p*—significance.

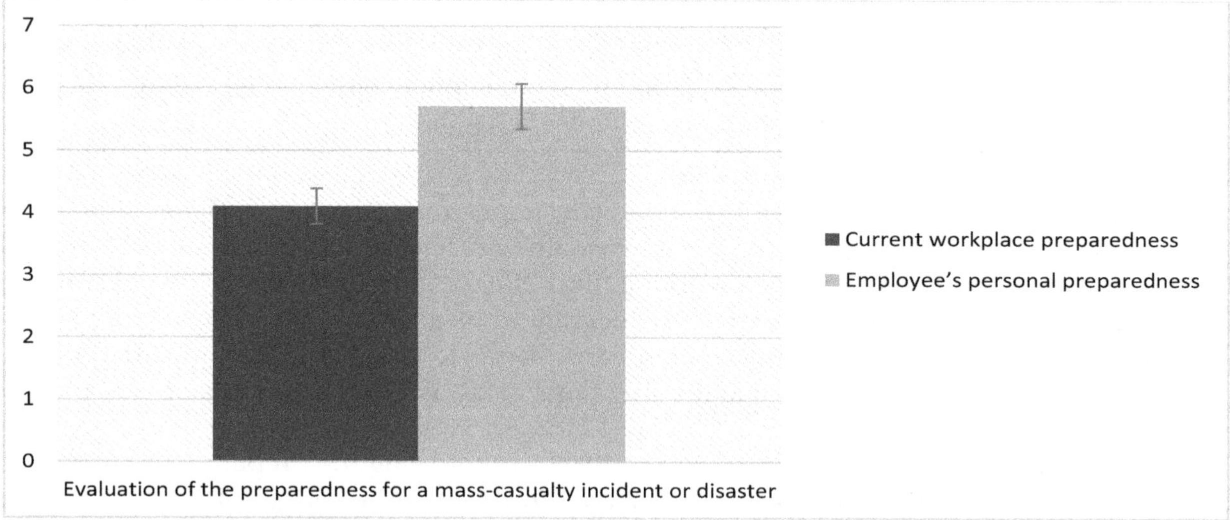

Figure 2. Average with a 95% confidence interval for the evaluation of preparedness for a mass-casualty incident or disaster for the current place of work, and one's own preparedness.

The test results indicate statistically significant differences. It turned out that the test subjects evaluate their own preparedness for mass-casualty incidents and disasters better than the preparedness of the current place of work. The strength of this effect is high.

4.4. Differences in the Evaluation of Preparedness for a Mass-Casualty Incident or Disaster Depending on Previous Participation in a Mass-Casualty Incident or Disaster as a Healthcare Professional

It was assessed whether the subjects who had previously been involved in a mass-casualty incident or disaster as a healthcare worker differ in their evaluation of preparedness for such situations from those who had not been involved in such an event. A Mann Whitney test was conducted due to the large numerical differences between the analyzed groups. The results are presented in Table 3.

Table 3. Differences between persons who have been involved in a mass-casualty incident or disaster as a healthcare worker, and persons who have not been involved in such an event in terms of their evaluation of preparedness for a mass-casualty incident or disaster.

	Have You Ever Been Involved in a Mass-Casualty Incident or Disaster as a Healthcare Professional?					
	Yes (n = 34)		No (n = 100)		Z	p
	Average Rank	*Me*	Average Rank	*Me*		
Evaluation of the preparedness of the current workplace for a mass-casualty incident or disaster	65.42	4.00	67.52	4.00	−0.28	0.783
Evaluation of one's own preparedness for a mass-casualty incident or disaster	86.12	7.00	61.17	5.00	−3.27	0.001

M—mean; *Me*—median; *SD*—standard deviation; *Bias.*—bias; *Kurt.*—kurtosis; *Min & Max.*—the lowest and highest value of distribution; *D*—Kolmogorov–Smirnov test result; *p*—significance.

The results of the tests indicate a statistically significant effect of moderate strength for the evaluation of one's own preparedness for mass-casualty incidents or disasters. As it turns out, respondents who took part in a mass-casualty incident or disaster as a healthcare worker evaluate their own preparedness much better than respondents who had not been involved in such an event.

4.5. Differences in the Evaluation of Preparedness for a Mass-Casualty Incident or Disaster Depending on the Organisation of Drills by the Institution and Whether They Were Attended by the Respondents

In order to check the differences in the evaluation of preparedness for mass-casualty incidents or disasters between respondents with different opinions concerning the organization of drills by the institution and depending on whether they took place, Student's t-tests for independent samples and Mann Whitney tests were performed. Initially, a Student's t-test for independent samples was conducted. It was decided to assess whether the respondents whose institution had organized drills regarding disaster management differed from those whose institution had not conducted such drills in relation to the evaluation of preparedness for such situations. The test results are presented in Table 2.

It was then assessed whether the evaluation of preparedness for such situations is impacted by the frequency of training on what to do in the event of a mass-casualty incident or disaster. Due to significant differences in the number of groups compared, Mann Whitney tests were performed.

The results of this test indicate a statistically significant and moderate effect for the evaluation of the preparedness of the current workplace for a mass-casualty incident or disaster. This results from the fact that the respondents, whose institution organized drills for such situations once every 3 years or more often, better evaluate the preparedness of the institution than the respondents whose institution organized trainings less frequently than once every 3 years. The results of the tests are presented in Table 4.

Table 4. Differences in the evaluation of preparedness for a mass-casualty incident or disaster, depending on the organization of drills by the institution, and whether they were attended by the respondents.

	Have There Been Any Disaster Management Drills Organized in the Facility Where you Currently Work?							
	Yes ($n = 60$)		**No ($n = 73$)**		t	p	**95% *CI***	
	M	*SD*	*M*	*SD*			*LL*	*UL*
Evaluation of the preparedness of the current workplace for a mass-casualty incident or disaster	4.43	1.58	3.82	1.72	2.12	0.036	0.04	1.18
Evaluation of one's own preparedness for a mass-casualty incident or disaster	6.49	1.67	5.11	2.33	3.99	< 0.001	0.70	2.07
	Less than once every 3 years ($n = 123$)		Once every 3 years or more often ($n = 11$)		Z	p		
	Average rank	*Me*	Average rank	*Me*				
Evaluation of the preparedness of the current workplace for a mass-casualty incident or disaster	64.28	4.00	97.18	6.00	−2.76	0.006		
Evaluation of one's own preparedness for a mass-casualty incident or disaster	66.19	6.00	82.18	7.00	−1.32	0.186		

M—mean; *Me*—median; *SD*—standard deviation; *Bias.*—bias; *Kurt.*—kurtosis; *Min & Max.*—the lowest and highest value of distribution; *D*—Kolmogorov–Smirnov test result; *p*—significance.

It was then assessed whether training in preparation for disasters impacts upon the evaluation of preparedness for mass-casualty incidents or disasters. Student's t-tests for independent tests were performed for this purpose.

The results of this test indicate significant differences for the evaluation of both one's own preparedness and also that of the institution. Both of these effects are of moderate strength. The analysis showed that after training, the respondents evaluate their own and the institution's preparedness for a mass-casualty incident or disaster better than the respondents without such training. Test results are presented in Figure 3.

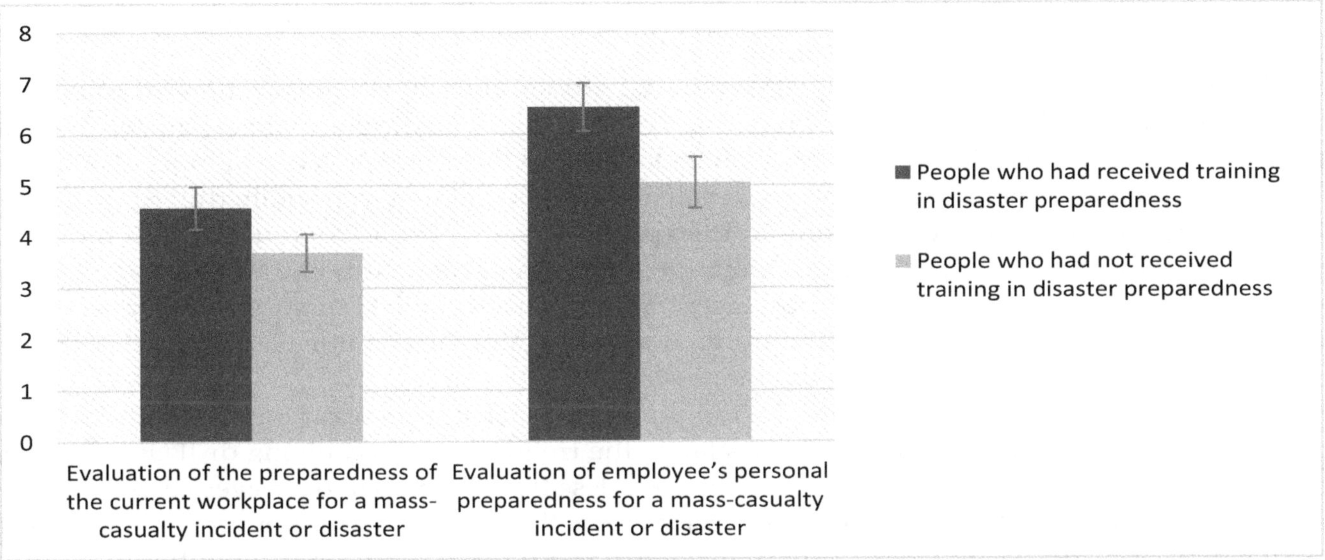

Figure 3. Average with a 95% confidence interval for evaluations of preparedness for mass-casualty incidents and disasters, categorized by participation in training related to preparation for such situations.

5. Discussion

The creation of hospital crisis management plans, evacuation plans and procedures in the event of mass-casualty incidents, and the necessity for staff to be familiar with them, is an important step towards preparing for such events. However, the lack of such plans may lead to chaos and complete disorientation [38–42].

The research shows that the majority of the respondents knew that the institution at which they currently worked had a plan for dealing with mass-casualty incidents and disasters. Moreover, over 70% of respondents reported that they knew who was responsible for the management of operations in crisis situations and were aware of the procedures to be followed during a disaster.

In mass-casualty incidents and disasters, due to the limited capacity and resources of the emergency services on site, it is not possible to provide medical assistance to all victims simultaneously. Some of them will have to wait for such assistance. In the first instance, medical assistance must be provided to victims who need it at that moment, i.e., people in immediate danger of death. This assistance must be effective. The aim is to provide maximum benefits to as many people as possible under specified conditions. The need to do what is best for victims of a mass-casualty incident or disaster makes it necessary to continuously apply medical segregation of the victims. Triage is one of the most important and often the only undertaking of rescue services providing quick control of the situation in the area of a mass-casualty incident or disaster [43].

In the study concerning triage, almost all respondents declared having the ability to conduct triage.

Each hospital should have its own evacuation plan, as every healthcare facility is different, with different architectural features, number of floors in the building, numbers of patients and their physical and mental condition, equipment, and many other features. Additionally, each event is different. Evacuation can take place in connection with a bomb threat when there are no obstacles in the form of smoke, fire, toxic products from combustion, problems with visibility, or time pressure—as happens in the case of fire. Proper evacuation of a hospital requires a well-thought-out strategy and good preparation and, in order to achieve this, drills carried out in advance [13].

The research demonstrates that the respondents are familiar with the procedures to be followed in case of evacuation in the event of a mass-casualty incident at their workplace. The developing of an evacuation plan for the healthcare facility, familiarizing the entire staff with it, and performing regular evacuation drills, are necessary to ensure the safety of patients and workers [13].

The impact of catastrophes can be avoided or reduced by adopting risk management measures, which should be implemented by taking advantage of local resources and taking appropriate actions in terms of planning, education and training [44,45].

The human factor is a significant problem in the proper, continuous preparation for emergency situations or disasters in healthcare organizations. The shortage of medical personnel [46], the overload of current work, the increasing amount of documentation, and the completion of a number of necessary formalities can make doctors reluctant to participate in such training, especially during prolonged periods of relative calm when there are no unexpected events. It can be a problem to force staff to familiarize themselves with the documentation, operating procedures and evacuation plans for mass-casualty events and disasters. In most cases, this consists of a quick, cursory, thoughtless review, because in times of prolonged security, people do not feel an approaching threat, so they do not have a strong motivation to prepare for crisis situations [47].

More than half of the respondents (54.5%) reported a lack of organization of drills concerning disaster management in their workplace. As far as the frequency of organizing drills is concerned, the majority indicated that such drills were organized less frequently than once every 3 years.

The challenges faced by the healthcare services force them to provide continuous training in the organization of responses to mass-casualty incidents and disasters, and in cooperation with other emergency services. Simulations and drills are organized from time to time, but this is not enough. It is worth remembering that every event, even seemingly simple to perform, is difficult, and not every scenario can be foreseen. There can never be too many drills. Only through continuous practice can the most appropriate procedures and skills to deal with crisis situations be developed. Besides having excellent equipment and access to appropriate personal protective equipment (e.g., in the case of a patient infected with the SARS-CoV-2 coronavirus), above all, working in accordance to safety procedures that have been prepared in advance is an example of exemplary disaster management [48].

The only drawback after the exercises is usually the lack of review and feedback for the participants. This problem was reported by the respondents in the conducted research.

Theory will never equate to practice. Only practiced procedures provide the opportunity to verify the knowledge and skills of staff, and make it possible to carry out an analysis of the speed and effectiveness of the drills, and if necessary to make corrections, eliminate errors and, above all, acquire habits that will guarantee proper behavior [49].

Each hospital should have properly prepared disaster management procedures. Such guidelines should be prepared well in advance. When a threat occurs, it should be sufficient enough to adapt them to the specific situation, so that there is no need to create everything from scratch.

Humanity has experienced many disasters and pandemics in the past, but these have been overcome (e.g., smallpox, plague, measles, polio, whooping cough, typhus, rabies and cholera).

The current pandemic has very clearly shown the speed with which even the best healthcare systems in different countries can be overwhelmed and devastated. These observations show that health should be at the top of the political agenda.

6. Limitations

The main limitation of this study was that only the employees of one hospital were studied. The COVID-19 pandemic proved to be a huge obstacle in further research. Despite these limitations, the study revealed some implementation and scientific gaps for researchers, but at the same time it is a chance to initiate discussion and become a small contribution to solving the crisis that disaster leads to. The experience gained from this study will form the basis for planned future studies with more hospitals, and a more comprehensive approach. It will also help to properly amend the questions, which will make it easier to design a future research tool.

7. Conclusions

The pilot study revealed that a properly designed questionnaire can be used to assess the relationship between hospital and staff preparedness and disaster response efficiency.

The knowledge and skills of health professionals in relation to specific events and their impact on people, as well as the appropriate treatment, are essential for the quality of healthcare services during disasters.

In order to achieve the level of preparedness and the effectiveness of the disaster response, it is necessary that every hospital has pre-prepared and validated procedures.

An experimental study involving a range of hospitals should be carried out, using more comprehensive assessment tools, to assess the correlation between the level of preparedness and performance of the hospital and the impact of the preparation of the hospital and its staff towards the survival of disaster victims.

Evaluation of the preparedness and effectiveness of disaster response is a means of identifying and removing possible gaps and weaknesses in the functioning and effective management of a hospital during mass-casualty incidents.

Author Contributions: Conceptualization: K.G.; data collection: K.G. and M.G.; formal Analysis: K.G. and M.G.; writing—original draft preparation: K.G. and M.G. All authors have read and agreed to the published version of the manuscript.

References

1. Djalali, A.; Carenzo, L.; Ragazzoni, L.; Azzaretto, M.; Petrino, R.; Della Corte, F.; Ingrassia, P.L. Does hospital disaster preparedness predict response performance during a full-scale exercise? A pilot study. *Prehospital Disaster Med.* **2014**, *29*, 441–447. [CrossRef] [PubMed]
2. Olivieri, C.; Ingrassia, P.L.; Della Corte, F.; Carenzo, L.; Sapori, J.M.; Gabilly, L.; Segond, F.; Grieger, F.; Arnod-Prin, P.; Larrucea, X.; et al. Hospital preparedness and response in CBRN emergencies: TIER assessment tool. *Eur. J. Emerg. Med.* **2017**, *24*, 366–370. [CrossRef] [PubMed]
3. Djalali, A.; Castren, M.; Khankeh, H.; Gryth, D.; Radestad, M.; Öhlen, G.; Kurland, L. Hospital disaster preparedness as measured by functional capacity: A comparison between Iran and Sweden. *Prehospital Disaster Med.* **2013**, *28*, 454–461. [CrossRef] [PubMed]
4. Adini, B.; Laor, D.; Hornik-Lurie, T.; Schwartz, D.; Aharonson-Daniel, L. Improving hospital mass casualty preparedness through ongoing readiness evaluation. *Am. J. Med. Qual.* **2012**, *27*, 426–433. [CrossRef]
5. Cagliuso, N. Stakeholders' experiences with US hospital emergency preparedness: Part 1. *J. Bus. Contin. Emerg. Plan.* **2014**, *8*, 156–168.
6. Gillett, B.; Silverberg, M.; Roblin, P.; Adelaine, J.; Valesky, W.; Arquilla, B. Computer-facilitated assessment of disaster preparedness for remote hospitals in a long-distance, virtual tabletop drill model. *Prehospital Disaster Med.* **2011**, *26*, 230–233. [CrossRef]
7. Higgins, W.; Wainright III, C.; Lu, N.; Carrico, R. Assessing hospital preparedness using an instrument based on the Mass Casualty Disaster Plan Checklist: Results of a statewide survey. *Am. J. Infect. Control* **2004**, *32*, 327–332. [CrossRef]
8. Mortelmans, L.J.; Gaakeer, M.I.; Dieltiens, G.; Anseeuw, K.; Sabbe, M.B. Are Dutch hospitals prepared for chemical, biological, or radionuclear incidents? A survey study. *Prehospital Disaster Med.* **2017**, *32*, 483–491. [CrossRef]

9. Nekoie-Moghadam, M.; Kurland, L.; Moosazadeh, M.; Ingrassia, P.L.; Della Corte, F.; Djalali, A. Tools and checklists used for the evaluation of hospital disaster preparedness: A systematic review. *Disaster Med. Public Health Prep.* **2016**, *10*, 781–788. [CrossRef]
10. Alruwaili, A.; Islam, S.; Usher, K. Disaster Preparedness in Hospitals in the Middle East: An Integrative Literature Review. *Disaster Med. Public Health Prep.* **2019**, *13*, 806–816. [CrossRef]
11. Lazar, E.J.; Cagliuso, N.V.; Gebbie, K.M. Are we ready and how do we know? The urgent need for performance metrics in hospital emergency management. *Disaster Med. Public Health Prep.* **2009**, *3*, 57–60. [CrossRef] [PubMed]
12. Ogedegbe, C.; Nyirenda, T.; DelMoro, G.; Yamin, E.; Feldman, J. Health care workers and disaster preparedness: Barriers to and facilitators of willingness to respond. *Int. J. Emerg. Med.* **2012**, *5*, 29. [CrossRef] [PubMed]
13. Goniewicz, K.; Misztal-Okońska, P.; Pawłowski, W.; Burkle, F.M.; Czerski, R.; Hertelendy, A.J.; Goniewicz, M. Evacuation from Healthcare Facilities in Poland: Legal Preparedness and Preparation. *International J. Environ. Res. Public Health* **2020**, *17*, 1779. [CrossRef] [PubMed]
14. Beerens, R.J.J.; Tehler, H. Scoping the field of disaster exercise evaluation—A literature overview and analysis. *Int. J. Disaster Risk Reduct.* **2016**, *19*, 413–446. [CrossRef]
15. Hodge, A.J.; Miller, E.L.; Skaggs, M.K.D. Nursing self-perceptions of emergency preparedness at a rural hospital. *J. Emerg. Nurs.* **2017**, *43*, 10–14. [CrossRef]
16. Kollek, D.; Cwinn, A.A. Hospital emergency readiness overview study. *Prehospital Disaster Med.* **2011**, *26*, 159–165. [CrossRef]
17. Cocco, C.; Thomas-Boaz, W. Preparedness planning and response to a mass-casualty incident: A case study of Sunnybrook Health Sciences Centre. *J. Bus. Contin. Emerg. Plan.* **2019**, *13*, 6–21.
18. Valesky, W.; Roblin, P.; Patel, B.; Adelaine, J.; Zehtabchi, S.; Arquilla, B. Assessing hospital preparedness: Comparison of an on-site survey with a self-reported, internet-based, long-distance tabletop drill. *Prehospital Disaster Med.* **2013**, *28*, 441–444. [CrossRef]
19. Adini, B.; Goldberg, A.; Cohen, R.; Bar-Dayan, Y. Relationship between equipment and infrastructure for pandemic influenza and performance in an avian flu drill. *Emerg. Med. J.* **2009**, *26*, 786–790. [CrossRef]
20. Skryabina, E.; Reedy, G.; Amlôt, R.; Jaye, P.; Riley, P. What is the value of health emergency preparedness exercises? A scoping review study. *Int. J. Disaster Risk Reduct.* **2017**, *21*, 274–283. [CrossRef]
21. Verheul, M.L.; Dückers, M.L.; Visser, B.B.; Beerens, R.J.; Bierens, J.J. Disaster exercises to prepare hospitals for mass-casualty incidents: Does it contribute to preparedness or is it ritualism? *Prehospital Disaster Med.* **2018**, *33*, 387–393. [CrossRef] [PubMed]
22. Foote, M.; Daver, R.; Quinn, C. Using "mystery patient" drills to assess hospital ebola preparedness in new York City, 2014–2015. *Health Secur.* **2017**, *15*, 500–508. [CrossRef] [PubMed]
23. Ali, M.; Williams, M.D. No-Notice Mystery Patient Drills to Assess Emergency Preparedness for Infectious Diseases at Community Health Centers in New York City, 2015-2016. *J. Community Health* **2019**, *44*, 387–394. [CrossRef] [PubMed]
24. Djalali, A.; Ardalan, A.; Ohlen, G.; Ingrassia, P.L.; Della Corte, F.; Castren, M.; Kurland, L. Nonstructural safety of hospitals for disasters: A comparison between two capital cities. *Disaster Med. Public Health Prep.* **2014**, *8*, 179–184. [CrossRef]
25. Arab, M.A.; Khankeh, H.R.; Mosadeghrad, A.M.; Farrokhi, M. Developing a hospital disaster risk management evaluation model. *Risk Manag. Healthc. Policy* **2019**, *12*, 287. [CrossRef]
26. Shabanikiya, H.; Jafari, M.; Gorgi, H.A.; Seyedin, H.; Rahimi, A. Developing a practical toolkit for evaluating hospital preparedness for surge capacity in disasters. *Int. J. Disaster Risk Reduct.* **2019**, *34*, 423–428. [CrossRef]
27. Lennquist Montán, K.; Riddez, L.; Lennquist, S.; Olsberg, A.; Lindberg, H.; Gryth, D.; Örtenwall, P. Assessment of hospital surge capacity using the MACSIM simulation system: A pilot study. *Eur. J. Trauma Emerg. Surg.* **2017**, *43*, 525–539. [CrossRef]
28. World Health Organization; Pan American Health Organization. *Hospital Safety Index: Guide for Evaluators*, 2nd ed.; World Health Organization: Geneva, Switzerland, 2015; Available online: https://apps.who.int/iris/handle/10665/258966 (accessed on 15 June 2020).
29. Fallah-Aliabadi, S.; Ostadtaghizadeh, A.; Ardalan, A.; Fatemi, F.; Khazai, B.; Mirjalili, M.R. Towards developing a model for the evaluation of hospital disaster resilience: A systematic review. *BMC Health Serv. Res.* **2020**, *20*, 64. [CrossRef]

30. Vichova, K.; Hromada, M. The Evaluation System to Ensure the Transport of Emergency Supplies of Fuel to the Hospitals. *Transp. Res. Procedia* **2019**, *40*, 1618–1624. [CrossRef]
31. Khankeh, H.; Mosadeghrad, A.M.; Abbasabadi Arab, M. Developing accreditation standards for disaster risk management: An approach for hospital preparedness improvement–editorial. *J. Mil Med.* **2019**, *20*, 574–576.
32. Martinez, D.; Talbert, T.; Romero-Steiner, S.; Kosmos, C.; Redd, S. Evolution of the Public Health Preparedness and Response Capability Standards to Support Public Health Emergency Management Practices and Processes. *Health Secur.* **2019**, *17*, 430–438. [CrossRef] [PubMed]
33. Veenema, T.G. (Ed.) *Disaster Nursing and Emergency Preparedness*; Springer Publishing Company: Berlin, Germany, 2018.
34. Gowing, J.R.; Walker, K.N.; Elmer, S.L.; Cummings, E.A. Disaster preparedness among health professionals and support staff: What is effective? An integrative literature review. *Prehospital Disaster Med.* **2017**, *32*, 321–328. [CrossRef] [PubMed]
35. Hussein, A.; Mahmoud, N. Emergency Preparedness and Perceived Competence in Disaster. *Alex. Sci. Nurs. J.* **2016**, *18*, 1–14.
36. Goniewicz, K.; Goniewicz, M.; Burkle, F.M. The Territorial Defence Force in disaster response in Poland: Civil-military collaboration during a state of emergency. *Sustainability* **2019**, *11*, 487. [CrossRef]
37. Goniewicz, K.; Burkle, F.M. Disaster early warning systems: The potential role and limitations of emerging text and data messaging mitigation capabilities. *Disaster Med. Public Health Prep.* **2019**, *13*, 709–712. [CrossRef]
38. Delshad, V.; Borhani, F.; Khankeh, H.; Abbaszadeh, A.; Sabzalizadeh, S.; Moradian, M.J.; Behzadi, M.J.R.; Abadi, M.G.; Farzinnia, B. The effect of activating early warning system on motahari hospital preparedness. *Health Emerg. Disasters Q.* **2015**, *1*, 3–8.
39. Amiri, M.; Chaman, R.; Raei, M.; Shirvani, S.D.N.; Afkar, A. Preparedness of hospitals in north of iran to deal with disasters. *Iran. Red Crescent Med. J.* **2013**, *15*, 519. [CrossRef]
40. Daneshmandi, M.; Amiri, H.; Vahedi, M.; Farshi, M. Assessing level of Preparedness for disaster in hospitals of a selected medical sciences university-1388. *J. Mil Med.* **2010**, *12*, 167–171.
41. Aladhrai, S.A.; Djalali, A.; Della Corte, F.; Alsabri, M.; El-Bakri, N.K.; Ingrassia, P.L. Impact of the 2011 revolution on hospital disaster preparedness in Yemen. *Disaster Med. Public Health Prep.* **2015**, *9*, 396–402. [CrossRef]
42. Jama, T.J.; Kuisma, M.J. Preparedness of Finnish emergency medical services for chemical emergencies. *Prehospital Disaster Med.* **2016**, *31*, 392–396. [CrossRef]
43. Christian, M.D.; Toltzis, P.; Kanter, R.K.; Burkle, F.M.; Vernon, D.D.; Kissoon, N. Treatment and triage recommendations for pediatric emergency mass critical care. *Pediatr. Crit. Care Med.* **2011**, *12*, S109–S119. [CrossRef] [PubMed]
44. Goniewicz, K.; Khorram-Manesh, A.; Hertelendy, A.J.; Goniewicz, M.; Naylor, K.; Burkle, F.M., Jr. Current Response and Management Decisions of the European Union to the COVID-19 Outbreak: A Review. *Sustainability* **2020**, *12*, 3838. [CrossRef]
45. Goniewicz, K.; Magiera, M.; Rucińska, D.; Pawłowski, W.; Burkle, F.M.; Hertelendy, A.J.; Goniewicz, M. Geographic Information System Technology: Review of the Challenges for Its Establishment as a Major Asset for Disaster and Emergency Management in Poland. *Disaster Med. Public Health Prep.* **2020**, 1–6. [CrossRef] [PubMed]
46. Dubas-Jakóbczyk, K.; Domagała, A.; Mikos, M. Impact of the doctor deficit on hospital management in Poland: A mixed-method study. *Int. J. Health Plan. Manag.* **2018**. [CrossRef]
47. Fox, J.H.; Burkle, F.M.; Bass, J.; Pia, F.A.; Epstein, J.L.; Markenson, D. The effectiveness of psychological first aid as a disaster intervention tool: Research analysis of peer-reviewed literature from 1990–2010. *Disaster Med. Public Health Prep.* **2012**, *6*, 247–252. [CrossRef]
48. Smith, N.; Fraser, M. Straining the System: Novel Coronavirus (COVID-19) and Preparedness for Concomitant Disasters. *Am J Public Health* **2020**, *110*, 648–649. [CrossRef]
49. Goniewicz, K.; Burkle, F.M. Challenges in implementing Sendai framework for disaster risk reduction in Poland. *Int. J. Environ. Res. Public Health* **2019**, *16*, 2574. [CrossRef]

7

Post-Traumatic Stress among Evacuees from the 2016 Fort McMurray Wildfires: Exploration of Psychological and Sleep Symptoms Three Months after the Evacuation

Genevieve Belleville *, Marie-Christine Ouellet and Charles M. Morin

School of Psychology, Laval University, Quebec, QC G1V 0A6, Canada; marie-christine.ouellet@psy.ulaval.ca (M.-C.O.); cmorin@psy.ulaval.ca (C.M.M.)

* Correspondence: genevieve.belleville@psy.ulaval.ca

Abstract: This study documents post-traumatic stress symptoms after the May 2016 wildfires in Fort McMurray (Alberta, Canada). A sample of 379 evacuees completed an online questionnaire from July to September 2016, and a subsample of 55 completed a psychiatric/psychological diagnostic interview. According to a self-report questionnaire, 62.5% of respondents had a provisional post-traumatic stress disorder (PTSD). The interview confirmed that 29.1% met criteria for PTSD, 25.5% for depression, and 43.6% for insomnia; in most cases, insomnia was definitely or probably related to the fires. Traumatic exposure may elicit or exacerbate sleep problems, which are closely associated with PTSD after a disaster.

Keywords: post-traumatic stress disorder; psychological distress; mental health; sleep

1. Introduction

Exposure to a natural disaster is a type of traumatic event that may lead to the development of post-traumatic stress disorder (PTSD). The wildfires that began on 1 May 2016 in Fort McMurray (Alberta, Canada) destroyed 1595 buildings, which contained 2600 housing units, and led to massive displacement of approximately 88,000 people. The fire, which was officially put out in August 2017, after 458 days, devastated a total of 5895 km^2. Although it caused no direct human fatality, during the evacuation, many individuals faced direct or potential threat to their life or health, or significant losses. Damage was estimated at $3.58 billion, making it the most expensive natural disaster in Canadian history. The inhabitants of the city were displaced at least one month. The city started rebuilding in June 2016, a process expected to take three to four years. Three months after the evacuation, families were still living through ongoing adversity and uncertainty as they adapted to new or temporary homes, schools and workplaces. Beyond the individual experience of the disaster, entire communities have experienced it collectively, facing a variety of challenges at the social, community and economic levels (e.g., housing issues, insurance claims, rebuilding). Both individual and collective stressors are known to contribute to psychological adjustment after a disaster [1].

Specific data on the consequences of major forest fires are not only rare, but their generalizability to other communities may be questioned. Data collected from victims of the 2003 California fires have revealed that two-thirds of the respondents had feared for their lives or the life of a loved one; three months later, a quarter met the criteria for PTSD, and a third met the criteria for major depression [2]. Another study with victims of the Australian bushfires of 1983 demonstrated that health conditions related to stress, including mental disorders, were much more common in this population than conditions unrelated to stress [3]. Three to four years after the Victorian Black Saturday bushfires in Australia (2009), 16–22% of highly affected communities had PTSD and 13% had major depression [4]. To date, two published studies have reported significant issues related to the mental health impacts of the Fort McMurray wildfires. One case-controlled study conducted 18 months after the wildfires showed elevated prevalence of probable self-reported mental health diagnoses (depression, anxiety, alcohol/substance use) in children [5]. The only study reporting mental health indicators in adults was conducted 6 months after the wildfires and focused on self-reported anxiety and alcohol/substance use: Almost 20% of the 486 surveyed participants had a probable diagnosis of generalized anxiety disorder, 14% had high risk of alcohol dependence, and 10% had high risk of drug dependence [6].

Most studies examining the mental health impacts of fires have focused on PTSD, depression, anxiety and substance use [7–9]. However, sleep problems—mostly in the form of insomnia and recurrent nightmares, but also sleep-related movement and breathing disorders—are closely associated with both PTSD [10] and depression [11]. Of the 160 studies on the impacts of disasters reviewed by Norris and collaborators (2002), only 10 measured sleep [12]. There is accumulating evidence that persistent sleep problems constitute an important predictor of psychopathology after a traumatic event [13]. Moreover, sleep disturbances appear to be among the most common reactions after a traumatic event: Severe problems with sleep were the most frequently reported complaints two to three weeks after the explosion of a fireworks storage facility in Enschede, The Netherlands, among a vast array of physical and mental health concerns including problems with daily functioning, pain, anxiety and depression [14].

Most people exposed to a disaster experience intense psychological reactions but will remit after some time [15,16]; in parallel, continued stressors contribute to enduring psychological distress, including PTSD [17,18]. Individual factors, such as appraisals of the event and coping strategies, may also influence mental health after a disaster. Ehlers and Clark's cognitive model suggests that post-traumatic symptoms persist when individuals process information in a way that produces a sense of imminent threat [19]. Two processes are thought to feed this perception of current threat: Recurrent negative appraisals of the trauma and its consequences and the disturbance of autobiographical memory. The latter process is potentiated by unhelpful coping strategies, such as avoidance. Avoidance may concern stimuli that are external (places, people) or internal (memories, thoughts); self-medication with alcohol or other substances may also be a form of avoidance. Sleep difficulties, such as insomnia and nightmares, may play a role as they contribute to physiological arousal and strong emotions, two aspects that may promote the perception of current threat.

In sum, both the wide range of symptoms (e.g., PTSD, anxiety, depression, sleep) and the timeline (e.g., when they occur, how long they persist) are important aspects to consider in the assessment of the mental health impact of a disaster on the affected community. Moreover, due to their unpredictable nature, it is exceptionally difficult to obtain empirical data about the impact of natural disasters. Methodological challenges must be faced: The main bias is often related to the retrospective nature of the data collected, i.e., when we ask people to remember their immediate post-traumatic reactions weeks or even years after the traumatic event [20] and the lack of baseline information on premorbid status. The objective of this research was thus to rapidly document post-traumatic stress symptoms, mental disorders and psychological difficulties in a sample of evacuees of the 2016 Fort McMurray wildfires. The goal was to collect data in the immediate aftermath, i.e., three months after the evacuation, to support self-reported symptoms with standardized clinical interviews, and to assess common mental health disorders (PTSD, depression, anxiety, substance use) as well as sleep problems. We also wanted to examine the associations between symptoms of post-traumatic stress and depression, sleep problems, post-traumatic cognitions and coping strategies. We wished to explore the differential contribution of sleep difficulties in post-traumatic stress severity once the severity of depression was accounted for, as well as the influence of cognitions and coping strategies once the severity of depression and sleep problems were accounted for.

2. Method

The Laval University institutional review board approved the research protocol, and participants provided informed consent.

2.1. Participants and Procedure

A sample of evacuees from the 2016 Fort McMurray wildfires were asked to complete an online questionnaire. To participate, they had to be aged 18 or older and be fluent in English. A subsample of these volunteers also underwent a standardized clinical interview. The clinical interviews were conducted in the business meeting room of a local hotel.

Two research assistants—doctoral students in clinical psychology—went to Fort McMurray from 25 July to 16 August 2016 to recruit participants and conduct the clinical interviews. They recruited volunteers in various public places (e.g., mall, grocery store). They distributed invitations to complete the online questionnaire, printed on business cards, and also participated in local radio broadcasts to discuss the project and its recruitment. The online questionnaire remained open from 25 July 25 to 5 September 2016. Appointments were taken with individuals interested to participate to the clinical interview, either later in the same day or in the following days. A snowball sampling methodology was also used where participants were invited to refer to the research team other potentially interested acquaintances. The research assistants were easily joinable by phone or email for the whole time of their stay in Fort McMurray.

The research assistants were supervised by the principal investigator (GB), a psychologist specialized in PTSD. They had access to phone supervision as needed for the entire duration of their stay.

2.2. Measures

The clinical interview merged two validated standardized diagnostic instruments: The Clinician-Administered PTSD Scale (CAPS) [21] to assess current PTSD, and the Mini International Neuropsychiatric Interview (MINI) [22] to assess current major depression, panic, agoraphobia, generalized anxiety, social phobia and obsessive-compulsive disorders, as well as drug and alcohol use disorders. These instruments provided a stringent examination of the fifth edition of the Diagnostic and Statistical Manual of Mental Disorders (DSM-5) [23] criteria for each disorder. Questions related to the CAPS item #E6 (sleep disturbance) were given a special attention, in order to be able to diagnose insomnia. An insomnia diagnosis was assigned to participants who met the following five criteria: (1) Difficulties falling or staying asleep or waking up too early, and these were (2) present at least three times a week, (3) associated with daytime disturbances, (4) present for at least three months, and (5) occurred despite adequate opportunity for sleep. Questions probing personal antecedents were asked at the end of the interview, i.e., "We just did an overview of the symptoms you have/might have had since the fires. Now I wonder if you have ever experienced problems similar in the past, before the fires. Have you ever had Depression/Insomnia/Recurrent Nightmares/Anxiety Disorder before?".

The online questionnaires were presented as aimed at studying post-traumatic stress among victims of the Fort McMurray fire. The first questions were open-ended and asked participants to describe their personal experience of the fire and the evacuation, as well as their consequences. Participants then proceeded to complete the PTSD Symptoms Checklist (PCL-5) [24], the Patient Health Questionnaire [25], the Insomnia Severity Index [26], the Pittsburgh Sleep Quality Index and its Addendum for PTSD (PSQI; PSQI-A) [27,28], the Post-Traumatic Cognitions Inventory (PTCI) [29] and the Ways of Coping Questionnaire (WCQ) [30].

The PCL-5 is a 20-item self-report measure that assesses PTSD symptoms in the past month. In this study, we used the PCL-5 to assess symptom severity and to make a provisional PTSD diagnosis. The symptom severity score ranges from 0–80, higher scores indicating more severe symptoms. A provisional PTSD diagnostic may be assigned to respondents who endorse 1 B item (questions 1–5),

1 C item (questions 6–7), 2 D items (questions 8–14), 2 E items (questions 15–20). A cutoff score of 33 is also proposed to discriminate between people with or without probable PTSD [31].

The PHQ is a 59-item questionnaire that was used as a screening tool for mental health disorders of depression, anxiety, alcohol, eating, and somatoform during the past four weeks. From the PHQ, we also used the PHQ-9, a subscale composed of 9 summed items to assess the severity of depressive symptoms [25].

The ISI is a 7-item questionnaire designed to assess the severity of both nighttime and daytime components of insomnia in the past month. Total score ranges from 0–21, higher scores indicating more severe insomnia. A cutoff score of 10 is optimal to detect insomnia in a community sample [32].

The PSQI is an 18-item questionnaire that assesses seven components of sleep quality in the past month: Subjective sleep quality, sleep latency, sleep duration, sleep efficiency, sleep disturbances, use of sleep medication, and impairment of daytime functioning. A global sleep quality score ranging from 0–21 is obtained by summing the seven component scores, higher scores indicating poorer sleep quality. A global sleep quality score higher than 5 is interpreted as poor sleep.

We also used the 7-item addendum to the PSQI, the PSQI-A, to assess the frequency of trauma-related sleep disturbances (hot flashes, general nervousness, memories or nightmares of traumatic experience, severe anxiety or panic not related to traumatic memories, bad dreams not related to traumatic memories, episodes of terror or screaming during sleep without fully awakening and episodes of acting out dreams) in the past month. Total score ranges from 0–21, higher scores indicating more frequent trauma-related sleep disturbances.

The PTCI is a 33-item questionnaire which assessed the degree to which respondents endorsed several post-traumatic cognitions (thoughts) in general on a 1–7 Likert-type scale. Three subscales constitute the PTCI. The Negative cognitions about the self subscale includes 21 items which depict a negative overall opinion of oneself, including a perception of the self as being incapable and weak (e.g., *I am a weak person*), permanently and negatively altered by the event (e.g., *I worsened forever*) and without hope for the future (e.g., *I have no future*). The Negative cognitions about the world/others subscale includes 7 items highlighting the world as a dangerous place and people as inherently unreliable (e.g., *You cannot trust anyone*). The self-blame subscale includes 5 items assessing blame for the occurrence of the traumatic event (e.g., *The event occurred because of the way I acted*). Each subscale score is the average 1-to-7 answer per statement.

Finally, a short version of the WCQ assessed the frequency of use of three coping strategies in the past week: Seeking social support (6 items), positive reappraisal/problem solving (9 items) and distancing/avoidance (6 items). Each item is rated on a 0–3 Likert-type scale. Subscale scores are computed by summing the score of each item, and higher scores indicate more frequent use of the strategy.

2.3. Data Analyses

To document post-traumatic stress symptoms, mental disorders and psychological difficulties, frequencies were computed for categorical variables, and means and standard deviations were computed for continuous variables. Lower and upper limits of 95% confidence interval for each mean and for each proportion were computed. Correlations between variables were examined by calculating Pearson's coefficients. To avoid overlap on the various questionnaires in the correlation and regression analyses, the PCL-5 total score was computed excluding the two sleep items (#2—repeated, disturbing dreams, and #20—trouble falling or staying asleep) and the PHQ-9 total score was computed excluding its sleep item (#3—trouble falling or staying asleep, or sleeping too much). To document the factors associated with the severity of PTSD symptoms, a hierarchical multiple regression analysis was performed, with PTSD symptom severity (PCL-5 total score) as the predicted variable. The observation of the Gaussian distribution of the studentized residuals along with a non-statistically significant Shapiro–Wilk test suggested that the residuals were normally distributed. The first block consisted of gender and age, and was entered with the standard method as a control for the potential effect of these sociodemographic characteristics on PTSD severity. The second block of variables was entered with the standard method and was composed of depressive symptoms (PHQ-9 total score excluding the sleep item). The third block was entered with the standard method and was composed of insomnia severity (ISI total score), global sleep quality (PSQI total score), and trauma-related sleep disturbances (PSQI-A total score). The fourth and final block was entered with the standard method and was composed of negative cognitions about the self (PTCI subscale), negative cognitions about the world (PTCI subscale), self-blame (PTCI subscale), seeking social support (WCQ subscale), problem-solving/positive reappraisal (WCQ subscale) and distancing/avoidance (WCQ subscale). Correlation and regression analyses were performed with SPSS 13.0 for Windows (SPSS Inc., Chicago, IL, USA).

3. Results

3.1. Sample Description

Three hundred and ninety-four (394) respondents registered to complete the online questionnaire, i.e., went on the website describing the study and clicked to begin the questionnaire. Fifteen questionnaires (3.8%) remained completely or mostly unanswered. Among the 379 completed questionnaires, between 0.02 and 8.4% of data were missing, depending on the question/variable. Missing data were not replaced. Participants were mostly female (77%). Mean age was 40.10 years old (SD = 12.20). Almost three quarters were married or in a common-law relationship (72%); 18% were single, and 7% were either separated, divorced or widowed. Most participants (61%) had children. Residence status in the regional municipality of Wood Buffalo (which includes the city of Fort McMurray) was permanent for 88% and temporary for 7%. Before the fires, most participants worked part or full time (77%); 4% were retired, 3% were on a sick or invalidity leave, and 2% were students. Nearly one participant in four (23%) reported a change in work status since the fires.

Fifty-six (56) respondents participated to the interview. One interview was excluded from the analyses because of incomplete responses: The interviewer suspected that the participant was intoxicated and/or suffering from psychotic symptoms, and redirected the interview to ensure the participant's safety and access to local mental health resources. The final subsample of 55 participants was practically equally distributed between males (49%) and females (51%). Mean age was 43.07 years old (SD = 14.67). About half were married or in a common-law relationship (49%); 31% were single, and 16% were either separated, divorced or widowed. Most participants (62%) had children. Residence status in the community of Wood Buffalo (which includes the city of Fort McMurray) was permanent for 95% and temporary for 4%. Before the fires, most participants worked part or full time (76%); 4% were retired, 18% were unemployed, and 2% were students. One participant in six (16%) reported a change in work status since the fires.

Although all participants of the clinical interview were invited to complete the online questionnaire, thirty-five (35) did so, representing 9.2% of the sample of completed questionnaires. Compared to respondents who only completed the online questionnaire (344), participants who completed the interview and the online questionnaire (35) were more likely to be male and older, and they showed an overall portrait of less severe mental health problems. They were less likely to have self-reported PTSD, somatoform disorder and major depressive disorder. They showed lower scores on measures of post-traumatic, insomnia and depressive symptoms. They reported less use of avoidance-based coping strategies, less endorsement of cognitions regarding the self, the world or self-blame, and better sleep quality.

3.2. Main Results

Data from the online survey showed that, three months after the fires, roughly 60% suffered from significant post-traumatic stress, i.e., they had a provisional PTSD diagnosis according to the PCL-5 or a PCL-5 score of 33 or higher (see Table 1). The most frequently reported symptoms were repeated disturbing memories, feeling upset when reminded of the stressful experience, and trouble falling or staying asleep. Table 2 presents scores obtained on the other self-report questionnaires. The PHQ showed high proportions of respondents endorsing the diagnostic criteria of major depressive disorder (33.1%), somatoform disorder (27.0%) and anxiety disorders other than panic (27.0%). High rates of panic disorder (17.4%), alcohol abuse disorder (17.1%) and binge eating disorder (15.1%) were also observed. Results showed overall high severity of depressive symptoms, insomnia and post-traumatic sleep disturbances, as well as poor sleep quality.

Data from the clinical interviews showed that in this subsample of 55 volunteer participants, 29.1% met the clinical diagnostic criteria for PTSD and 25.5% met the clinical diagnostic criteria for major depression disorder (see Table 3). Among the anxiety disorders, panic disorder and generalized anxiety disorder were the most frequent. Substance use disorders, especially drug use disorder, were diagnosed in 16.7% of the sample. The most frequently encountered diagnosis in this sample was insomnia disorder, with a proportion of 43.6%. Participants were asked whether their sleep difficulties started or got worse after the fires; in most cases, the insomnia disorder was definitely (68%) or probably (16%) related to the fires. Most people with current insomnia (78%) reported having experienced insomnia in the past. PTSD was associated with current insomnia ($X^2(1) = 17.65$, $p < 0.001$), but not with insomnia antecedents ($X^2(1) = 0.432$, $p = 0.511$).

Table 4 presents the associations between the different variables under study. More severe PTSD symptoms was associated with more severe depression and insomnia symptoms, poorer sleep quality and more severe trauma-related sleep disturbances, stronger endorsement of negative cognitions concerning the self, others and self-blame, and with more frequent use of avoidance strategies. PTSD symptom severity was also negatively correlated with age, that is, more severe in younger people.

Results from hierarchical multiple regression analyses indicated that the final model accounted for 77.0% of PTSD symptom severity variance, $F(8, 340) = 146.722$, $p < 0.001$ (Table 5). Sex and age did not contribute significantly to the model (although age was positively associated with symptom severity when no other variable than sex was included in the model). Significant predictors included depressive and insomnia symptoms, trauma-related sleep disturbances, post-traumatic cognitions concerning the others or the world as untrustworthy or dangerous, avoidance-based coping strategies and problem-solving/reappraisal coping strategies.

Table 1. Proportion of respondents reporting post-traumatic stress disorder (PTSD) symptoms according to the PTSD symptoms checklist (PCL-5) (n = 374–379 [a]).

Symptom	Number of Respondents Who Endorsed the Symptom (Rated as 2 = "Moderately" or Higher)	Proportion of Respondents Who Endorsed the Symptom (Rated as 2 = "Moderately" or Higher)	95% CI
1. Repeated, disturbing memories (n = 376)	291	77.39	[72.90–81.35]
2. Repeated, disturbing dreams (n = 374)	203	54.28	[49.21–59.26]
3. Suddenly feeling as if the stressful experience was happening again (n = 376)	206	54.79	[49.74–59.75]
4. Feeling very upset when reminded of the stressful experience (n = 377)	289	76.66	[72.13–80.65]
5. Strong physical reactions when reminded of the stressful experience (n = 377)	250	66.31	[61.40–70.90]
6. Avoidance of memories, thoughts or feelings related to the stressful experience (n = 375)	247	65.87	[60.93–70.49]
7. Avoidance of external reminders of the stressful experience (n = 376)	226	60.11	[55.08–64.93]
8. Trouble remembering important parts of the stressful experience (n = 374)	167	44.65	[39.69–49.72]
9. Strong negative feelings about oneself, other people or the world (n = 377)	145	38.46	[33.69–43.46]
10. Blaming oneself or someone else for the stressful experience (n = 376)	155	41.22	[36.36–46.26]
11. Strong negative feelings (n = 376)	225	59.84	[54.81–64.67]
12. Loss of interest (n = 378)	229	60.58	[55.57–65.38]
13. Feeling distant or cut off (n = 378)	253	66.93	[62.04–71.48]
14. Trouble experiencing positive feelings (n = 378)	197	52.12	[47.09–57.11]
15. Irritable behaviors (n = 376)	226	60.11	[55.08–64.93]
16. Taking too many risks (n = 377)	72	19.10	[15.45–23.37]
17. Being "superalert" (n = 377)	265	70.29	[65.49–74.68]
18. Easily startled (n = 378)	229	60.58	[55.57–65.38]
19. Difficulty concentrating (n = 378)	262	69.31	[64.49–73.75]
20. Trouble falling or staying asleep (n = 378)	274	72.49	[67.78–76.75]
Provisional PTSD diagnosis [b] (n = 379)	237	62.53	[57.55–67.25]
PCL-5 Total Score 33 or higher (n = 379)	226	59.63	[54.62–64.45]

Note: [a] On each of the 379 completed PCL-5, between 1 and 5 questions were left unanswered. Missing data were not replaced. [b] Proportion of respondents who have endorsed 1 B item (questions 1–5), 1 C item (questions 6–7), 2 D items (questions 8–14), 2 E items (questions 15–20).

Table 2. Results on self-report questionnaires (n = 347–378 [a]).

Questionnaire	n	%	95% CI
PHQ—Somatoform Disorder (n = 378)	102	26.98	[22.75–31.67]
PHQ—Major Depression Disorder (n = 378)	125	33.07	[28.52–37.96]
PHQ—Panic Disorder (n = 379)	66	17.41	[13.92–21.55]
PHQ—Other Anxiety Disorder (n = 378)	102	26.98	[22.75–31.67]
PHQ—Bulimia (n = 377)	14	3.71	[2.22–6.13]
PHQ—Binge Eating Disorder (n = 377)	57	15.12	[11.86–19.09]
PHQ—Alcohol Abuse (n = 375)	64	17.07	[13.06–21.21]
	M	SD	95% CI
Depressive Symptoms (PHQ-9) (n = 378)	10.72	6.65	[10.05–11.39]
Insomnia Symptoms (ISI) (n = 375)	15.50	7.75	[14.72–16.28]
Trauma-Related Sleep Disturbances (PSQI-A) (n = 375)	5.52	4.72	[5.04–6.00]
Global sleep Quality (PSQI) (n = 375)	11.76	4.98	[11.26–12.26]
Sleep Quality (PSQI) (n = 375)	1.90	0.85	[1.81–1.99]
Sleep Latency (PSQI) (n = 375)	2.01	1.10	[1.90–2.12]
Sleep Duration (PSQI) (n = 370)	1.76	1.03	[1.66–1.86]
Sleep Efficiency (PSQI) (n = 370)	1.61	1.28	[1.48–1.74]
Sleep Disturbances (PSQI) (n = 375)	1.92	0.76	[1.84–2.00]
Use of Sleep Medications (PSQI) (n = 374)	0.99	1.28	[0.86–1.12]
Daytime Dysfunction (PSQI) (n = 375)	1.62	0.95	[1.52–1.72]
Post-Traumatic Cognitions (PTCI) (n = 347)	48.05	43.06	[43.55–52.55]
Self (PTCI) (n = 359)	1.40	1.43	[1.25–1.55]
World (PTCI) (n = 359)	2.25	1.66	[2.08–2.42]
Self-Blame (PTCI) (n = 359)	0.55	0.99	[0.45–0.65]
Seeking Social Support (WCQ) (n = 358)	6.70	4.02	[6.28–7.12]
Problem-Solving / Positive Re-Appraisal (WCQ) (n = 358)	10.24	6.07	[9.61–10.87]
Distancing / Avoidance (WCQ) (n = 359)	6.82	4.15	[6.39–7.25]

Note: [a] Among the 379 completed questionnaires, between 1 and 32 data were missing per variable. Missing data were not replaced. M = mean; PHQ = Patient Health Questionnaire; SD = standard deviation.

Table 3. Proportions of respondents diagnosed with PTSD or other mental disorders according to clinical interviews [a] (n = 54 or 55 [b]).

Diagnosis	Number of Respondents	Proportion of Respondents	95% CI
PTSD (n = 55)	16	29.09	[18.77–42.14]
Major Depression Disorder (n = 55)	14	25.45	[15.81–38.30]
Panic Disorder (n = 55)	13	23.64	[14.37–36.35]
Agoraphobia (n = 55)	7	12.73	[6.31–24.02]
Generalized Anxiety Disorder (n = 55)	13	23.64	[14.37–36.35]
Social Phobia (n = 55)	5	9.09	[3.95–19.58]
Obsessive-Compulsive Disorder (n = 55)	0	0.00	–
Drug Use Disorder (n = 54)	7	12.96	[6.42–24.42]
Alcohol Use Disorder (n = 54)	2	3.70	[1.02–12.53]
Insomnia Disorder (n = 55)	24	43.64	[31.38–56.73]

Note: [a] PTSD diagnosed with the Clinician-Administered PTSD Scale for DSM-5 (CAPS), Insomnia Disorder diagnosed with questions from the Insomnia Interview Schedule adapted according to the DSM-5 criteria, all other disorders diagnosed with the Mini International Neuropsychiatric Interview (MINI). [b] One participant did not provide information to assess alcohol use and another one did not provide information to assess alcohol use.

Table 4. Correlation coefficients between variables (n = 354–374).

	PTSD	Sex	Age	Depression	Insomnia	Sleep Quality	Sleep Disturbances	Self	World	Self-Blame	Support	Problem-Solving
PTSD												
Sex	0.088											
Age	−0.122 *	−0.177 **										
Depression	0.808 **	0.023	−0.056									
Insomnia	0.673 **	0.082	−0.022	0.726 **								
Sleep Quality	0.564 **	0.107 *	0.044	0.624 **	0.803 **							
Sleep Disturbances	0.702 **	0.118 *	−0.033	0.671 **	0.634 **	0.592 **						
Self	0.730 **	0.028	−0.166 **	0.733 **	0.529 **	0.425 **	0.639 **					
World	0.638 **	−0.042	−0.116 *	0.568 **	0.408 **	0.347 **	0.543 **	0.768 **				
Self-Blame	0.501 **	−0.094	−0.056	0.508 **	0.353 **	0.289 **	0.462 **	0.680 **	0.596 **			
Support	0.053	0.150 **	−0.054	0.100	0.088	0.066	0.115 *	−0.025	0.064	0.043		
Problem-Solving	−0.096	0.012	0.078	−0.090	−0.053	−0.052	0.010	−0.180 **	0.022	−0.014	0.622 **	
Avoidance	0.532 **	0.153 **	−0.248 **	0.464 **	0.414 **	0.351 **	0.444 **	0.505 **	0.445 **	0.351 **	0.196 **	0.134 *

* $p < 0.05$; ** $p < 0.01$; Note: Avoidance: distancing/avoidance (WCQ subscale); Depression: depressive symptoms (PHQ-9 total score excluding the #3 sleep item); Insomnia: insomnia severity (ISI total score); Problem-Solving: problem-solving/positive reappraisal (WCQ subscale); PTSD: post-traumatic symptom severity (PCL-5 total score excluding the #2 and #20 sleep items); Sleep Disturbances: trauma-related sleep disturbances (PSQI-A total score); Sleep Quality: global sleep quality (PSQI total score); Self: negative cognitions about the self (PTCI subscale); Self-Blame: self-blame (PTCI subscale); Support: seeking social support (WCQ subscale), World: negative cognitions about the world (PTCI subscale).

Table 5. Multiple regression analyses predicting PTSD symptom severity (excluding sleep items) ($n = 344$).

	Variables	B	SE B	β	Adjusted R^2	R^2 Change
Step 1					0.023 **	0.23 **
	Sex	4.778	2.377	0.102		
	Age	−0.176	0.077	−0.123 *		
Step 2					0.680 **	0.654 **
	Sex	2.403	1.363	0.055		
	Age	−0.125	0.044	−0.087 **		
	Depressive symptom severity (PHQ-9 excluding sleep item)	2.439	0.092	0.811 **		
Step 3					0.721 **	0.043 **
	Sex	0.853	1.296	0.019		
	Age	−0.126	0.042	−0.088 **		
	Depressive symptom severity (PHQ-9 excluding sleep item)	1.732	0.138	0.576 **		
	Global sleep quality (PSQI)	−0.141	0.173	−0.040		
	Insomnia symptom severity (ISI)	0.291	0.126	0.128 *		
	Post-traumatic sleep disturbances (PSQI-A)	0.932	0.154	0.249 **		
Step 4					0.753 **	0.035 **
	Sex	1.555	1.263	0.035		
	Age	−0.064	0.041	−0.045		
	Depressive symptom severity (PHQ-9 excluding sleep item)	1.393	0.153	0.465 **		
	Global sleep quality (PSQI)	−0.121	0.164	−0.034		
	Insomnia symptom severity (ISI)	0.287	0.119	0.126 *		
	Post-traumatic sleep disturbances (PSQI-A)	0.646	0.155	0.173 **		
	Negative cognitions about the self (PTCI)	0.227	0.736	0.018		
	Negative cognitions about the world/others (PTCI)	1.827	0.463	0.172 **		
	Self-blame (PTCI)	0.046	0.681	0.002		
	Seeking social support (WCQ)	−0.166	0.157	−0.038		
	Positive reappraisal/Problem solving (WCQ)	−0.107	0.107	−0.037		
	Distancing/Avoidance (WCQ)	0.461	0.145	0.109 **		

* $p < 0.05$; ** $p < 0.01$. B = beta weight; SE B = standard error of the beta weight.

4. Discussion

The objective of this study was to rapidly document post-traumatic stress symptoms, mental disorders and psychological difficulties in a sample of evacuees in the immediate aftermath of the 2016 Fort McMurray wildfires. Result showed that roughly 60% of respondents to an online questionnaire reported significant post-traumatic stress symptoms, or could be given a provisional PTSD diagnosis according to their responses to a validated self-report questionnaire (PCL-5). This is similar to what was observed among the residents of Enschede, The Netherlands, two or three weeks after the explosion of a fireworks storage facility in a residential area, where more than 50% reported anxious and depressive symptoms of anxiety and sleeping problems, and nearly 75% reported disaster-related reactions of intrusion and avoidance [14]. Four months after a devastating tornado struck the town of Albion, PA in 1985, 76% of its residents also showed high levels of post-traumatic stress [33].

The most frequently reported post-traumatic stress symptoms were repeated disturbing memories (reported by 77.4% of the sample), feeling upset when reminded of the stressful experience (76.7%), and trouble falling or staying asleep (72.5%). The widespread presence of sleep disturbances is a finding consistent with that of studies with larger and more representative samples exposed to a disaster: Rates of severe problems with sleep were threefold that of the general population in the residents of Enschede, The Netherlands, after the fireworks storage facility explosion [14].

Self-report questionnaires suggested alarmingly elevated rates of clinically significant symptoms of major depressive disorder (one in three respondents), but also of somatoform, anxiety and panic disorders, alcohol abuse and binge eating. Respondents reported overall high severity of depressive symptoms, insomnia symptoms and trauma-related sleep disturbances, as well as poor sleep quality. This highlights the relevance to include various outcomes in the assessment of the impact of a disaster on mental health. Because this study did not benefit neither from a comparison with a non-exposed control group nor from an estimation of pre-traumatic mental health of the Fort McMurray population, we cannot directly attribute the observed symptoms to the experience of the fires and of the evacuation. However, all of the observed values were largely greater than prevalence rates of mental health disorders reported in the general population: For example, according to the 2002 Canadian Community Health Survey on Mental Health and Well-Being, the 12-month prevalence of any anxiety disorder is 4.8%, and any mood disorder is 5.3% [34].

We also analyzed data from a subsample of 55 evacuees who participated in a clinical interview where a stringent examination of DSM criteria was conducted. This more rigorous and conservative approach indicated that 29.1% fulfilled the DSM-5 criteria for PTSD. Prevalence of PTSD was somewhat more elevated than that assessed with a DSM-IV-based clinical interview in a sample of individuals three months after an earthquake in North China (18.8%) [35]. However, in the latter study, when researchers calculated the prevalence of PTSD without the requirement for presence of both avoidance and numbing symptoms (DSM-IV's Criterion C), as is it now the case in DSM-5, they obtained an estimated closer to the one we obtained (27.4%). Almost half of participants with PTSD in the present study (43.6%) could be considered as having an insomnia disorder (recurrently having significant trouble falling or staying asleep). This is about three times higher than in the general Canadian population where the prevalence of insomnia disorder is estimated to be 13.4% [36]. Moreover, although 78% of the subsample reported having had insomnia episodes before the fires, the current insomnia episode was presumably trauma-related, i.e., definitely/probably started or got worse after the fires, in 84% of the cases.

We also wanted to explore the association between of symptoms of post-traumatic stress, and depression, sleep problems, post-traumatic cognitions and coping strategies as assessed three months after the fires. After controlling for sex and age, significant factors associated with post-traumatic stress symptom severity included, depressive symptoms, trauma-related sleep disturbances, post-traumatic cognitions (perceiving other people or the world as untrustworthy or dangerous), insomnia symptoms, avoidance-based coping strategies and problem-solving/reappraisal coping strategies. The observed associations were consistent with the role of cognitions and coping strategies in producing a sense of imminent threat that contribute to maintain and exacerbate post-traumatic stress symptoms [19]. These preliminary findings also suggest that sleep problems, either sleep disturbances or insomnia, are closely associated with PTSD in the aftermath of a disaster, beyond the expected association due to the presence of depressive symptoms. Sleep difficulties may be present before the traumatic event or occur as a result of trauma, and their persistence several days or weeks after the traumatic event may act as a specific risk factor for PTSD [37]. They may constitute symptoms of PTSD, but they may also develop into difficulties concomitant with PTSD, but still different in their nature and their response to treatment [38,39]. Inversely, the treatment of trauma-related sleep problems may have a positive impact on other post-traumatic stress symptoms [40,41]. Interventions to protect or restore sleep after exposure to a disaster are likely to be useful, but the efficacy of sleep management strategies to prevent the development of other mental health problems after traumatic exposure has yet to be studied.

These findings are to be interpreted with caution, as they were assessed very early in the aftermath of the fires and the evacuation, i.e., approximately three months after the evacuation. Some of the respondents had not yet returned home. Furthermore, it is possible that individuals feeling distress could have been more motivated to participate compared to persons with no particular mental health symptoms. Previous findings have shown that resilience, namely the ability to maintain at a stable, healthy level of psychological and physical functioning [15], is to be expected in the majority of individuals. In a study of the aftermath of Hurricane Ike [42], it was found that 75% of the population never developed PTSD when they were evaluated in the 18-month period following the disaster. In addition, between 45–58% did not develop depression, functional impairment, or report days of poor health. Recovery, whereby persons may experience some levels of psychopathology (such as anxiety, depression or sleep problems) but gradually return to pre-event levels of functioning [16], is another common trajectory, where some level of psychological symptoms could be expected as a "normal" reaction to a severely abnormal event, but where symptoms eventually subside. Data collected three to four years after the Victorian Black Saturday bushfires in Australia (February 2009) indicated that more than 80% recovered from symptoms of psychological distress without developing significant mental health problems in the long run [4]. However, studies of resilience and recovery have focused on PTSD and depression, and have not included the assessment of sleep difficulties. Longitudinal follow-ups of the Fort McMurray community will be needed to assess the longer-term evolution of the all of the psychological impacts that were highlighted in these results.

5. Conclusions

This study represented a preliminary effort to guide future investigations on the mental health of the Fort McMurray community. A study of the natural history of PTSD, depression and sleep disorders is currently in progress to document the prevalence of psychopathology in the long-term (e.g., three years post-disaster), and to examine the impact of sociodemographic characteristics (e.g., sex/gender, age, ethnicity, income and membership in a First Nation) and degree of loss caused by the fires on prevalence rates. This ongoing study will examine the longitudinal predictors of the course of post-traumatic adaptation, by determining the sociodemographic, psychopathological, cognitive, behavioural and social factors longitudinally associated with not only distress, but also resilience and post-traumatic growth. Finally, we perceived an urgent need in our pool of respondents to be heard about their mental health service needs. Although evidence has shown that patients usually prefer psychological treatment to medication to treat anxiety and depression problems, gender, age and ethnicity greatly influence beliefs and perceived needs in terms of mental health [43]. Data on mental health needs after a disaster from the patients' perspective are needed to guide the development of large-scale interventions that are accessible and relevant to the affected community.

Author Contributions: Data curation, G.B.; Formal analysis, G.B.; Funding acquisition, G.B., M.-C.O. and C.M.M.; Investigation, G.B.; Methodology, G.B., M.-C.O. and C.M.M.; Project administration, G.B.; Supervision, M.-C.O.; Writing—original draft, G.B.; Writing—review & editing, G.B., M.-C.O. and C.M.M.

References

1. Norris, F.H.; Friedman, M.J.; Watson, P.J.; Byrne, C.M.; Diaz, E.; Kaniasty, K. 60,000 disaster victims speak: Part I. An empirical review of the empirical literature, 1981–2001. *Psychiatry* **2002**, *65*, 207–239. [CrossRef] [PubMed]
2. Marshall, G.N.; Schell, T.L.; Elliott, M.N.; Rayburn, N.R.; Jaycox, L.H. Psychiatric disorders among adults seeking emergency disaster assistance after a wildland-urban interface fire. *Psychiatr. Serv.* **2007**, *58*, 509–514. [CrossRef] [PubMed]
3. Clayer, J.R.; Bookless-Pratz, C.; Harris, R.L. Some health consequences of a natural disaster. *Med. J. Aust.* **1985**, *143*, 182–184.
4. Bryant, R.A.; Waters, E.; Gibbs, L.; Gallagher, H.C.; Pattison, P.; Lusher, D.; MacDougall, C.; Harms, L.; Block, K.; Snowdon, E.; et al. Psychological outcomes following the Victorian Black Saturday bushfires. *Aust. N. Z. J. Psychiatry* **2014**, *48*, 634–643. [CrossRef] [PubMed]
5. Brown, M.R.G.; Agyapong, V.; Greenshaw, A.J.; Cribben, I.; Brett-MacLean, P.; Drolet, J.; McDonald-Harker, C.; Omeje, J.; Mankowsi, M.; Noble, S.; et al. After the Fort McMurray wildfire there are significant increases in mental health symptoms in grade 7–12 students compared to controls. *BMC Psychiatry* **2019**, *19*. [CrossRef]

6. Agyapong, V.I.O.; Hrabok, M.; Juhas, M.; Omeje, J.; Denga, E.; Nwaka, B.; Akinjise, I.; Corbett, S.E.; Moosavi, S.; Brown, M.; et al. Prevalence rates and predictors of generalized anxiety disorder symptoms in residents of Fort McMurray six months after a wildfire. *Front. Psychiatry* **2018**, *9*. [CrossRef] [PubMed]
7. Fergusson, D.M.; Horwood, L.J.; Boden, J.M.; Mulder, R.T. Impact of a major disaster on the mental health of a well-studied cohort. *JAMA Psychiatry* **2014**, *71*, 1025–1031. [CrossRef] [PubMed]
8. Goldmann, E.; Galea, S. Mental health consequences of disasters. *Annu. Rev. Public Health* **2014**, *35*, 169–183. [CrossRef] [PubMed]
9. Laugharne, J.; Van de Watt, G.; Janca, A. After the fire: The mental health consequences of fire disasters. *Curr. Opin. Psychiatry* **2011**, *24*, 72–77. [CrossRef] [PubMed]
10. Miller, K.E.; Brownlow, J.A.; Woodward, S.; Gehrman, P.R. Sleep and Dreaming in Posttraumatic Stress Disorder. *Curr. Psychiatry Rep.* **2017**, *19*, 71. [CrossRef]
11. Murphy, M.J.; Peterson, M.J. Sleep disturbances in depression. *Sleep Med. Clin.* **2015**, *10*, 17–23. [CrossRef]
12. Norris, F.H.; Sherrieb, K.; Galea, S. Prevalence and consequences of disaster-related illness and injury from Hurricane Ike. *Rehabil Psychol* **2010**, *55*, 221–230. [CrossRef]
13. Babson, K.A.; Feldner, M.T. Temporal relations between sleep problems and both traumatic event exposure and PTSD: A critical review of the empirical literature. *J. Anxiety Disord.* **2010**, *24*, 1–15. [CrossRef] [PubMed]
14. van Kamp, I.; van der Velden, P.G.; Stellato, R.K.; Roorda, J.; van Loon, J.; Kleber, R.J.; Gersons, B.B.; Lebret, E. Physical and mental health shortly after a disaster: First results from the Enschede firework disaster study. *Eur. J. Public Health* **2006**, *16*, 253–259. [CrossRef] [PubMed]
15. Bonanno, G.A. Loss, trauma, and human resilience: Have we underestimated the human capacity to thrive after extremely aversive events? *Am. Psychol.* **2004**, *59*, 20–28. [CrossRef] [PubMed]
16. Bonanno, G.A.; Mancini, A.D. Beyond resilience and PTSD: Mapping the heterogeneity of responses to potential trauma. *Psychol. Trauma* **2012**, *4*, 74–83. [CrossRef]
17. Math, S.B.; Nirmala, M.C.; Moirangthem, S.; Kumar, N.C. Disaster Management: Mental Health Perspective. *Indian J. Psychol. Med.* **2015**, *37*, 261–271. [CrossRef] [PubMed]
18. Tempest, E.L.; Carter, B.; Beck, C.R.; Rubin, G.J. Secondary stressors are associated with probable psychological morbidity after flooding: A cross-sectional analysis. *Eur. J. Public Health* **2017**, *27*, 1042–1047. [CrossRef]
19. Ehlers, A.; Clark, D.M. A cognitive model of posttraumatic stress disorder. *Behav. Res. Ther.* **2000**, *38*, 319–345. [CrossRef]
20. Frissa, S.; Hatch, S.L.; Fear, N.T.; Dorrington, S.; Goodwin, L.; Hotopf, M. Challenges in the retrospective assessment of trauma: Comparing a checklist approach to a single item trauma experience screening question. *BMC Psychiatry* **2016**, *16*. [CrossRef]
21. Blake, D.D.; Weathers, F.W.; Nagy, L.M.; Kaloupek, D.G.; Gusman, F.D.; Charney, D.S.; Keane, T.M. The development of a Clinician-Administered PTSD Scale. *J. Trauma Stress* **1995**, *8*, 75–90. [CrossRef]
22. Sheehan, D.V.; Lecrubier, Y.; Sheehan, K.H.; Amorim, P.; Janavs, J.; Weiller, E.; Hergueta, T.; Baker, R.; Dunbar, G.C. The Mini-International Neuropsychiatric Interview (M.I.N.I.): The development and validation of a structured diagnostic psychiatric interview for DSM-IV and ICD-10. *J. Clin. Psychiatry* **1998**, *59* (Suppl. 20), S22–S33.
23. American Psychiatric Association. *Diagnostic and Statistical Manual of Mental Disorders: DSM-5™*, 5th ed.; American Psychiatric Publishing, Inc.: Arlington, VA, USA, 2013.
24. Forbes, D.; Creamer, M.; Biddle, D. The validity of the PTSD checklist as a measure of symptomatic change in combat-related PTSD. *Behav. Res. Ther.* **2001**, *39*, 977–986. [CrossRef]
25. Kroenke, K.; Spitzer, R.L.; Williams, J.B. The PHQ-9: Validity of a brief depression severity measure. *J. Gen. Intern. Med.* **2001**, *16*, 606–613. [CrossRef]
26. Bastien, C.H.; Vallieres, A.; Morin, C.M. Validation of the Insomnia Severity Index as an outcome measure for insomnia research. *Sleep Med.* **2001**, *2*, 297–307. [CrossRef]
27. Buysse, D.J.; Reynolds, C.F.; Monk, T.H.; Berman, S.R.; Kupfer, D.J. The Pittsburgh Sleep Quality Index: A new instrument for psychiatric practice and research. *Psychiatry Res.* **1989**, *28*, 193–213. [CrossRef]
28. Germain, A.; Hall, M.; Krakow, B.; Shear, M.K.; Buysse, D.J. A brief sleep scale for Posttraumatic Stress Disorder: Pittsburgh Sleep Quality Index Addendum for PTSD. *J. Anxiety Disord.* **2005**, *19*, 233–244. [CrossRef]
29. Foa, E.B.; Ehlers, A.; Clark, D.M.; Tolin, D.F.; Orsillo, S.M. The Posttraumatic Cognitions Inventory (PTCI): Development and validation. *Psychol. Assess.* **1999**, *11*, 303–314. [CrossRef]

30. Folkman, S.; Lazarus, R.S. *Manual for the Ways of Coping Questionnaire*; Consulting Psychologists Press: Palo Alto, CA, USA, 1988.
31. Weathers, F.W.; Litz, B.T.; Keane, T.M.; Palmieri, P.A.; Marx, B.P.; Schnurr, P.P. The PTSD Checklist for DSM-5 (PCL-5). National Center for PTSD; 2013. Available online: https://www.ptsd.va.gov/professional/assessment/adult-sr/ptsd-checklist.asp (accessed on 27 February 2019).
32. Morin, C.M.; Belleville, G.; Belanger, L.; Ivers, H. The insomnia severity index: Psychometric indicators to detect insomnia cases and evaluate treatment response. *Sleep* **2011**, *34*, 601–608. [CrossRef]
33. Steinglass, P.; Gerrity, E. Natural disasters and post-traumatic stress disorder: Short-term versus long-term recovery in two disaster-affected communities. *J. Appl. Soc. Psychol.* **1990**, *20*, 1746–1765. [CrossRef]
34. Statistics Canada. Canadian Community Health Survey: Mental Health and Well-Being 2003. Available online: https://www150.statcan.gc.ca/n1/daily-quotidien/030903/dq030903a-eng.htm (accessed on 27 February 2019).
35. Wang, J.; Smailes, E.; Sareen, J.; Fick, G.H.; Schmitz, N.; Patten, S.B. The prevalence of mental disorders in the working population over the period of global economic crisis. *Can. J. Psychiatry* **2010**, *55*, 598–605. [CrossRef]
36. Morin, C.M.; LeBlanc, M.; Bélanger, L.; Ivers, H.; Mérette, C.; Savard, J. Prevalence of insomnia and its treatment in Canada. *Can. J. Psychiatry* **2011**, *56*, 540–548. [CrossRef]
37. Koren, D.; Arnon, I.; Lavie, P.; Klein, E. Sleep complaints as early predictors of posttraumatic stress disorder: A 1-year prospective study of injured survivors of motor vehicle accidents. *Am. J. Psychiatry* **2001**, *159*, 855–857. [CrossRef]
38. Belleville, G.; Guay, S.; Marchand, A. Persistence of sleep disturbances following cognitive-behavior therapy for posttraumatic stress disorder. *J. Psychosom. Res.* **2011**, *70*, 318–327. [CrossRef]
39. Galovski, T.E.; Monson, C.; Bruce, S.E.; Resick, P.A. Does cognitive-behavioral therapy for PTSD improve perceived health and sleep impairment? *J. Trauma Stress* **2009**, *22*, 197–204. [CrossRef]
40. Casement, M.D.; Swanson, L.M. A meta-analysis of imagery rehearsal for post-trauma nightmares: Effects on nightmare frequency, sleep quality, and posttraumatic stress. *Clin. Psychol. Rev.* **2012**, *32*, 566–574. [CrossRef]
41. Talbot, L.S.; Maguen, S.; Metzler, T.J.; Schmitz, M.; McCaslin, S.E.; Richards, A.; Perlis, M.L.; Posner, D.A.; Weiss, B.; Ruoff, L.; et al. Cognitive behavioral therapy for insomnia in posttraumatic stress disorder: A randomized controlled trial. *Sleep* **2014**, *37*, 327–341. [CrossRef]
42. Lowe, S.R.; Joshi, S.; Pietrzak, R.H.; Galea, S.; Cerdá, M. Mental health and general wellness in the aftermath of Hurricane Ike. *Soc. Sci. Med.* **2015**, *124*, 162–170. [CrossRef]
43. Prins, M.A.; Verhaak, P.F.; Bensing, J.M.; van der Meer, K. Health beliefs and perceived need for mental health care of anxiety and depression—The patients' perspective explored. *Clin. Psychol. Rev.* **2008**, *28*, 1038–1058. [CrossRef]

8

Forecasting of Landslide Displacement Using a Probability-Scheme Combination Ensemble Prediction Technique

Junwei Ma [1], Xiao Liu [1,*], Xiaoxu Niu [1], Yankun Wang [2], Tao Wen [3], Junrong Zhang [2] and Zongxing Zou [1]

1 Three Gorges Research Center for Geo-Hazards of the Ministry of Education, China University of Geosciences, Wuhan 430074, China; majw@cug.edu.cn (J.M.); nxx@cug.edu.cn (X.N.); zouzongxing@cug.edu.cn (Z.Z.)
2 Faculty of Engineering, China University of Geosciences, Wuhan 430074, China; yankun_wang@cug.edu.cn (Y.W.); zjr@cug.edu.cn (J.Z.)
3 School of Geosciences, Yangtze University, Wuhan 430100, China; wentao200840@yangtzeu.edu.cn
* Correspondence: liuxiao@cug.edu.cn

Abstract: Data-driven models have been extensively employed in landslide displacement prediction. However, predictive uncertainty, which consists of input uncertainty, parameter uncertainty, and model uncertainty, is usually disregarded in deterministic data-driven modeling, and point estimates are separately presented. In this study, a probability-scheme combination ensemble prediction that employs quantile regression neural networks and kernel density estimation (QRNNs-KDE) is proposed for robust and accurate prediction and uncertainty quantification of landslide displacement. In the ensemble model, QRNNs serve as base learning algorithms to generate multiple base learners. Final ensemble prediction is obtained by integration of all base learners through a probability combination scheme based on KDE. The Fanjiaping landslide in the Three Gorges Reservoir area (TGRA) was selected as a case study to explore the performance of the ensemble prediction. Based on long-term (2006–2018) and near real-time monitoring data, a comprehensive analysis of the deformation characteristics was conducted for fully understanding the triggering factors. The experimental results indicate that the QRNNs-KDE approach can perform predictions with perfect performance and outperform the traditional backpropagation (BP), radial basis function (RBF), extreme learning machine (ELM), support vector machine (SVM) methods, bootstrap-extreme learning machine-artificial neural network (bootstrap-ELM-ANN), and Copula-kernel-based support vector machine quantile regression (Copula-KSVMQR). The proposed QRNNs-KDE approach has significant potential in medium-term to long-term horizon forecasting and quantification of uncertainty.

Keywords: landslide displacement; predictive uncertainty; ensemble prediction; probability combination scheme; quantile regression neural networks (QRNNs); kernel density estimation (KDE)

---

1. Introduction

As one of the most common natural hazards in the world, landslides pose a significant threat to public health and safety. According to statistics, landslides have affected 4.8 million people and caused 18,275 deaths during the period of 2009–2019 [1]. Landslide displacement prediction, which provides the necessary information to determine the extent of ongoing hazard, has proven to be the most cost-saving risk reduction measure [2–4]. However, landslide displacement prediction is complex and remains a key challenge in natural hazard research. This challenge arises because landslides are nonlinear, dynamic systems, and the associated movements can be induced by different causes, such as geological factors [5], hydrological factors [6,7], morphological factors, and human activities [4,8].

A large number of efforts in the literature have focused on the precise prediction of landslide displacement [9]. Currently, approaches used for landslide displacement prediction are categorized as physical modelling approaches and data-driven approaches [10]. Physical models (also known as white-box models), which rely on detailed descriptions of landslide mechanism processes, can provide clear physical explanations of landslides. The commonly used physical models include the tertiary creep model [11], the Hayashi model [12], and the general creep model [13]. Those physical models require numerous expensive geotechnical characterizations of the materials involved in landslides and therefore may be applicable only in limited cases [14].

Data-driven models differ from physical models because a characterization of the actual landslide mechanism processes is not fully required. Thus, the data-driven models are also known as black-box models. The main advantage of data-driven models is that the trained models can be easily updated on the basis of new and more recent data.

Data-driven models include but are not limited to statistical methods, artificial neural networks (ANNs), support vector machines (SVMs) [15], and extreme learning machines (ELMs) [16]. Owing to their capacity to approximate arbitrary, nonlinear, and dynamic systems with high precision, data-driven models achieve good model performance in the prediction of landslide displacement.

Despite their widespread application, the output of most existing data-driven models is a single estimate for each prediction horizon. These single estimates, which provide deterministic values, are referred to as point predictions [3]. The defining characteristic of a point prediction is its accessibility with regard to understanding and operation. The main drawback of point prediction is that it only provides the prediction error, with no information regarding the associated predictive uncertainties, which limits the use of point prediction in decision-making applications.

The predictive uncertainties consisting primarily of input uncertainty, parameter uncertainty, and model uncertainty could be substantial. It is highly desirable to know the degree of uncertainty that is associated with a particular point prediction and convert the point prediction into informative resources for emergency landslide risk management [3,17]. Only limited studies have examined the quantification of uncertainty associated with landslide displacement prediction by constructing prediction intervals (PIs). The output of a PI is an interval composed of upper and lower bounds, where we expect the predictive value of the series to fall within some (prespecified) probability, which is deemed the PI nominal confidence (PINC). A hybrid approach based on an echo state network and mean-variance estimation was proposed by Yao et al. [18] to measure the uncertainty in landslide deformation prediction and perform interval prediction. A bootstrap-based approach was proposed by Ma et al. [4] to perform interval prediction of landslide displacement. Wang et al. [2] proposed a direct interval prediction using least squares support vector machines or the construction of PIs of landslide displacement. Kernel-based support vector machine quantile regression (KSVMQR) was utilized in [3] for quantification of the predictive uncertainty of landslide displacement.

However, the traditional methods have certain disadvantages in displacement prediction and quantification of predictive uncertainty. For example, the bootstrap-based approach requires significantly high computational costs, especially for large datasets [2]. Additionally, the performances of SVM-based approaches are sensitive to the choice of kernel type and parameter values [19]. Therefore, more efforts still need to be made for the improvement of prediction performance and quantification of the predictive uncertainty.

Ensemble prediction, a state-of-the-art artificial intelligence technique, aims to improve prediction robustness and accuracy and uncertainty quantification [20,21]. Ensemble prediction has been successfully applied in a variety of fields, including prediction performance improvement and uncertainty quantification of remaining useful life [22], bankruptcy [23], shear capacity of reinforced-concrete deep beams [24], residential electricity consumption [25], wind power [26], flood susceptibility [27,28], and landslide susceptibility [29].

In this study, a probability-scheme combination ensemble prediction that employs quantile regression neural networks and kernel density estimation (QRNNs-KDE) was proposed for robust and accurate prediction and uncertainty quantification of landslide displacement. The Fanjiaping landslide with long-term and near real-time monitoring data was selected as a case study to explore the performance of the QRNNs-KDE approach. The deformation characteristics were clarified for fully understanding the triggering factors.

2. Methodology

2.1. Description of Uncertainty Sources

Predictive uncertainty in data-driven models consists primarily of input uncertainty, parameter uncertainty, and model uncertainty [30–32].

The input uncertainty is related to the input data uncertainty and the input variable section uncertainty. The input data uncertainty is primarily due to measurement and sampling error and environmental noise. The input variable section uncertainty accounts for uncertainty inherent in the selection of input variables from the candidate data set. For physical models, the required inputs are pre-determined, being consistent with considered rheological models. However, for data-driven models, the selection of input variables is problem-dependent and cannot be determined in advance. Only major and relevant variables are selected as final inputs to train the data-driven model. The selection of the variables to include in a data-driven model from the original data set is inherently uncertain, especially when the input candidate pool is very large. For example, in data-driven models that utilize decomposition algorithms, only a portion of the decomposed sub-components are selected as input variables. The candidate input pool, which consists of sub-components, increases very quickly with the decomposition level and potentially increases the input variable selection uncertainty.

The parameter uncertainty refers to the uncertainty in the model parameter vector and mainly arises from the inability to identify a unique set of best parameters for the model [33].

Model uncertainty arises primarily from the model structure uncertainty and model error. Model structure uncertainty is associated with the specific model setting of learning algorithms, such as the polynomial order in polynomial regression models, the number of hidden nodes in an ANN or ELM, and the type of kernel function in an SVM. The input uncertainty may also account for model structure uncertainty, because different input variables “automatically" produce different model structures. Model error refers to the difference between two model estimates with respect to the corresponding target and is caused by the inability to reproduce the real processes.

2.2. Ensemble Prediction

Ensemble prediction is not a specific learning algorithm but a strategic combination of multiple predictions into a single output with a model combination process [21]. Based on the selection of the learning algorithm, ensemble prediction models can be further classified into homogeneous and heterogeneous ensemble models (Figure 1). A homogeneous ensemble model generates multiple learners with the same learning algorithm on different training datasets, which are produced by manipulating the original training data (schematic illustrated in Figure 1a). Bootstrap aggregation, also known as bagging for short, is the most straightforward and widely used method of manipulating the training dataset. By contrast, a heterogeneous ensemble model generates multiple learners with different learning algorithms on the same training data set (schematic illustrated in Figure 1b).

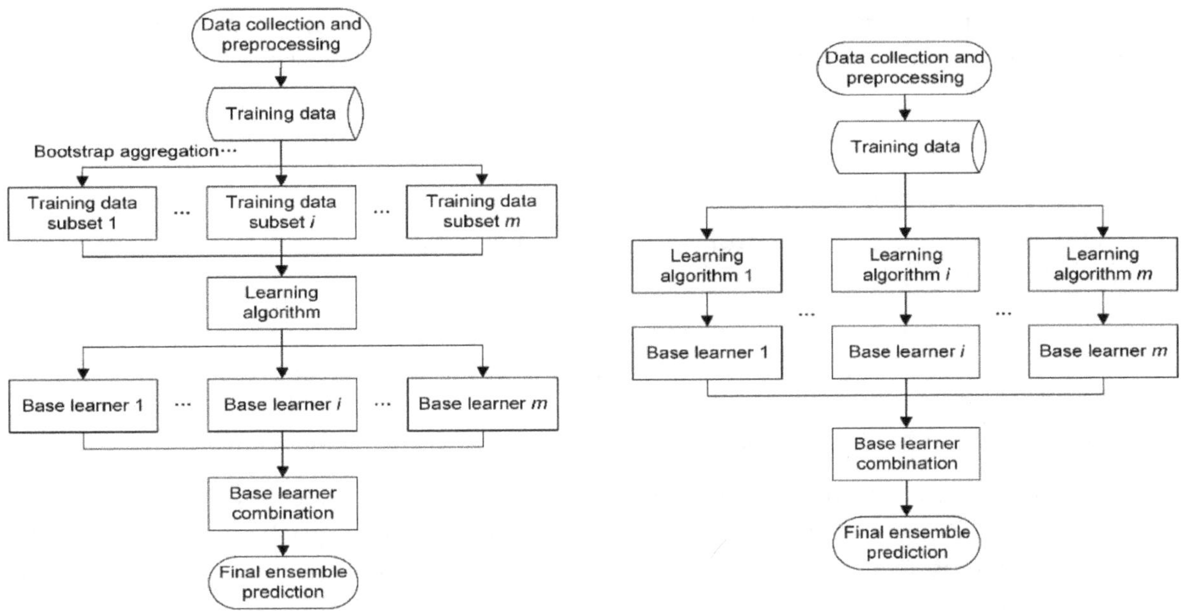

(a) Homogeneous ensemble mode (b) Heterogeneous ensemble mode

Figure 1. General framework for ensemble prediction models. (**a**) Homogeneous ensemble model and (**b**) heterogeneous ensemble model.

The base learner combination is the main step in the ensemble prediction model. Summation and averaging are simple combination schemes. A more general approach involves assigning a weight to each base learner. In the present study, a heterogeneous ensemble model was built based on QRNNs and KDE. QRNNs serve as base learning algorithms to produce multiple base learners, and the probability combination scheme based on KDE is used to combine the base learners into the final ensemble prediction.

2.3. *Quantile Regression Neural Network*

2.3.1. Quantile Regression

Quantile regression is a common statistical technique for conducting inferences concerning conditional quantile functions [34,35]. More formally, any real-valued random variable Y may be characterized by its distribution function as follows:

$$F(y) = \text{Prob}(Y \leq y) \tag{1}$$

whereas for any $0 < \tau < 1$,

$$Q(\tau) = \inf\{y : F(y) \geq \tau\} \tag{2}$$

is called the τth quantile of Y.

Given a data set $(x_i(t), Y(t))$ for $i = 1, 2, \cdots, I$ and $t = 1, 2, \cdots, N$, the linear quantile regression can be expressed as follows:

$$\hat{Y}_\tau(t) = \sum_{i=1}^{I} \theta_i x_i(t) + b \tag{3}$$

where $0 < \tau < 1$ is the quantile, and b is an error with zero expectation.

The estimated parameters θ_i can be approximated by minimizing a sum of the asymmetrically weighted absolute residual cost functions, which are expressed as follows:

$$E_\tau = \frac{1}{N}\sum_{t=1}^{N} \rho_\tau(Y(t) - \hat{Y}_\tau(t)) \tag{4}$$

where $Y(t)$ is the observation at time t and ρ_τ is the check function, which is also known as the pinball loss function and is defined as follows:

$$\rho_\tau(x) = \begin{cases} \tau x & \text{if } x \geq 0 \\ (\tau - 1)x & \text{if } x < 0 \end{cases} \tag{5}$$

2.3.2. Quantile Regression Neural Network

Given inputs $x_i(t)$ and an output $Y(t)$, the output from a QRNN is calculated as follows:

Consider a hidden-layer transfer function $h(\cdot)$; the output from the j-th hidden-layer node $g_j(t)$ is given by applying the hidden-layer transfer function to the inner product between $x_i(t)$ and hidden-layer weights $w_{ij}^{(h)}$ plus the hidden-layer bias $b_j{}^{(h)}$, which can be calculated as follows:

$$g_j(t) = h(\sum_{i=1}^{I} x_i(t) w_{ij}^{(h)} + b_j^{(h)}) \tag{6}$$

An estimate of the conditional τ-quantile $\hat{y}_\tau(t)$ is

$$\hat{Y}_\tau(t) = f(\sum_{j=1}^{J} g_j(t) w_j^{(o)} + b^{(o)}) \tag{7}$$

where $w_j^{(o)}$ are the output-layer weights, $b^{(o)}$ is the output-layer bias, and $f(\cdot)$ is the output-layer transfer function. The transfer function $h(\cdot)$ and $f(\cdot)$ are usually set as the hyperbolic tangent sigmoidal and linear function, respectively [36].

As an alternative method to prevent overfitting, weight delay regularization for the magnitude of the input-hidden layer weight can be applied by setting a penalty with a nonzero value.

2.4. Kernel Density Estimation (KDE)

Nonparametric density estimation is the process of fitting a parametric density model of a random variable without making the assumption that the density belongs to a particular parametric family [37,38]. Various methods have been proposed for nonparametric density estimation, e.g., k-nearest neighbors method, Parzen windows, histogram, and KDE [38]. In the domain of nonparametric density estimation, the K-nearest neighbors method has a very limited scope of practical applications due to its very poor performance. The Parzen windows method presents slightly better performance but also produces discontinuities (stair-like curves) that are quite annoying in practice [38]. A histogram is a simple form of the nonparametric density estimation. However, it suffers serious and noticeable drawbacks. First, the resulting visualization strongly depends on the choice of binning. Second, the natural feature of the histogram is discontinuity, which causes extreme difficulty if derivatives of the estimates are required.

Fortunately, those abovementioned drawbacks can be easily eliminated by using KDE [38,39]. In fact, KDE has been extensively studied and has become the most popular method in nonparametric density estimation. Given a random sample $Y_1, Y_2, \cdots, Y_m$, the value of the density at the point y estimated by the KDE method is given by the following:

$$\hat{f}(y,h) = \frac{1}{mh}\sum_{i=1}^{m} K(\frac{y-Y_i}{h}) \tag{8}$$

where h is the bandwidth with positive real value and $K(\cdot)$ is the kernel function. In this study, the most effective Epanechnikov kernel [38] was adopted and expressed as

$$K(y) = \frac{3}{4}(1-y^2)\mathbb{R}(|y| \leq 1) \tag{9}$$

where $\mathbb{R}(\cdot)$ is the indicator function, that is, $\mathbb{R}(y \in A) = 1$ for $y \in A$ and $\mathbb{R}(y \in A) = 0$ for $y \notin A$.

The selection of bandwidth parameter is a crucial issue in KDE. The bandwidth parameter influences the smoothness of the KDE curve and also determines the tradeoff between the bias and variance. In general, the smaller the bandwidth, the smaller the bias, and the larger the variance. A number of methods have been proposed to find the optimal bandwidth, such as Silverman's rule of thumb and the Sheather-Jones method. Silverman's rule of thumb bandwidth with a Gaussian kernel and Epanechnikov kernel can be computed as follows:

$$h^{optimal} \approx 1.06\hat{\sigma}n^{-\frac{1}{5}} \tag{10}$$

$$h^{optimal} \approx 2.34\hat{\sigma}n^{-\frac{1}{5}} \tag{11}$$

where $\hat{\sigma}$ is the estimation of σ (standard deviation of the input data) [38].

2.5. Ensemble Prediction Employing QRNNs and KDE

The proposed ensemble prediction employing QRNNs and KDE is shown in Figure 2. The QRNNs-KDE approach consists of four stages: (1) data splitting and normalization, (2) QRNN modelling, (3) probability density function (PDF) estimation by KDE, and (4) final ensemble prediction.

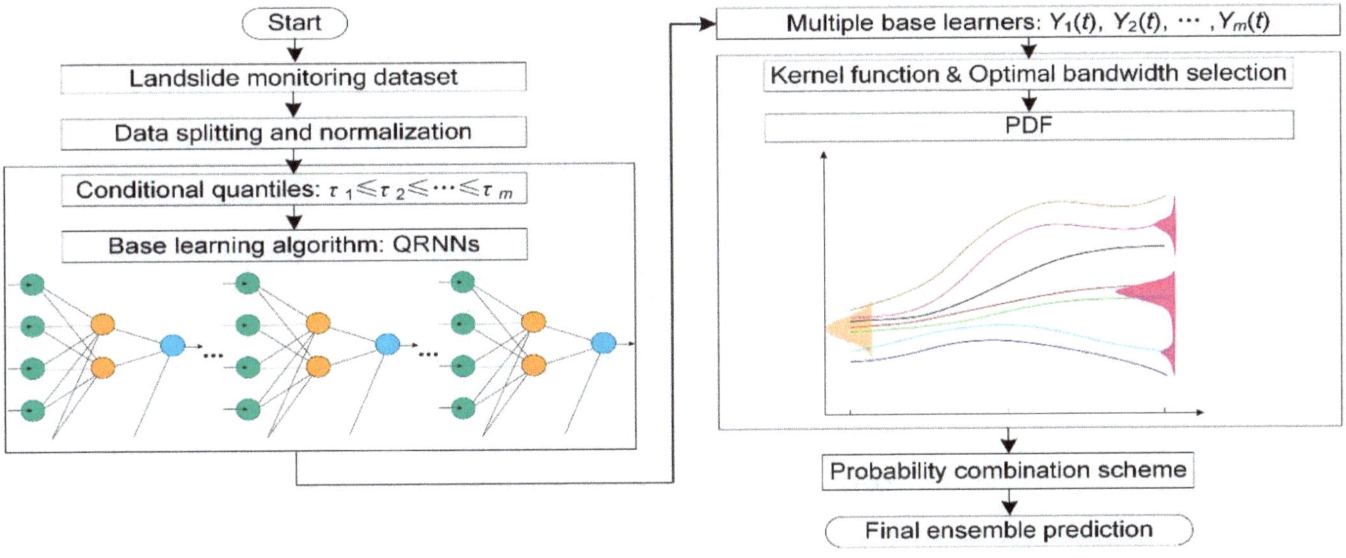

Figure 2. The overall flowchart of ensemble prediction based on the quantile regression neural networks and kernel density estimation (QRNNs-KDE) approach.

Data splitting and normalization: The original landslide monitoring dataset is divided into training data and testing data. The training data are used for model construction, and the testing data are used to evaluate the performance of the constructed model. To eliminate the influence of dimensional data, the training data and testing data are first normalized in the range of 0 to 1.

QRNNs modelling: QRNNs serve as base learning algorithms to generate multiple base learners $Y_1(t), Y_2(t), \cdots, Y_m(t)$ by applying a finite number of conditional quantities $\tau_1 \le \tau_2 \le \cdots \le \tau_m$ within the domain $0 < \tau < 1$, e.g., $\tau = 0.01, 0.02, \ldots, 0.98, 0.99$. The base learners of landslide displacement are obtained after renormalizing the outputs from the QRNNs approach. To avoiding overfitting in QRNNs modelling, a penalty parameter with nonzero value is applied.

PDF estimation by KDE: Multiple base learners from the QRNNs base model are treated as the input for KDE to estimate the probability density function (PDF) of the base learners. The kernel function and bandwidth influence the shape of the KDE curve. An appropriate kernel function and an optimal bandwidth should be chosen to best match the features of the original dataset.

Final ensemble prediction: In the present study, the final ensemble prediction was obtained through a probability combination scheme as follows:

$$u_t = \sum_{i=1}^{m} p_i(t) Y_i(t) \tag{12}$$

where $p_i(t)$ is the probability value of the i-th base learner and $Y_i(t)$ is obtained from the KDE for monitoring period t.

2.6. Evaluation Metrics and Uncertainty Quantification

In this study, five indices—coefficient of determination (R^2) MSE, RMSE, NRMSE, and MAPE—were applied to assess the performance of point prediction. R^2, MSE, RMSE, NRMSE, and MAPE are defined as

$$R^2 = \left[\frac{\sum_{t=1}^{N} (u_t - \overline{u})(\hat{u}_t - \overline{\hat{u}})}{\sqrt{\sum_{t=1}^{N} (u_t - \overline{u})^2 (\hat{u}_t - \overline{\hat{u}})^2}} \right]^2 \tag{13}$$

$$MSE = \frac{\sum_{t=1}^{N} (\hat{u}_t - u_t)^2}{N} \tag{14}$$

$$RMSE = \sqrt{\frac{\sum_{t=1}^{N} (\hat{u}_t - u_t)^2}{N}} \tag{15}$$

$$NRMSE = \sqrt{\frac{\sum_{t=1}^{N} (\hat{u}_t - u_t)^2}{\sum_{t=1}^{N} u_t{}^2}} \tag{16}$$

$$MAPE = \frac{1}{N} \left(\sum_{t=1}^{N} \left| \frac{\hat{u}_t - u_t}{u_t} \right| \right) \times 100\% \tag{17}$$

where $\hat{u}_t$ and u_t denote the t-th predictive value and observation, respectively, and $\overline{u}$ and $\overline{\hat{u}}$ denote the mean of the observation and the mean of the predictive value, respectively.

In the present study, the associated predictive uncertainties were quantified with PIs. After the above procedures, full PDFs of the future landslide displacement were achieved. An interval prediction with a $(1 - \alpha) \times 100\%$ confidence interval can be obtained from the $\alpha/2$ and $1 - \alpha/2$ quantiles of the obtained PDF. The α level, also called the significance level, ranges from 0 to 1 and is the probability of not capturing the value of the parameter. The predictive values of the $\alpha/2$ quantity and $1-\alpha/2$ quantity are set as the upper bound ($U_t^{1-\alpha}$) and lower bound ($L_t^{1-\alpha}$), respectively. For example, a 90% central PI can be obtained from the 0.05 and 0.95 quantiles of the PDF. The upper bound and lower bound of the 90% confidence level correspond to the predictive values of the 0.95 and 0.05 quantiles of the obtained PDF.

The prediction interval coverage probability (PICP), normalized mean PI width (NMPIW), and coverage width-based criterion (CWC) are three indices for evaluating the correctness of the approximated PIs. The PICP reflects the degree of reliability of PIs and is defined as

$$\text{PICP} = \frac{1}{N}\sum_{t=1}^{N} I_t^{1-\alpha} \tag{18}$$

where $I_t^{1-\alpha}$ is defined as follows:

$$I_t^{1-\alpha} = \begin{cases} 1 & u_t \in [L_t^{1-\alpha}, U_t^{1-\alpha}] \\ 0 & u_t \notin [L_t^{1-\alpha}, U_t^{1-\alpha}] \end{cases} \tag{19}$$

NMPIW measures the width of the PI; it is defined as

$$NMPIW = \frac{1}{N\varsigma}\sum_{t=1}^{N} (U_t^{1-\alpha} - L_t^{1-\alpha}) \tag{20}$$

where ς is the range of the underlying targets.

For high-quality PIs, narrow PIs (smaller NMPIW) with a high coverage probability (large PICP close to 100%) have great value [40,41]. Theoretically, NMPIW and PICP are conflicting. Therefore, CWC, which is a new balance criterion between PICP and NMPIW [42], is proposed to give a comprehensive assessment of PIs. CWC is defined as

$$CWC = (NMPIW + \psi)e^{\frac{\gamma(PICP-\mu)}{2\delta^2}} \tag{21}$$

where ψ is a small positive value within the range of (0.1%, 0.5%), μ corresponds to the nominal confidence level associated with PIs that is usually set to $1-\alpha$, and δ is a small positive value less than 1. γ is set to 1 during the training process; for testing, it is defined by the following step function:

$$\gamma = \begin{cases} 1, & PICP \geq \mu \\ 0, & PICP < \mu \end{cases} \tag{22}$$

3. Case Study: Fanjiaping Landslide

3.1. Features of the Fanjiaping Landslide

The Fanjiaping landslide is located on the southern bank of the Yangtze River and upstream of the Baishuihe landslide and downstream of the well-known Huangtupo landslide, which is approximately 56 km northwest of the Three Gorges Reservoir Dam (see Figure 3 for location). The Fanjiaping landslide is an ancient landslide [43,44] composed of two blocks: the Muyubao landslide and Fanjiaping landslide. The entire planar area of the landslide is approximately 1.96 million square meters, and the landslide volume is approximately 106 million cubic meters. The thickness of the Fanjiaping landslide ranges from 40 to 139.16 m. The Muyubao landslide is approximately 1500 m long and 1200 m wide. The average thickness of the Muyubao landslide body is approximately 50 m, and its estimated volume is 90 million m^3.

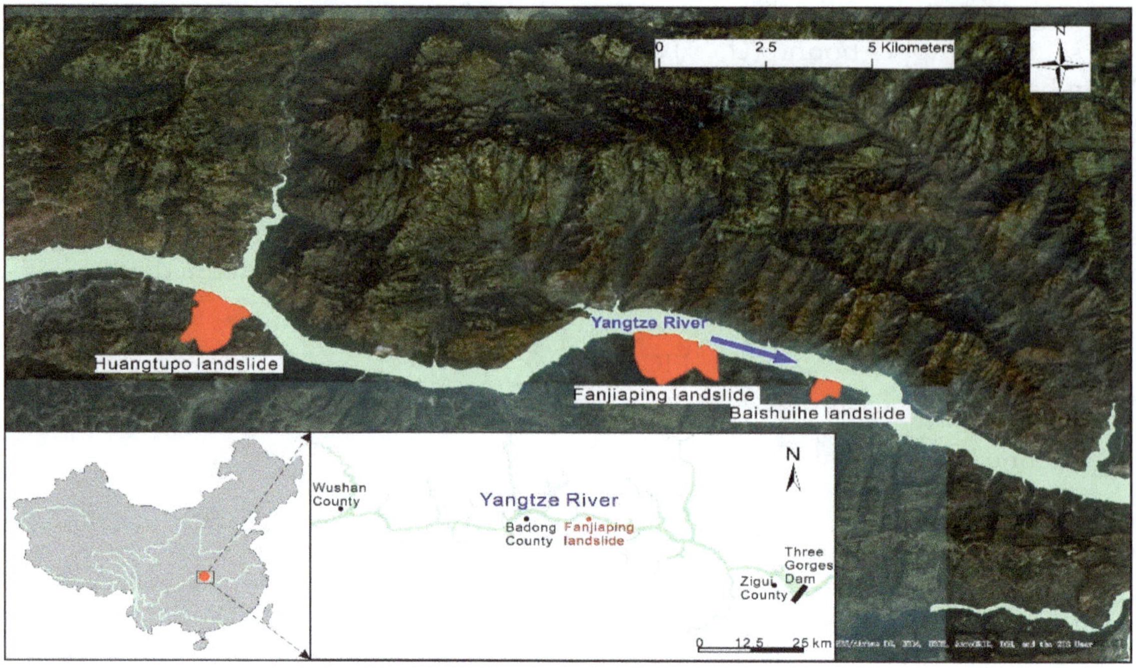

Figure 3. Location of the landslide site.

The Muyubao landslide extends from an elevation of 100 m at the toe to 520 m at the crown (Figure 4a,b). The slope surface consists of alternating gentle and comparatively steep landforms. The sliding direction of the landslide is 20°. The Tanjiahe landslide, located on the downstream of the Muyubao landslide, is approximately 1000 m long and 400 m wide. The average thickness of the Tanjiahe landslide body is approximately 40 m, and its estimated volume is 16 million m^3. The Tanjiahe landslide extends from an elevation of 135 m at the toe to 420 m at the crown (Figure 4c,d). The slope surface consists of alternating gentle and comparatively steep landforms. The sliding direction of the landslide is 345°.

The site-specific investigation shows that the landslide materials are arranged in two different layers: a colluvial deposit at the upper surface and highly disturbed sandstone at the lower surface. The cataclastic sandstone is underlaid by sandstone and mudstone of the Jurassic Xiangxi formation (J1x) with an average dip direction of 10–25° and a dip angle of 27–36° (Figure 4b,d). Soft coal layers are prevalent in the J1x formation, and many landslides have developed along the soft coal layers. The borehole data indicates that the landslide mass of the Muyubao and Tanjiahe landslide slide along a soft coal layer with a thickness ranging from 0.1 to 0.3 m. According to laboratory testing of sliding zone soil obtained from the borehole, the natural moisture content of the soil is 12.6%, and the natural density is 1.9 g/cm^3.

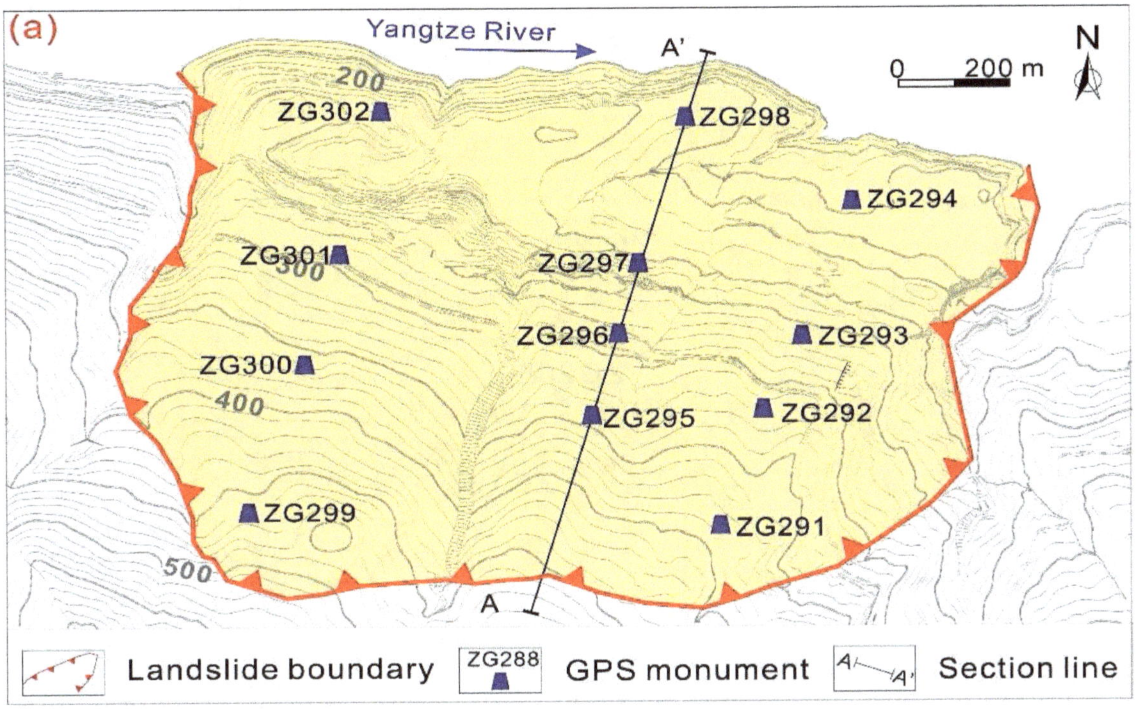

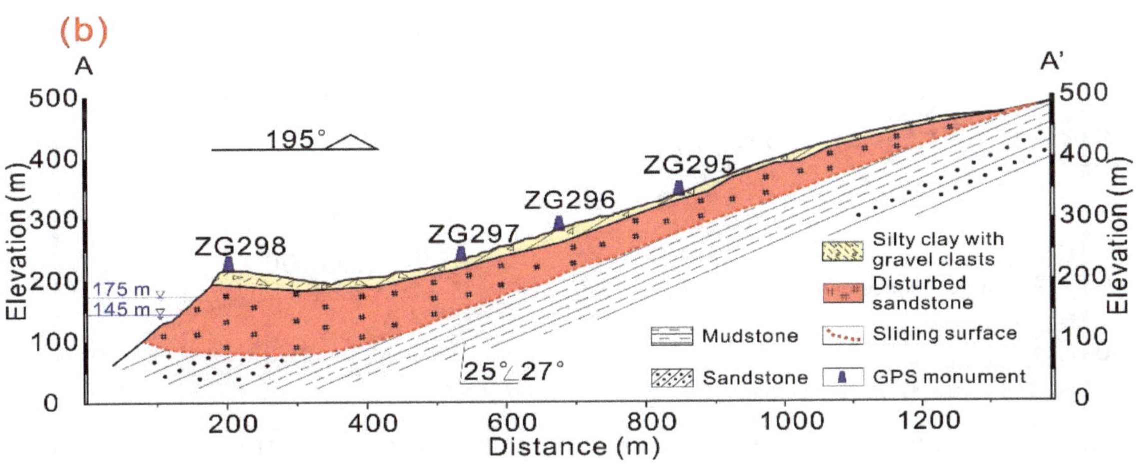

Figure 4. *Cont.*

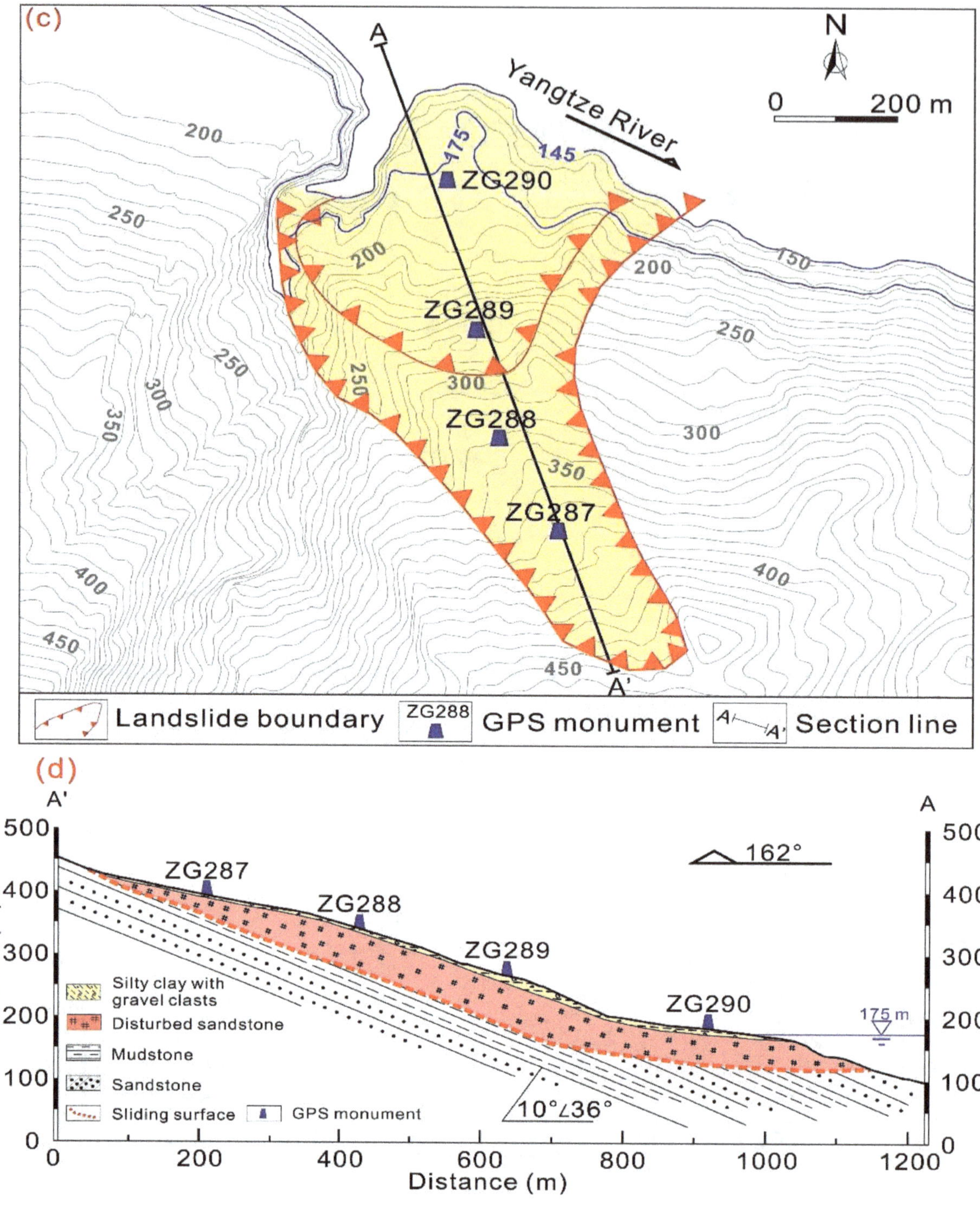

Figure 4. Topographic map and geological profile of the Fanjiaping landslide. (**a**) Topographic map of the Muyubao landslide. (**b**) Geological profile of the Muyubao landslide along sections A-A′, as recorded with monitoring instruments. (**c**) Topographic map of the Tanjiahe landslide. (**d**) Geological profile of the Tanjiahe landslide along sections B-B′, as recorded with monitoring instruments.

3.2. Input Data

A total of sixteen GPS beacons were installed on the landslide mass to monitor the landslide movements in September 2006 (see Figure 4 for the GPS locations): four on the Tanjiahe landslide and twelve on the Muyubao landslide. The GPS monuments were manually surveyed once a month. In April 2016, four GPS monitoring points, ZG295, ZG296, ZG297, and ZG298, were updated to near real-time monitoring. At most, thirteen years' worth of monitoring data were obtained. Figure 5 shows the monthly rainfall intensity obtained from the Shazhenxi Meteorological Station near the Fanjiaping landslide, the reservoir water level, and the displacement from GPS survey monuments over the thirteen-year period from October 2006 to March 2018. The available data indicate that the landslide was unstable and continuously deforming during the entire monitoring period. The landslide exhibits a step-like deformation behavior because of the periodic fluctuations in the reservoir water level and heavy precipitation. The monitoring data from both Muyubao and Tanjiahe show that larger displacements occurred in the upper middle part of the landslide mass. From the sequence of the surface cracks and displacement magnitude, we speculate that the movement occurred first at the rear part and progressed downslope. Based on a previous study on the relations between slip-surface geometry, material structures, and deformational structures [45,46], the observed kinematic behaviors are expected independent of the characteristics of the landslide material. However, more work is needed to confirm these findings.

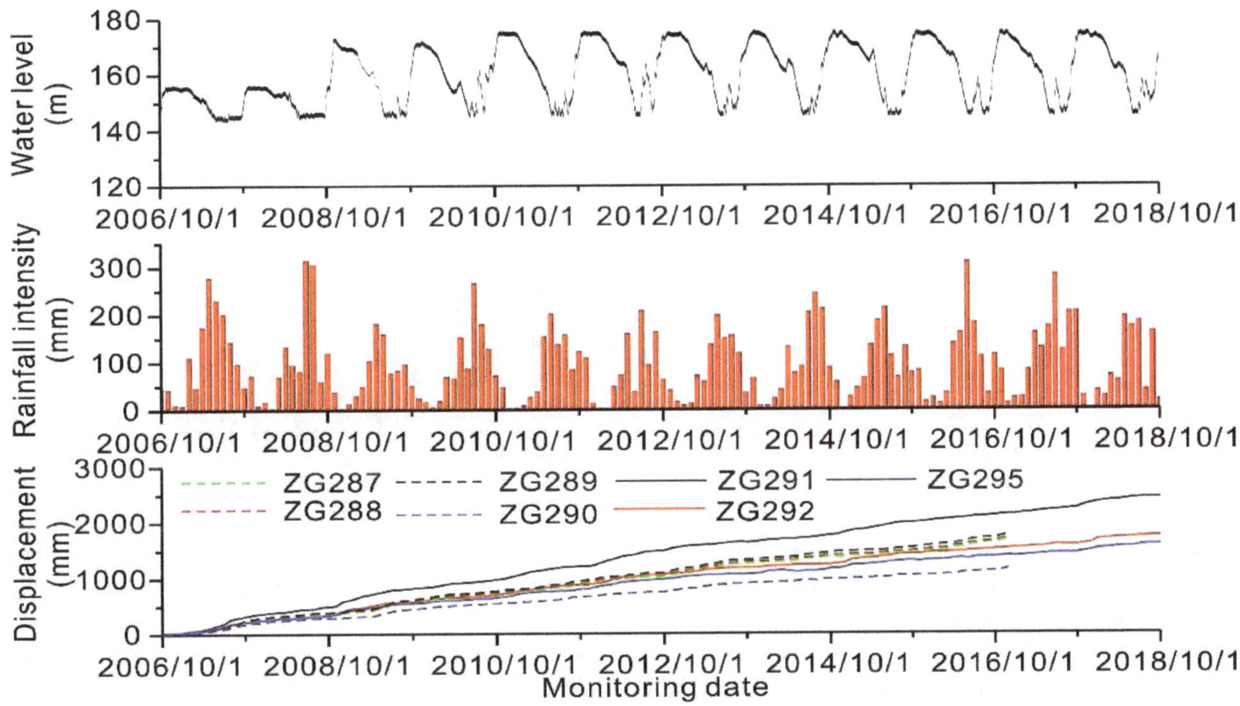

Figure 5. Reservoir water level, monthly rainfall intensity, and cumulative displacement from the Fanjiaping landslide area.

3.3. *Triggering Factors of the Landslide Movements*

Although the Fanjiaping landslide is one of the largest landslides in the TGRA, very few publications have reported detailed information on the triggering factors of the landslide movements. Fully understanding the triggering factors is critical for landslide mitigation and early warning. In this study, long-term and near real-time monitoring data were used to comprehensively analyze the landslide movements. The cumulative displacement at monitoring point ZG295, monthly rainfall intensity, and reservoir water levels in 2009, 2011, 2012, 2015 are shown in Figure 6a–d. The available data shows the following trends:

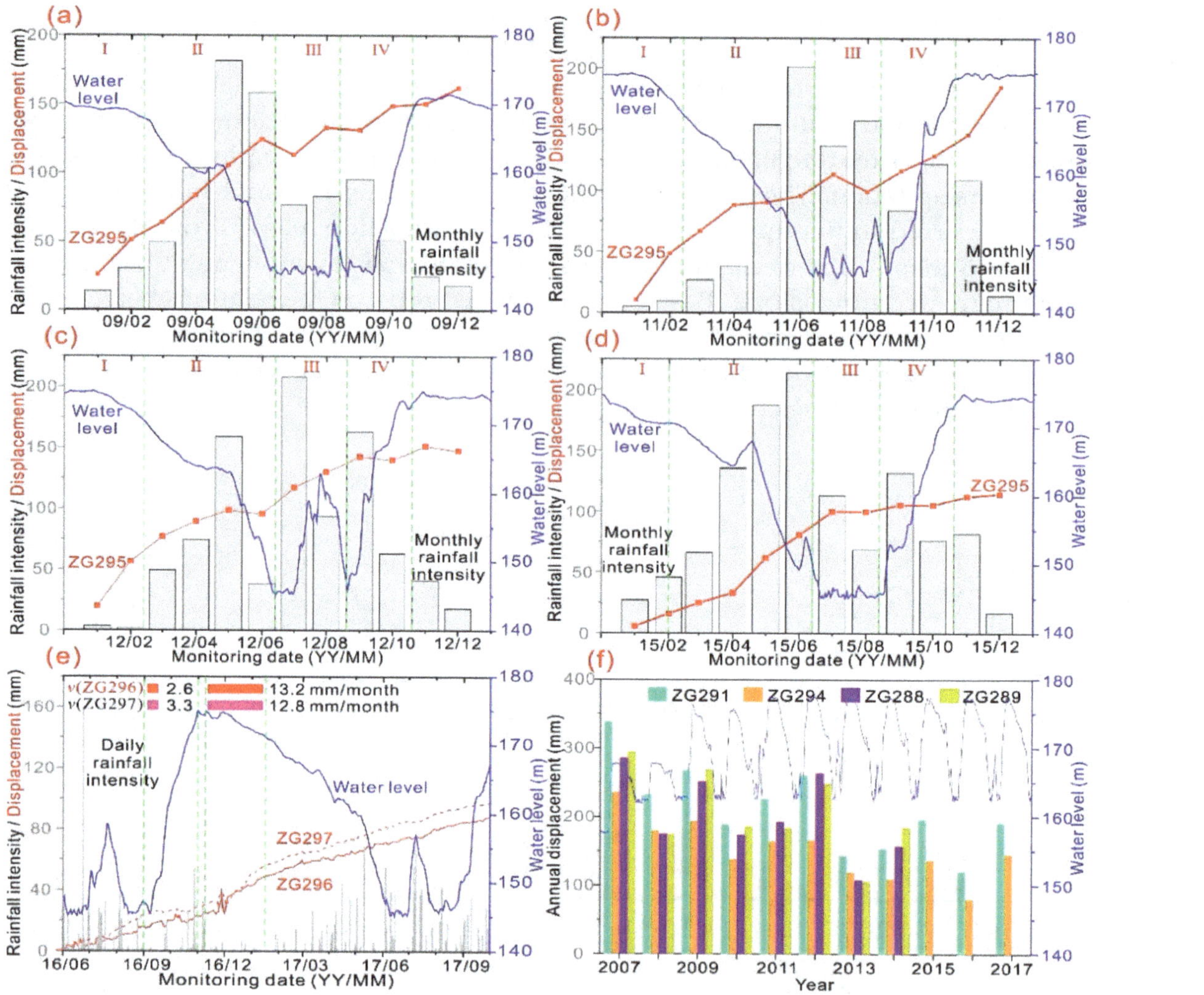

Figure 6. (**a–d**) Cumulative displacement at monitoring point ZG295, monthly rainfall intensity, and reservoir water level spanning the period of 2009, 2011, 2012, and 2015. (**e**) Cumulative displacement at monitoring points ZG296 and ZG297, daily rainfall intensity, and reservoir water level spanning the period of June 2016 to October 2017. (**f**) Annual displacement at monitoring point ZG291, ZG294, ZG288, and ZG289, and reservoir water level spanning the period of 2007 to 2017.

(1) When the reservoir water level first rose from 135 to 156 m at the end of 2006, a significant annual displacement of 330 mm occurred at monitoring point ZG291 in 2007. Similarly, an annual displacement of 260 mm occurred at monitoring point ZG291 in 2009 when the reservoir water level rose from 156 to 172 m at the end of 2008. After 2009, the annual displacements shows a decreasing trend (Figure 6f). The results of the above analysis suggest that landslide deformation occurred at the preliminary operation phase, and more significant movement is likely to occur when the reservoir water level reaches a new higher level.

(2) A large deformation occurred when the reservoir water level slightly dropped from 175 m to 170 m in November to February (I in Figure 6). During 2009 to 2015, the monthly deformation rate during this drawdown period was greater than 20 mm per month (Figure 6a–d). For example, when the reservoir water level dropped from 174 m to 172.21 m in January 2012 to February 2012, the displacements measured at monitoring points ZG295, ZG296, ZG297, and ZG298 were 38.98, 26.39, 35.12, and 41.78 mm, respectively (Figure 6c). However, when the reservoir water level significantly dropped from 170 m to 145 m in February to June (II in Figure 6), the monthly deformation rate decreased to less than 20 mm per month.

(3) When the reservoir level remained at 145 m in July to September (III in Figure 6) and the landslide area suffered a heavy rainfall event, the landslide deformation was likely to be suspended except for 2012. The maximum monthly rainfall intensity during those suspended activities was 158 mm. In July 2012, the landslide area suffered from a heavy rainfall event with a monthly rainfall intensity of 208 mm, and the monitoring point deformed at a high rate. From those comparative analyses, we can speculate than the minimum triggering threshold consists of episodes lasting one month with cumulative rainfall exceeding 158 mm.

(4) When the reservoir rose from 145 m to 175 m in September to November (IV in Figure 6), monthly deformation rate decreased to a small positive (less than 10 mm per month) or even negative value.

(5) The near real-time monitoring data also showed the abovementioned trends: when the reservoir water level rose from 147.25 to 174.42 m on August 31 2016 to October 27 2016, the monthly deformation rates for ZG296 and ZG297 were 2.6 and 3.3 mm/month, respectively. When the reservoir dropped from 174.45 to 171.18 m on November 9 2016 to January 16 2017, deformations of 24.07 and 26.46 mm occurred at ZG296 and ZG297, respectively. The corresponding monthly deformation rates were 12.8 and 13.2 mm/month, respectively.

From the above analysis we can conclude that landslide movement was especially pronounced under prolonged periods of dropping reservoir levels, especially during periods of slight dropdown at the highest reservoir level, and the minimum triggering threshold consisted of episodes lasting one month, with cumulative rainfall exceeding 158 mm.

3.4. *QRNNs-KDE-Based Method for Ensemble Prediction*

3.4.1. Data Splitting and Normalization

The available data (Figure 5) indicate that for the two active blocks, the largest displacements were observed at monitoring points ZG289 and ZG291, respectively. Therefore, monitoring points ZG289 and ZG291 were selected to establish a prediction model for the Fanjiaping landslide.

Previous correlation analysis in [3] revealed that weak to very strong correlations exist between landslide displacement and triggering and state variables. Therefore, based on triggering factor analysis and previous work on correlation analysis in [3], seven variables including four trigger variables and three state variables were selected as the inputs: rainfall intensity over the past month ($x_1(t)$), rainfall intensity over the past two months ($x_2(t)$), average reservoir water level in the current month ($x_3(t)$), variation in the reservoir water level in the current month ($x_4(t)$), displacement over the past one month ($x_5(t)$), displacement over the past two months ($x_6(t)$), and displacement over the past three months ($x_7(t)$). In addition, the displacement in the current month ($Y(t)$) was selected as the output. A data set $(x_i(t), Y(t)), i = 1, 2, \cdots, 7$ was generated based on the inputs and corresponding outputs. For the Tanjiahe landslide, the data from October 2006 to January 2015 with a size of 100 were treated as the training set, and the data from February 2015 to June 2015 with a size of 5 were used as the testing set. For the Muyubao landslide, the data from October 2006 to January 2015 with a size of 133 were treated as the training set, and the data from November 2017 to October 2018 with a size of 12 were used as the testing set.

3.4.2. QRNN Modelling

Two nonlinear models with a sigmoidal transfer function and linear transfer function for $\tau = 0.01$, 0.02, ... , 0.98, 0.99 with an interval of 0.01 were trained for monitoring points ZG289 and ZG291 to generate multiple base learners. The number of hidden nodes in the QRNNs model was set to 5. The penalty for weight delay regularization was set to 1 to prevent overfitting in QRNNs model construction. For each monitoring period, a total of 99 base learners were obtained at conditional quantities ranging from 0.01 to 0.99 based on the QRNNs. The main parameters applied in the modelling of QRNNs are shown in Table 1.

Table 1. The parameters utilized in the QRNNs modeling for the Fanjiaping landslide.

Parameter	Value	Parameter	Value
Maximum number of iterations	5000	Penalty for weight decay regularization	1
Number of quantiles	99	Number of input nodes	7
Number of repeated trials	5	Number of hidden nodes	5

3.4.3. PDF Estimation by KDE

The multiple base learners from QRNNs were employed as inputs of Epanechnikov KDE to estimate the PDF. The optimal bandwidths for PDF estimation were calculated based on Silverman's rule of thumb. The optimal bandwidths for PDF estimation of testing data at ZG289 were set to 7.98, 8.05, 5.66, 7.05, and 9.26. The optimal bandwidths for PDF estimation of testing data at ZG291 were set to 5.28, 8.61, 7.77, 5.62, and 5.30.

3.4.4. Final Ensemble Prediction

Final ensemble predictions for the Fanjiaping landslide were generated through a probability combination scheme. PIs were constructed from the obtained PDF to estimate the predictive uncertainty. For the purpose of aiding decision-making, it is preferable to have prediction information with high confidence levels to reduce risks. Therefore, PIs at a high PINC value of 90% were obtained and analyzed in the study.

4. Results

PDFs: The PDFs of predictive displacement at ZG289 and ZG291 constructed by the proposed QRNNs-KDE approach are shown in Figures 7 and 8. The fast movement is the main concern in landslide displacement prediction. Here, only a portion of the prediction describing the fast landslide is selected and shown. Figures 7 and 8 show that rather than a single estimate, the range and complete PDF of the predictive displacement are provided by the proposed approach. All landslide displacement observations are distributed in the middle of the PDFs with high probability in addition to the observations of May and June at ZG289, which appear at the tail of the probability density curve. The small fraction falling into the right tail follows the increase in the prediction period; here, there are more uncertainties associated with longer-term landslide predictions.

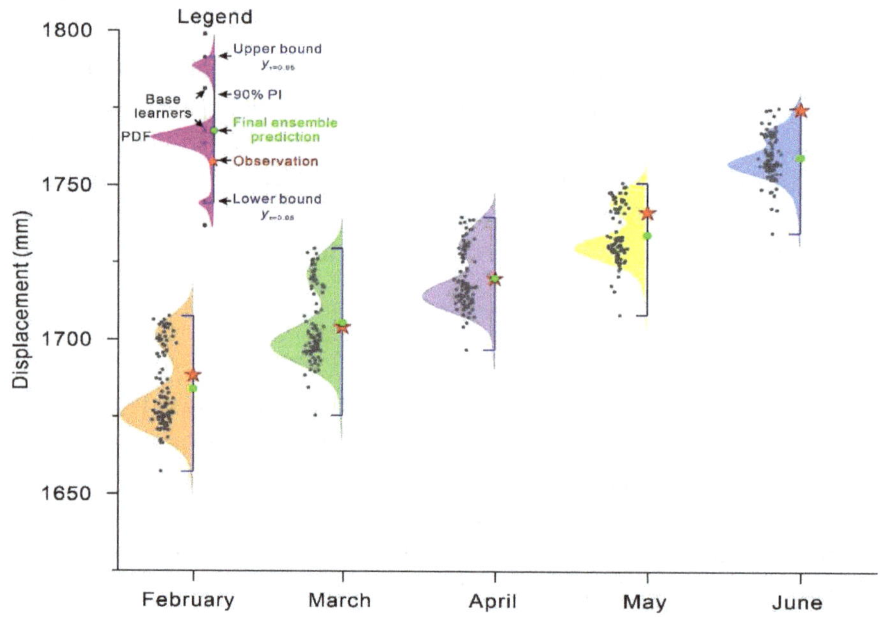

Figure 7. Probability density functions (PDFs) for the Fanjiaping landslide at ZG289 from February 2015 to June 2015.

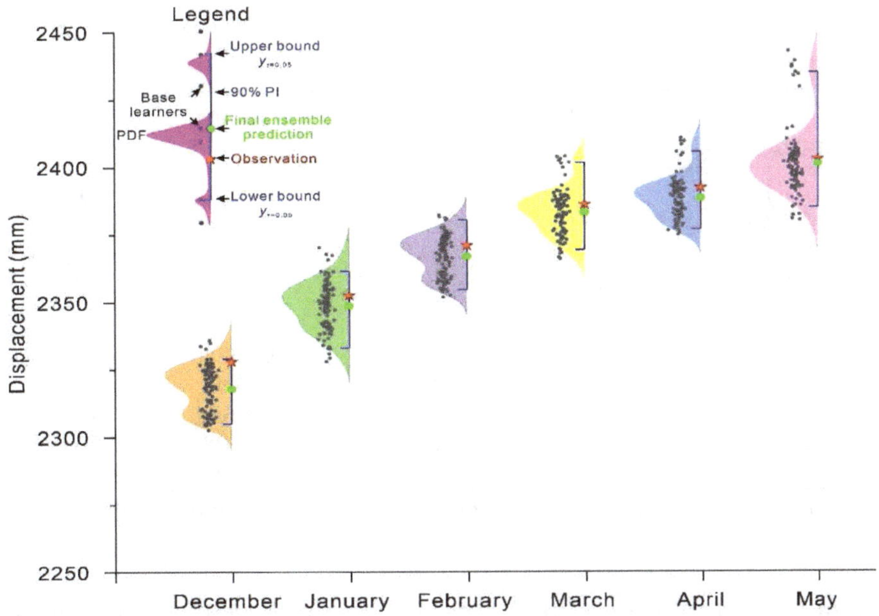

Figure 8. PDFs for the Fanjiaping landslide at ZG291 from December 2017 to May 2018.

Final ensemble prediction: Figure 9 shows the final ensemble predictions. As shown in Figure 9, the ensemble predictions obtained via the probability combination scheme showed a high degree of consistency in the landslide displacement observations, with coefficient of determination values of 0.999932 and 0.999944. To further evaluate the prediction performances of ensemble prediction based on the QRNNs-KDE, the evaluation metrics of the BP, RBF, ELM, and SVM approaches are shown in Table 2. As shown in Table 2, the final ensemble predictions using the QRNNs-KDE approach outperformed the persistence methods with the smallest MSE, RMSE, NRMSE, and MAPE and the largest R^2. Moreover, compared with predictions at monitoring point ZG289 using the Copula-KSVMQR approach in [3], the QRNNs-KDE approach provided more accurate prediction with smaller MAPE and RMSE.

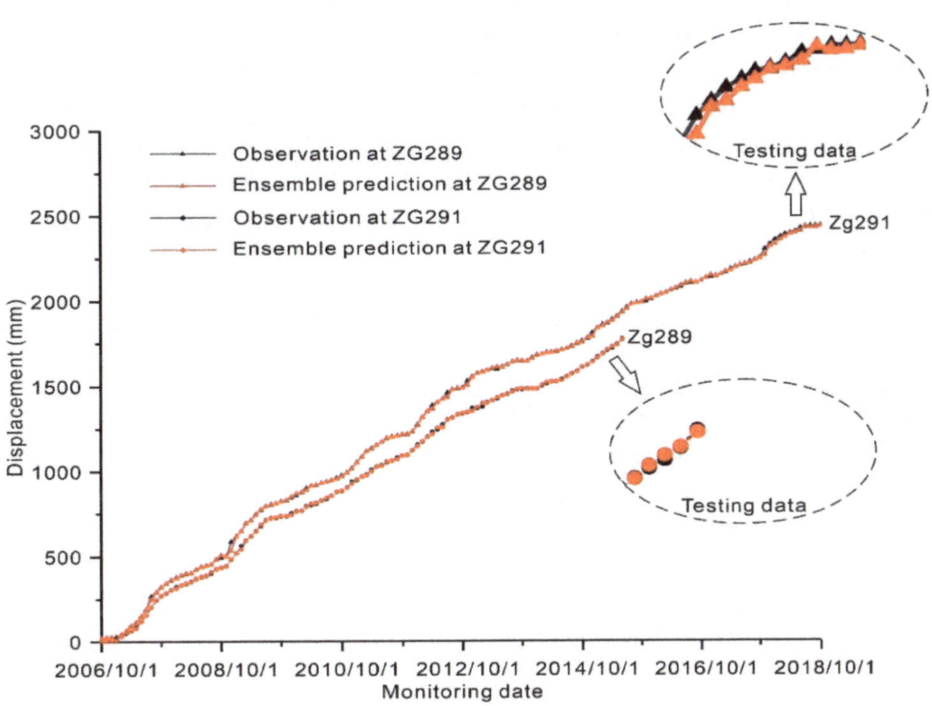

Figure 9. Comparisons of the final ensemble predictions and observations for the Fanjiaping landslide at ZG289 and ZG291.

Table 2. Comparisons of predictions obtained from QRNNs-KDE, BP, RBF, ELM, and SVM for the Fanjiaping landslide.

Monitoring Point	Model / Index	BP	RBF	ELM	SVM	QRNNs-KDE
ZG289	R^2	0.99730	0.99992	0.99785	0.99993	***0.99997***
	MSE	3192.07	99.54	2538.74	78.12	***30.69***
	RMSE	56.50	9.98	50.39	8.84	***5.54***
	NRMSE	0.032263	0.005697	0.028772	0.005047	***0.003163***
	MAPE	2.74	2.00	1.57	1.27	***1.17***
ZG291	R^2	0.99991	0.99759	0.99991	0.99995	***0.99997***
	MSE	206.32	5684.98	215.41	119.75	***70.15***
	RMSE	14.36	75.40	14.68	10.94	***8.38***
	NRMSE	0.005953	0.031251	0.006083	0.004536	***0.003471***
	MAPE	3.97	1.96	2.59	2.33	***0.41***

Note: The most accurate prediction results are shown in bold italics.

Uncertainty quantification: Based on the PDFs shown in Figures 7 and 8, PIs at a high confidence level (90%) were constructed for ZG289 and ZG291 (Figure 10a,c, respectively). To evaluate the prediction performances based on the QRNNs-KDE approach, 90% PIs were constructed based on the bootstrap-ELM-ANN approach (Figure 10b,d). The corresponding evaluation metrics are shown in Table 3. As shown in Figure 10 and Table 3, the constructed PIs based on the QRNNs-KDE approach perfectly covered the observations with a high percentage, and the QRNNs-KDE approach outperformed the bootstrap-ELM-ANN approach with smaller NMPIW and CWC. For example, the performance indices NPIW and CWC of 90% PIs at ZG289 were 0.0215 and 0.1661, respectively, which were lower than those obtained using the bootstrap-ELM-ANN approach. The normalized mean PI width using the QRNNs-KDE approach was approximately 90% narrower than that for the bootstrap-ELM-ANN approach.

The experimental results show that the final ensemble predictions based on the QRNNs-KDE approach outperformed the traditional BP, RBF, ELM, SVM, and Copula-KSVMQR algorithms with regard to deterministic point prediction. The QRNNs-KDE approach was more informative than traditional algorithms because it provided the likely range of landslide displacement. The landslide observations were distributed in the middle of the prediction range with high probability. Moreover, regarding the aspect of uncertainty quantification, the QRNNs-KDE provided more satisfactory PIs than the bootstrap-ELM-ANN approach. Therefore, we believe that the final ensemble predictions based on the QRNNs-KDE approach have the advantages of accurate prediction and uncertainty quantification of landslide displacement.

Table 3. Comparisons of 90% PIs obtained from Bootstrap-ELM-ANN and QRNNs-KDE for the Fanjiaping landslide.

Monitoring Point	Index / Model	PICP	NPIW	CWC
ZG289	Bootstrap-ELM-ANN	100%	0.27	0.2071
	QRNNs-KDE	***100%***	***0.0215***	***0.1661***
ZG291	Bootstrap-ELM-ANN	99%	0.024	0.143
	QRNNs-KDE	***99%***	***0.018***	***0.085***

Note: The prediction results with a narrower PI range are shown in bold italics.

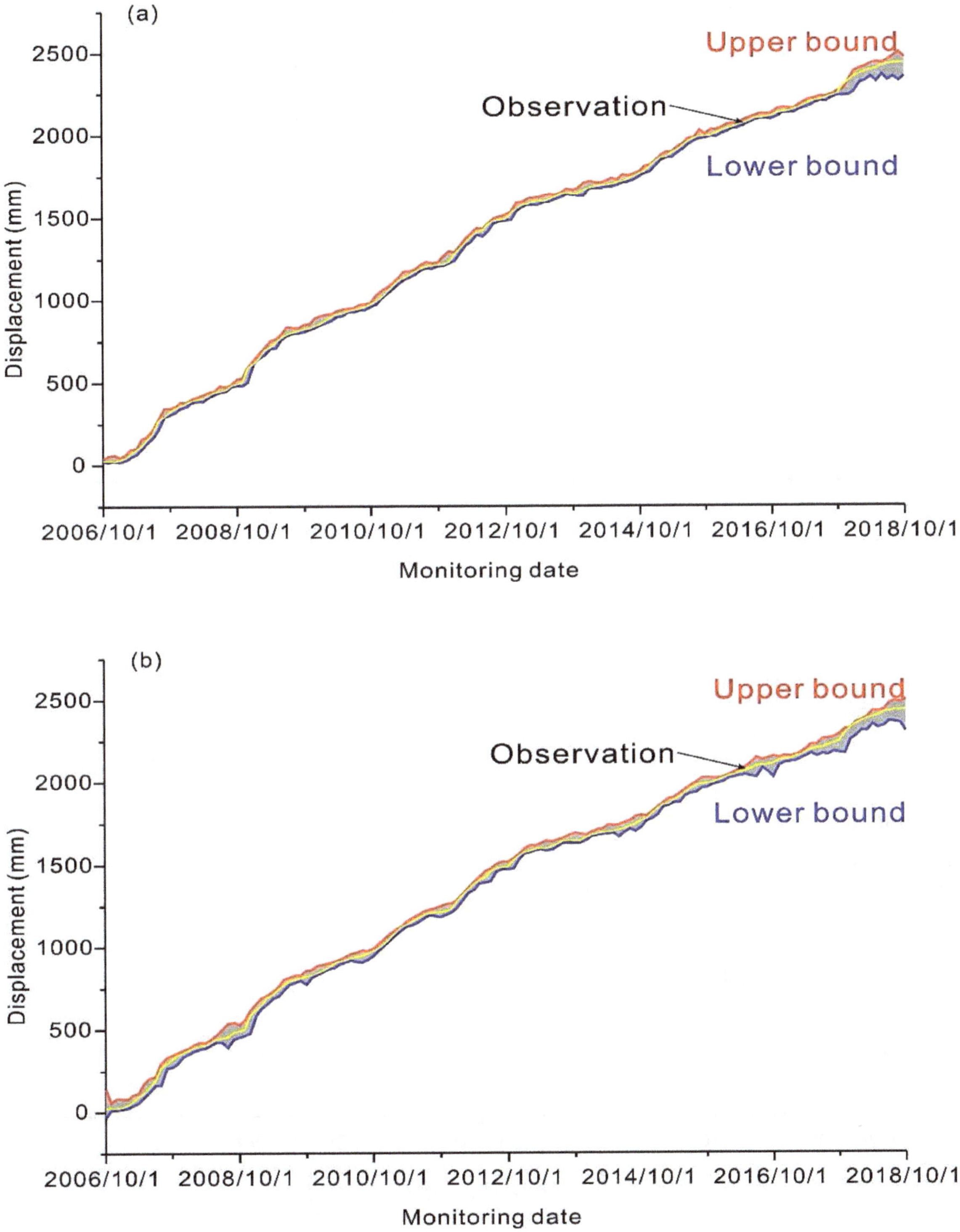

Figure 10. *Cont.*

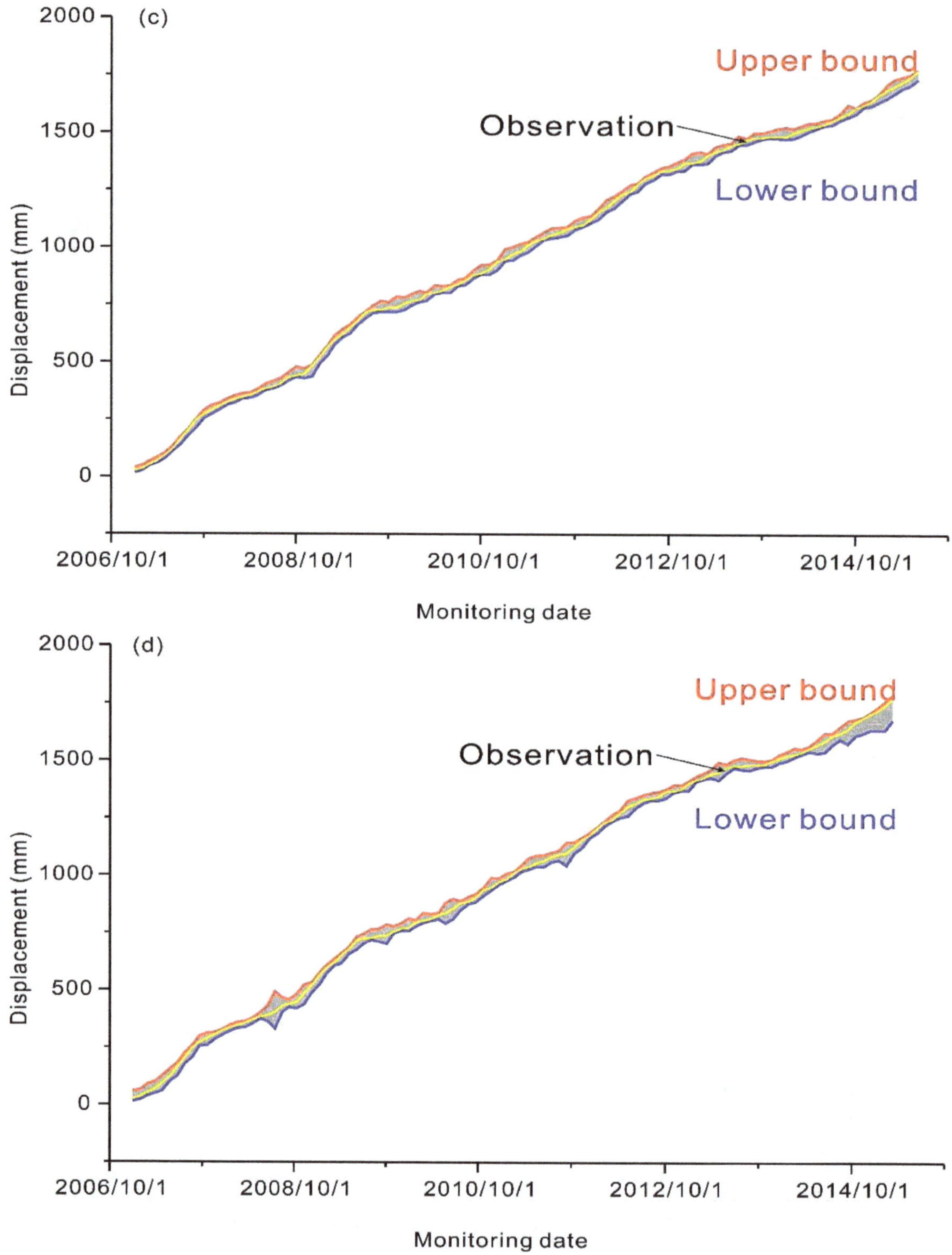

Figure 10. Comparisons of the observations and the constructed PIs at a 90% confidence level for the Fanjiaping landslide at ZG289 and ZG291 using QRNNs-KDE and bootstrap-ELM-ANN. (**a**) 90% PIs at ZG291 using QRNNs-KDE; (**b**) 90% PIs at ZG291 using bootstrap-ELM-ANN; (**c**) 90% PIs at ZG289 using QRNNs-KDE, (**d**) 90% PIs at ZG289 using bootstrap-ELM-ANN.

5. Discussion

In this study, with regard to point prediction, the probability-scheme combination ensemble prediction, which employs QRNNs-KDE, provided the best prediction. The fundamental reasons behind this can be explained from statistical, computational, and representational perspectives [47].

From a statistical perspective, the available training data set may not be able to provide sufficient information for training the true model (h^* in Figure 11). Constructing an ensemble model (h' in Figure 11) might not be better than the single best prediction model h^*, but it does reduce the risk of choosing a bad learner with poor generalizability (schematic in Figure 11a). From a computational perspective, in a single model the training algorithms might get stuck in lock optima by only performing a local search. Constructing an ensemble model by searching from different starting positions might be a better alternative (schematic in Figure 11b). From a representational perspective, it is possible that the searched hypothesis space might not contain the true model h^*. Constructing an ensemble model might expand the representable space (schematic in Figure 11c).

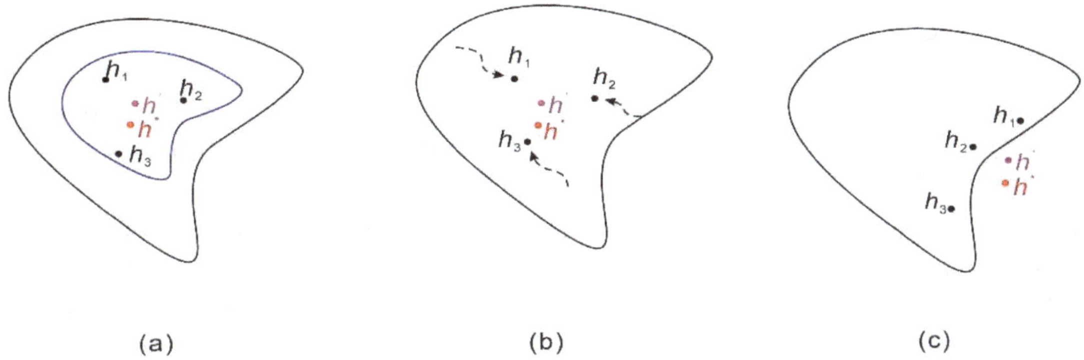

Figure 11. Schematic that shows the fundamental benefits of the ensemble prediction model from statistical (**a**), computational (**b**), and representational (**c**) perspectives. h^* is the true prediction model; h_1, h_2, and h_3 are single prediction models; and h' is the ensemble prediction model obtained by combining the single prediction models h_1, h_2, and h_3. The outer black curve is the hypothesis space of all possible models. The inner blue curve denotes the subset of hypotheses that give reasonable accuracy with the available training data (modified from [47]).

In the proposed QRNNs-KDE approach, the probability combination scheme is employed to combine 99 base learners into one final ensemble to improve the model performance. However, a concern about computational time may be associated with this ensemble strategy. The required computational time is highly related to the number of base learners. For the case of ZG 291, the required computation time is 191.85 s to train 99 base learners in RStudio Version 1.2.5042 on an Intel(R) Xeon(R) E-2176M @ 2.70 GHz CPU with 64 GB RAM. Thus, we believe that the proposed approach is computationally efficient.

Nevertheless, the probability-scheme combination ensemble prediction, which employ QRNNs and KDE, also holds inherent limitations associated with data-driven models, such as the lack of an explicit input-output relationship, and the requirement of large training data to maintain the model performance.

In practical applications, the main motivation for the construction of predictive range and complete PDF is to quantify the likely predictive uncertainty in the deterministic point predictions. Availability of range and complete PDF of the predictive displacement allows the researchers and practitioners to efficiently quantify the level of predictive uncertainty with the deterministic point predictions and to consider a multiple of solutions/scenarios for the best and worst conditions. Wide ranges are an indication of presence of a high level of uncertainty in the operation. This information can guide the researchers and practitioners to avoid the selection of risky actions under uncertain conditions. In contrast, narrow range means that decisions can be made more confidently with less chance of confronting an unexpected condition in the future, for example, if a sharp displacement increment with a wider range was predicted for the further. An alert should be carefully determined whether reaching tertiary creep stage by researchers and practitioners through comprehensive analysis. Under this circumstance, time-of-failure forecasting should be run in parallel, and a multiple of solutions/scenarios should be considered until either failure precursors are identified or the movements suspended.

The proposed QRNNs-KDE approach is suitable for medium-term to long-term horizon forecasting. Results from previous studies [2,48] have shown that the performance of data-driven models varies for landslides with different deformation behaviors. Usually, for landslides with drastic step-like deformation, the prediction accuracy is lower, and the corresponding prediction error is larger. Therefore, in practical applications of medium-term to long-term horizon forecasting, when predicting landslides with drastic deformation, the proposed QRNNs-KDE approach should be applied with caution. To achieve excellent performance, sufficient data are recommended and needed for model training.

6. Conclusions

In this study, a QRNNs-KDE approach was proposed to improve the prediction accuracy and uncertainty quantification of landslide displacement. The Fanjiaping landslide in the TGRA was selected as a case study to explore the performance of the QRNNs-KDE approach. The following conclusions from the study were obtained:

The movements of the Fanjiaping landslide was especially pronounced under prolonged periods of dropping reservoir levels, especially during periods of slight dropdown at the highest reservoir level, and the minimum triggering threshold consists of episodes lasting one month, with cumulative rainfall exceeding 158 mm.

The QRNNs-KDE approach achieves perfect performance and outperforms the traditional BP, RBF, ELM, SVM, bootstrap-ELM-ANN, and Copula-KSVMQR methods. Additionally, the proposed approach is more informative by providing the likely range and complete PDFs of landslide displacement. The landslide displacement observations are distributed in the middle of the prediction range with high probability.

In practical application, the proposed QRNNs-KDE approach is suitable for medium-term to long-term horizon forecasting. The range and complete PDF of the predictive displacement can supplement final point predictions for decision making.

Author Contributions: The work was carried out in collaboration between all the authors. J.M. and X.L. guided and supervised this research; X.N., Y.W., T.W., J.Z., and Z.Z. performed the field investigation; J.M. wrote the original draft; and J.M. and X.L. reviewed and edited the draft. All authors have contributed to, seen, and approved the manuscript. All authors have read and agreed to the published version of the manuscript.

References

1. CRED. EM-DAT: International Disaster Database. Available online: https://public.emdat.be/data (accessed on 9 June 2020).
2. Wang, Y.; Tang, H.; Wen, T.; Ma, J. Direct Interval Prediction of Landslide Displacements Using Least Squares Support Vector Machines. *Complexity* **2020**, *2020*, 7082594. [CrossRef]
3. Ma, J.W.; Niu, X.X.; Tang, H.M.; Wang, Y.K.; Wen, T.; Zhang, J.R. Displacement Prediction of a Complex Landslide in the Three Gorges Reservoir Area (China) Using a Hybrid Computational Intelligence Approach. *Complexity* **2020**, *2020*, 2624547. [CrossRef]
4. Ma, J.W.; Tang, H.M.; Liu, X.; Wen, T.; Zhang, J.R.; Tan, Q.W.; Fan, Z.Q. Probabilistic forecasting of landslide displacement accounting for epistemic uncertainty: A case study in the Three Gorges Reservoir area, China. *Landslides* **2018**, *15*, 1145–1153. [CrossRef]
5. Pinto, F.; Guerriero, L.; Revellino, P.; Grelle, G.; Senatore, M.R.; Guadagno, F.M. Structural and lithostratigraphic controls of earth-flow evolution, Montaguto earth flow, Southern Italy. *J. Geol. Soc. Lond.* **2016**, *173*, 649. [CrossRef]

6. Guerriero, L.; Diodato, N.; Fiorillo, F.; Revellino, P.; Grelle, G.; Guadagno, F.M. Reconstruction of long-term earth-flow activity using a hydroclimatological model. *Nat. Hazards* **2015**, *77*, 1–15. [CrossRef]
7. Hu, X.; Bürgmann, R.; Schulz, W.H.; Fielding, E.J. Four-dimensional surface motions of the Slumgullion landslide and quantification of hydrometeorological forcing. *Nat. Commun.* **2020**, *11*, 2792. [CrossRef]
8. Ma, J.W.; Tang, H.M.; Hu, X.L.; Bobet, A.; Zhang, M.; Zhu, T.W.; Song, Y.J.; Ez Eldin, M.A.M. Identification of causal factors for the Majiagou landslide using modern data mining methods. *Landslides* **2017**, *14*, 311–322. [CrossRef]
9. Corominas, J.; Moya, J.; Ledesma, A.; Lloret, A.; Gili, J.A. Prediction of ground displacements and velocities from groundwater level changes at the Vallcebre landslide (Eastern Pyrenees, Spain). *Landslides* **2005**, *2*, 83–96. [CrossRef]
10. Li, S.H.; Wu, L.Z.; Chen, J.J.; Huang, R.Q. Multiple data-driven approach for predicting landslide deformation. *Landslides* **2020**, *17*, 709–718. [CrossRef]
11. Saito, M. Forecasting the time of occurrence of a slope failure. In Proceedings of the 6th International Congress of Soil Mechanics and Foundation Engineering, Montreal, QC, Canada, 8–15 September 1965; pp. 537–541.
12. Hayashi, S.; Komamura, F.; Park, B.W.; Yamamori, T. On the forecast of time to failure of slope-Approximate forecast in the early period of the tertiary creep. *J. Jpn. Landslide Soc.* **1988**, *25*, 11–16. [CrossRef]
13. Federico, A.; Popescu, M.; Fidelibus, C.; Interno, G. On the prediction of the time of occurrence of a slope failure: A review. In Proceedings of the 9th International Symposium on Landslides, Rio de Janeiro, Brazil, 28 June–2 July 2004; pp. 979–983.
14. Ma, J.W.; Tang, H.M.; Liu, X.; Hu, X.L.; Sun, M.J.; Song, Y.J. Establishment of a deformation forecasting model for a step-like landslide based on decision tree C5.0 and two-step cluster algorithms: A case study in the Three Gorges Reservoir area, China. *Landslides* **2017**, *14*, 1275–1281. [CrossRef]
15. Wen, T.; Tang, H.M.; Wang, Y.K.; Lin, C.Y.; Xiong, C.R. Landslide displacement prediction using the GA-LSSVM model and time series analysis: A case study of Three Gorges Reservoir, China. *Nat. Hazards Earth Syst. Sci.* **2017**, *17*, 2181–2198. [CrossRef]
16. Huang, F.M.; Yin, K.L.; Zhang, G.R.; Gui, L.; Yang, B.B.; Liu, L. Landslide displacement prediction using discrete wavelet transform and extreme learning machine based on chaos theory. *Environ. Earth Sci.* **2016**, *75*, 1376. [CrossRef]
17. Zhang, J.; Wang, Z.P.; Zhang, G.D.; Xue, Y.D. Probabilistic prediction of slope failure time. *Eng. Geol.* **2020**, *271*, 105586. [CrossRef]
18. Yao, W.; Zeng, Z.G.; Lian, C. Generating probabilistic predictions using mean-variance estimation and echo state network. *Neurocomputing* **2017**, *219*, 536–547. [CrossRef]
19. Tehrany, M.S.; Pradhan, B.; Jebur, M.N. Flood susceptibility mapping using a novel ensemble weights-of-evidence and support vector machine models in GIS. *J. Hydrol.* **2014**, *512*, 332–343. [CrossRef]
20. Zhu, Y.J. Ensemble forecast: A new approach to uncertainty and predictability. *Adv. Atmos. Sci.* **2005**, *22*, 781–788. [CrossRef]
21. Wang, Z.Y.; Srinivasan, R.S. A review of artificial intelligence based building energy use prediction: Contrasting the capabilities of single and ensemble prediction models. *Renew. Sust. Energ. Rev.* **2017**, *75*, 796–808. [CrossRef]
22. Rigamonti, M.; Baraldi, P.; Zio, E.; Roychoudhury, I.; Goebel, K.; Poll, S. Ensemble of optimized echo state networks for remaining useful life prediction. *Neurocomputing* **2018**, *281*, 121–138. [CrossRef]
23. Kim, M.-J.; Kang, D.-K. Ensemble with neural networks for bankruptcy prediction. *Expert Syst. Appl.* **2010**, *37*, 3373–3379. [CrossRef]
24. Prayogo, D.; Cheng, M.-Y.; Wu, Y.-W.; Tran, D.-H. Combining machine learning models via adaptive ensemble weighting for prediction of shear capacity of reinforced-concrete deep beams. *Eng. Comput. Ger.* **2019**, *36*, 1135–1153. [CrossRef]
25. Chen, K.; Jiang, J.; Zheng, F.; Chen, K. A novel data-driven approach for residential electricity consumption prediction based on ensemble learning. *Energy* **2018**, *150*, 49–60. [CrossRef]
26. Lee, D.; Baldick, R. Short-Term Wind Power Ensemble Prediction Based on Gaussian Processes and Neural Networks. *IEEE Trans. Smart Grid* **2014**, *5*, 501–510. [CrossRef]

27. Choubin, B.; Moradi, E.; Golshan, M.; Adamowski, J.; Sajedi-Hosseini, F.; Mosavi, A. An ensemble prediction of flood susceptibility using multivariate discriminant analysis, classification and regression trees, and support vector machines. *Sci. Total Environ.* **2019**, *651*, 2087–2096. [CrossRef] [PubMed]
28. Chen, J.; Li, Q.; Wang, H.; Deng, M. A Machine Learning Ensemble Approach Based on Random Forest and Radial Basis Function Neural Network for Risk Evaluation of Regional Flood Disaster: A Case Study of the Yangtze River Delta, China. *Int. J. Environ. Res. Public Health* **2020**, *17*, 49. [CrossRef]
29. Di Napoli, M.; Carotenuto, F.; Cevasco, A.; Confuorto, P.; Di Martire, D.; Firpo, M.; Pepe, G.; Raso, E.; Calcaterra, D. Machine learning ensemble modelling as a tool to improve landslide susceptibility mapping reliability. *Landslides* **2020**. [CrossRef]
30. Srivastav, R.K.; Sudheer, K.P.; Chaubey, I. A simplified approach to quantifying predictive and parametric uncertainty in artificial neural network hydrologic models. *Water Resour. Res.* **2007**, *43*, W10407. [CrossRef]
31. Tiwari, M.K.; Chatterjee, C. Development of an accurate and reliable hourly flood forecasting model using wavelet-bootstrap-ANN (WBANN) hybrid approach. *J. Hydrol.* **2010**, *394*, 458–470. [CrossRef]
32. Kasiviswanathan, K.S.; He, J.; Sudheer, K.P.; Tay, J.-H. Potential application of wavelet neural network ensemble to forecast streamflow for flood management. *J. Hydrol.* **2016**, *536*, 161–173. [CrossRef]
33. Zhang, J.; Tang, W.H.; Zhang, L.M.; Huang, H.W. Characterising geotechnical model uncertainty by hybrid Markov Chain Monte Carlo simulation. *Comput. Geotech.* **2012**, *43*, 26–36. [CrossRef]
34. Cannon, A.J. Quantile regression neural networks: Implementation in R and application to precipitation downscaling. *Comput. Geosci. UK* **2011**, *37*, 1277–1284. [CrossRef]
35. Xu, Q.F.; Liu, X.; Jiang, C.X.; Yu, K.M. Quantile autoregression neural network model with applications to evaluating value at risk. *Appl. Soft Comput.* **2016**, *49*, 1–12. [CrossRef]
36. Donaldson, R.G.; Kamstra, M. Forecast combining with neural networks. *J. Forecast.* **1996**, *15*, 49–61. [CrossRef]
37. Charlton, T.S.; Rouainia, M. Probabilistic capacity analysis of suction caissons in spatially variable clay. *Comput. Geotech.* **2016**, *80*, 226–236. [CrossRef]
38. Gramacki, A. *Nonparametric Kernel Density Estimation and Its Computational Aspects*; Springer: New York, NY, USA, 2017.
39. Zhang, S.; Ma, J.W.; Tang, H.M. Estimation of Risk Thresholds for a Landslide in the Three Gorges Reservoir Based on a KDE-Copula-VaR Approach. *Geofluids* **2020**, *2020*, 8030264. [CrossRef]
40. Wan, C.; Xu, Z.; Pinson, P.; Dong, Z.Y.; Wong, K.P. Probabilistic forecasting of wind power generation using extreme learning machine. *IEEE Trans. Power Syst.* **2014**, *29*, 1033–1044. [CrossRef]
41. Wan, C.; Xu, Z.; Wang, Y.L.; Dong, Z.Y.; Wong, K.P. A hybrid approach for probabilistic forecasting of electricity price. *IEEE Trans. Smart Grid* **2014**, *5*, 463–470. [CrossRef]
42. Wang, Y.K.; Tang, H.M.; Wen, T.; Ma, J.W. A hybrid intelligent approach for constructing landslide displacement prediction intervals. *Appl. Soft Comput.* **2019**, *81*, 105506. [CrossRef]
43. Zhang, L.; Liao, M.S.; Balz, T.; Shi, X.G.; Jiang, Y.N. Monitoring landslide activities in the Three Gorges area with multi-frequency satellite SAR data sets. In *Modern Technologies for Landslide Monitoring and Prediction*; Scaioni, M., Ed.; Springer Berlin Heidelberg: Berlin/Heidelberg, Germany, 2015; pp. 181–208. [CrossRef]
44. Fan, J.H.; Qiu, K.T.; Xia, Y.; Li, M.; Lin, H.; Zhang, H.T.; Tu, P.F.; Liu, G.; Shu, S.Q. InSAR monitoring and synthetic analysis of the surface deformation of Fanjiaping landslide in the Three Gorges Reservoir area. *Geol. Bull. China* **2017**, *36*, 1665–1673.
45. Guerriero, L.; Coe, J.A.; Revellino, P.; Grelle, G.; Pinto, F.; Guadagno, F.M. Influence of slip-surface geometry on earth-flow deformation, Montaguto earth flow, southern Italy. *Geomorphology* **2014**, *219*, 285–305. [CrossRef]
46. Guerriero, L.; Bertello, L.; Cardozo, N.; Berti, M.; Grelle, G.; Revellino, P. Unsteady sediment discharge in earth flows: A case study from the Mount Pizzuto earth flow, southern Italy. *Geomorphology* **2017**, *295*, 260–284. [CrossRef]
47. Dietterich, T.G. Ensemble Methods in Machine Learning. In Proceedings of the Multiple Classifier Systems, Cagliari, Italy, 21–23 June 2000; pp. 1–15.
48. Du, J.; Yin, K.L.; Lacasse, S. Displacement prediction in colluvial landslides, Three Gorges Reservoir, China. *Landslides* **2013**, *10*, 203–218. [CrossRef]

9

Psychosocial Management Before, During and After Emergencies and Disasters—Results from the Kobe Expert Meeting

Mélissa Généreux [1,2,*], Philip J. Schluter [3,4], Sho Takahashi [5,6], Shiori Usami [7], Sonoe Mashino [8], Ryoma Kayano [9] and Yoshiharu Kim [10]

1 Sherbrooke Hospital University Centre, Eastern Townships Integrated University Centre in Health and Social Services, Sherbrooke, QC J1J 3H5, Canada
2 Department of Community Health Sciences, Faculty of Medicine and Health Sciences, Université de Sherbrooke, Sherbrooke, QC J1G 1B1, Canada
3 School of Health Sciences, University of Canterbury—Te Whare Wānanga o Waitaha, Christchurch 8140, New Zealand; philip.schluter@canterbury.ac.nz
4 Primary Care Clinical Unit, School of Clinical Medicine, The University of Queensland, Brisbane QLD 4006, Australia
5 Department of Disaster Psychiatry, University of Tsukuba, Tsukuba 305-8575, Japan; takahashi.sho.fn@u.tsukuba.ac.jp
6 Ibaraki Prefectural Medical Center of Psychiatry, Kasama 309-1717, Japan
7 Department of Mental Health and Psychiatric Nursing, Faculty of Life Sciences, Kumamoto University, Kumamoto 860-8555, Japan; susami@kumamoto-u.ac.jp
8 Research Institute of Nursing Care for People and Community, University of Hyōgo, Akashi 673-8588, Japan; sonoe_mashino@cnas.u-hyogo.ac.jp
9 World Health Organization Centre for Health Development, Kobe 651-0073, Japan; kayanor@who.int
10 National Institute of Mental Health, National Center for Neurology and Psychiatry, Kodaira 187-0031, Japan; kim@ncnp.go.jp
* Correspondence: melissa.genereux@usherbrooke.ca

Abstract: Emergencies and disasters typically affect entire communities, cause substantial losses and disruption, and result in a significant and persistent mental health burden. There is currently a paucity of evidence on safe and effective individual- and community-level strategies for improving mental health before, during, and after such events. In October 2018, the World Health Organization (WHO) Centre for Health Development (WHO Kobe Centre) convened a meeting bringing together leading Asia Pacific and international disaster research experts. The expert meeting identified key research needs in five major areas, one being "Psychosocial management before, during, and after emergencies and disasters". Experts for this research area identified critical gaps in observational research (i.e., the monitoring of long-term psychological consequences) and interventional research (i.e., the development and evaluation of individual- and community-level interventions). Three key research issues were identified. First, experts underscored the need for a standardized and psychometrically robust instrument that classified the mental health/psychosocial risk of people within both a clinical and community setting. Then, the need for a standardization of methods for prevention, screening, diagnosis, and treatment for affected people was highlighted. Finally, experts called for a better identification of before, during, and after emergency or disaster assets associated with greater community resilience.

Keywords: health emergency and disaster risk management (Health-EDRM); Sendai Framework for Disaster Risk Reduction; WHO Thematic Platform for Health-EDRM Research Network; post-traumatic stress disorder; mental health impacts; psychosocial management; community resilience

1. Introduction

Large-scale emergency and disaster events, resulting from natural, technological, or human causes, often affect entire communities. They invariably yield significant human and capital injuries and losses coupled with prolonged social and infrastructure disruption. Moreover, emergencies and disasters typically place a significant and persistent mental health burden on those directly and indirectly affected, together with those who respond and their associated services. As a result, public health organizations are charged with intervening and helping citizens and communities cope in the aftermath of emergencies and disasters. The public health response during and after emergencies and disasters has historically focused on protecting populations from immediate threats [1]. However, the role of public health and health systems in providing sustained psychosocial support for directly and indirectly affected victims, the long-term monitoring of psychological profiles, and delivering ongoing strategies for enhancing resilience may be just as important [2].

In October 2018, the World Health Organization (WHO) Centre for Health Development (WHO Kobe Centre) convened a meeting in order to identify key emergency and disaster research needs. A panel of invited experts from the WHO, WHO Thematic Platform for Health Emergency and Disaster Risk Management (Health-EDRM) Research Network (TPRN), World Association for Disaster and Emergency Medicine, and the Japan International Cooperation Agency, along with delegates to the Asia Pacific Conference for Disaster Medicine 2018, was convened [3]. The panel was informed by multiple sources, including the progress and implementation of the Sendai Framework on Disaster Risk Reduction 2015–2030 [4], documentation from the 3rd UN World Conference on Disaster Risk Reduction (including the establishment of TPRN), and literature on the recommended Health-EDRM research activities [5–8]. After a review of these documents, together with appraising existing projects and activities, five major areas of research need were identified. These were clustered and named under the following banners: (i) Health data management before, during, and after emergencies and disasters; (ii) Psychosocial management before, during, and after emergencies and disasters, and other medium- and long-term effects on the public health and health systems, the topic of this paper; (iii) Community emergency and disaster risk management, including risk literacy and addressing needs of sub-populations; (iv) Health workforce development for health emergency and disaster risk management; and, (v) Research methods and ethics.

2. Material and Methods

The content of this discussion paper arises from the WHO Kobe Centre convened panel's deliberations, based on available evidence and their expertise in psychosocial management before, during, and after emergencies and disasters. The lead discussant (Yoshiharu Kim), the rapporteur (Mélissa Généreux), and the other experts who participated to the discussion ($n = 7$) primarily sought to (i) identify critical gaps in scientific evidence in this major area of research, as well as (ii) discuss concrete research questions and issues, with the aim of potentially resolving these gaps through collaboration among Asian Pacific regional and global researchers and related stakeholders. Additionally, the panel aimed to assess knowledge-to-practice gaps in order to better integrate current expertise and research in this area for each disaster management phase.

3. Results

A consensus emerged among the expert panel that there is currently a paucity of evidence on safe and effective individual- and community-level strategies for monitoring and improving psychosocial health and building resilience before, during, and after emergencies and disasters.

3.1. Critical Research Gap Identification

The discussion on critical gaps in scientific evidence led to the identification of three priorities in research, namely the monitoring of long-term psychological consequences; the need for individual-level interventions; and the need for community-level interventions. Each of these identified gaps are now described in turn.

3.1.1. Monitoring of the Long-Term Psychological Consequences

In order to strengthen current psychosocial strategies to promote health and wellbeing before, during, and after emergencies and disasters, the monitoring of people's psychological profile needs to be harmonized or standardized. Such standardized monitoring enables population patterns to be followed over time, across the phases of the emergency or disaster, and provides an empirical characterization of recovery for the whole population and various important subgroups. Moreover, it would enable national and international comparisons to be drawn and facilitate a better understanding of community-level psychosocial wellbeing. Ideally, any standardized instrument would be derived from routinely collected information, thereby reducing participant burden and also being available before, during, and after emergencies and disasters. Many studies have reported both persistent adverse outcomes (notably post-traumatic stress disorders (PTSD) or symptoms (PTSS), anxiety, and depression) and positive outcomes (e.g., post-traumatic growth, and closer sense of community) for years following exposure to natural or anthropogenic disasters. Moreover, these positive and negative effects have been observed among those directly affected by the emergency or disaster, and also among those peripherally affected, such as workers and caregivers, and the wider population. However, community-level profiles are often left unmeasured prior to emergencies or disasters, making longitudinal recovery patterns difficult to fully ascertain. This is further compounded by the fact that specific sub-groups are often disproportionally impacted, may have differential recovery periods, and that the impact may vary greatly according to exposure type and intensity [9–15]. Children and youth, the elderly, those socioeconomically deprived, and disabled people frequently carry this disproportionate burden. Although standardization of exposure and outcome measures is desirable and central, this should not preclude the additional use and reporting of other culturally or geographically specific measures. Various indigenous and other groups of people around the globe define health and wellbeing in different but equally valid ways, and this should be acknowledged and respected in any form of reporting or monitoring.

3.1.2. Individual-Level Interventions

To better understand the psychosocial risks, vulnerabilities, and capacities following an emergency or disaster, a wide range of individual-level interventions need to be developed and evaluated, both in clinical and community-based settings. Such interventions should include, but are not limited to, self-care programs, humanitarian support, psychological first aid, prevention, screening and diagnosis tools for both health and non-health workers, and medication required for various types of sequelae mental health problems [16,17]. Preventive interventions are thought to be especially important to reduce the risk of PTSD and depression among workers who are acutely exposed [18], including first responders (e.g., fire, police, emergency medical staff). It is also critical to ensure that validated clinical interventions and tools can be shared and used more widely, through training, guidelines, repositories, and communication and dissemination strategies. Guidelines for the appropriate use of the interventions and tools must be clearly articulated, and their misuse must be avoided.

3.1.3. Community-Level Interventions

In a similar vein to the above, there is a need to further develop and evaluate community-level strategies, such as psychosocial education (before emergency or disaster), addressing the unmet psychosocial needs through self-help groups and dynamic group psychotherapy (after emergency or disaster), cultivating community resilience, empowering the citizens, and mobilizing the community (before, during, and after emergency or disaster) [19–22]. An evidence base of interventions that have empirically demonstrated successful implementation and efficacy needs to be developed and established. As for individual-level interventions, there is an added need for enhanced knowledge translation strategies so that lessons learned from community-level interventions can be pooled, shared, and used on a broader basis.

3.2. Proposed Research Questions and Issues

Concrete research questions were proposed to meet each of the identified knowledge gaps. The first question pertained to the classification of people exposed to a disaster according to their level of psychosocial need. Currently, multiple and often inconsistent definitions are employed. It was advocated that an epidemiological tool (i.e., a standardized and psychometrically robust instrument) should be developed and validated for the classification of risk (e.g., high-risk, mid-risk, and low-risk) for people exposed to an emergency or disaster. Drawing on the social determinants of health framework, a wide range of risks and assets previously documented in the scientific literature should underpin the construction of this tool [23–25]. Broadly, it is likely to include the following:

- Before emergency or disaster: pre-existing risk and protective factors;
- During emergency or disaster: exposure to primary stressors, human and material losses;
- After emergency or disaster: exposure to secondary stressors, and access and use of local resources.

As the emergency or disaster impacts invariably extend beyond the clinical setting, the tool should be suitable for patients within that setting but also for persons within the wider community (e.g., conducting a community health survey). As such, it is likely the tool will have robust screening rather than definitive clinical exposure diagnostic properties. The validation of this tool should be performed using longitudinal and multi-centric studies, and should focus on its ability to predict various outcomes, like PTSD, other psychological symptoms (including psychological distress, anxiety, and depressive symptoms), maladaptive behaviors (including alcohol and drug abuse), self-care, quality of life, and positive outcomes (including post-traumatic growth).

The need to standardize interventions delivered to people exposed to a disaster using evidence-based best practices was also stressed. Panel members suggested the development and validation of methods to screen, diagnose, and treat people exposed to a disaster in clinical and community-based settings. Such clinical tools should frame emerging practices, such as risk screening by community members, by ensuring that they are both effective and safe, and by underlining the conditions for success of such methods.

Finally, panel members called for a better identification of what makes a community resilient, through an assessment of before, during, and after emergency or disaster assets (i.e., characteristics, strengths, and resources) that are associated with greater community resilience. Local knowledge should be considered in the same manner as scientific knowledge. Having been through a unique and informative experience, the local health workforce involved in psychosocial management must draw and share lessons in the aftermath of a disaster (in close collaboration with researchers and community members) through case studies. Guidelines for their reporting of these studies should include the following.

- What were the needs and assets in the local community?
- How and by whom were these needs and assets addressed?
- What were the barriers and the success factors for sustaining resilience and recovery?

Standards (or format) to report case studies should facilitate the pooling and the sharing of such local evidence. Moreover, respective roles of health and non-health sectors need to be clarified, as community resilience absolutely requires a cross-sectoral approach. In time, these case studies could be subjected to meta-analyses in order to distill common features that transcend each unique emergency or disaster-ravaged community.

4. Discussion

The current research gaps and priorities in psychosocial management after emergencies and disasters identified by the expert panel are, perhaps unsurprisingly, mirrored within the literature. The lack of long-term observational and interventional research [8,26–28], challenges in systematically collating and delivering lessons learned from events, and difficulties in creating and sustaining effective community engagement [29–31] have all been described before. However, this paper is among the first that attempts to draw the various threads of these research needs together.

Although the before, during, and after phases of emergency and disaster management are all important, the panel asserted that local efforts in psychosocial management are mostly oriented toward the short-term after the event. Once the emergency or disaster is over, medical, psychosocial, and public health teams are often required to revert to and resume their regular tasks as quickly as possible. Long-term psychosocial recovery is perhaps the most challenging task because of the burden on professionals (e.g., accumulating workload) and organizational factors (e.g., weakening political commitment). As a result of this fatigue, monitoring of long-term psychological health consequences is not usually done (with a few exceptions) [25,32], much less in a standardized manner.

Another critical area that is typically overlooked in the post-event landscape is the evaluation of psychosocial interventions provided during the recovery phase of an emergency or disaster, which are typically not routinely carried out. Such evaluations would provide the necessary evidence for establishing standards and best practices [26]. Due to the often unpredictable nature of emergencies or disasters, it is often impossible to conduct randomized or prospective cohort studies that capture the before, during, and after phases of the event. Instead, within this emergency or disaster setting, interventional research should exploit apposite tailored natural experiment designs. These will often be shaped by pragmatic considerations, such as resources, expertise, and data availability, but are likely to include pre–post, interpreted time series, and change point study designs. Together with the standard cross-sectional or repeated measure studies often initiated following an event, a richer empirical evidence base will emerge. With the increasing availability of routinely collected data and greater ability for matching and tracking individuals over time, these data sources are likely to have increased utility in emergency and disaster research. With data sufficiency, the psychosocial profiles within affected communities could be monitored by measuring changes before, during, and after the emergency or disaster and comparing these patterns to unaffected control communities [33]. Finally, learning from past events should be systematized, notably through case studies, as they are likely to inform the identification and sharing of common international problems and solutions.

The importance of identifying and leveraging existing assets at the community level was also raised. Working from existing capacities was strongly valued among the panel. However, communities typically remain poorly engaged in disaster management. Indeed, often after an emergency or disaster, various sectors within the community, particularly those disproportionately affected, experience heightened barriers which contribute to further physical and social exclusion, and pursuant disengagement. Evidence-based efficacious strategies to mobilize local knowledge and expertise before, during, and after a disaster are yet to be developed [34].

Finally, the discussion of our expert panel on solutions to fill psychosocial management knowledge and knowledge-to-practice gaps before, during, and after emergencies and disasters aligned with the priorities set by the 2015–2030 Sendai Framework for Disaster Risk Reduction [35]. Indeed, the Sendai Framework emphasizes the requirement for *"improving the knowledge of government representatives at all levels through the sharing of experiences, lessons learned and good practices"* (Paragraph 24g) and *"ensuring that local knowledge and practices complete, as appropriate, scientific knowledge of disaster risk assessment"* (Paragraph 24i) [4].

5. Conclusions

It is hoped that this delineation and discussion on key research issues in psychosocial management will contribute to the identification and implementation of concrete solutions that foster the creation and the use of knowledge for psychosocial support and resilience building before, during, and after emergencies and disasters. As for other major Health-EDRM research areas, psychosocial management requires collaboration between experts, decision makers, practitioners, and communities in order to facilitate coordinated responses when and where they are most needed. It is critical that psychosocial strategies developed to support victims and communities affected by emergencies and disasters are validated and that knowledge gained from these experiences is shared and used as much as possible.

Author Contributions: Conceptualization: M.G., Y.K.; Methodology: M.G., Y.K.; Original Draft Preparation: M.G.; Writing—Review and Editing: Y.K., P.J.S., S.T., S.U., S.M., R.K.; Project Administration: R.K.

Acknowledgments: The opinions contained in the paper are those of its authors and, except where specifically stated, are not intended to represent the official policies or positions of the WHO.

References

1. Généreux, M.; Petit, G.; Maltais, D.; Roy, M.; Simard, R.; Boivin, S.; Shultz, L.M.; Pinsonneault, L. The public health response during and after the Lac-Mégantic train derailment tragedy: A case study. *Disaster Health* **2015**, *2*, 1–8.
2. Spittlehouse, J.K.; Joyce, P.R.; Vierck, E.; Schluter, P.J.; Pearson, J.F. Ongoing adverse mental health impact of the earthquake sequence in Christchurch, New Zealand. *Aust. N. Z. J. Psychiatry* **2014**, *48*, 756–763. [CrossRef] [PubMed]
3. Asian Pacific Conference for Disaster Medicine 2018. Available online: http://www.apcdm2018.org/index.html (accessed on 31 January 2019).
4. Sendai Framework for Disaster Risk Reduction 2015–2030. Available online: https://www.unisdr.org/we/inform/publications/43291 (accessed on 31 January 2019).
5. WHO Thematic Platform for Health Emergency and Disaster Risk Management. Available online: http://www.who.int/hac/techguidance/preparedness/WHO-Thematic-Platform-Health-EDRM-Terms-Reference-2018.pdf?ua=1 (accessed on 31 January 2019).
6. WHO Thematic Platform for Health Emergency and Disaster Risk Management Research Network. Available online: http://www.who.int/hac/techguidance/preparedness/WHO-Thematic-Platform-Health-EDRM-Research-Network-2018.pdf?ua=1 (accessed on 31 January 2019).
7. Chan, E.Y.Y.; Murray, V. What are the health research needs for the Sendai Framework. *Lancet* **2017**, *390*, E35–E36. [CrossRef]
8. Lo, C.T.T.; Chan, E.Y.Y.; Chan, G.K.W.; Murray, V.; Abrahams, J.; Ardalan, A.; Kayano, R.; Chung, J.; Yau, W. Health Emergency and Disaster Risk Management (Health-EDRM): Developing the Research Field within the Sendai Framework Paradigm. *Int. J. Disaster Risk Sci.* **2017**, *8*, 145–149. [CrossRef]
9. Galea, S. The long-term health consequences of disasters and mass traumas. *CMAJ* **2007**, *176*, 1293–1294. [CrossRef]
10. Galea, S.; Nandi, A.; Vlahov, D. The epidemiology of post-traumatic stress disorder after disasters. *Epidemiol. Rev.* **2005**, *27*, 78–91. [CrossRef]
11. Goldmann, E.; Galea, S. Mental health consequences of disasters. *Ann. Rev. Public Health* **2014**, *35*, 169–183. [CrossRef]
12. Neria, Y.; Nandi, A.; Galea, S. Post-traumatic stress disorder following disasters: A systematic review. *Psychol. Med.* **2008**, *38*, 467–480. [CrossRef]
13. Hull, A.M.; Alexander, D.A.; Klein, S. Survivors of the Piper Alpha oil platform disaster: Long-term follow-up study. *Br. J. Psychiatry* **2002**, *181*, 433–438. [CrossRef] [PubMed]
14. Bromet, E.J.; Havenaar, J.M.; Guey, L.T. A 25 year retrospective review of the psychological consequences of the Chernobyl accident. *Clin. Oncol.* **2011**, *23*, 297–305. [CrossRef] [PubMed]
15. Généreux, M.; Maltais, D. Three years after the tragedy: How the Le Granit community is coping. *Bull. Vis. Santé Publique* **2017**, *34*, 1–8.

16. Usami, U.; Takahashi, N.; Kayano, R. Development of specific care strategies to maintain and recover survivors' health after disasters-intervention program to prevent PTSD and depression after Kumamoto earthquake: Case report. In Proceedings of the International Conference on Nursing, Pharmacy, Traditional Medicine and Health Cciences, TKP Conference, Osaka, Japan, 28–30 September 2018.
17. Kim, Y. Great East Japan earthquake and early mental-health-care response. *Psychiatry Clin. Neurosci.* **2011**, *65*, 539–548. [CrossRef] [PubMed]
18. Suzuki, Y.; Fukasawa, M.; Obara, A.; Kim, Y. Mental health distress and related factors among prefectural public servants seven months after the great East Japan earthquake. *J. Epidemiol.* **2014**, *24*, 287–294. [CrossRef] [PubMed]
19. Usami, S. Kumamoto earthquake, certified nurse specialist in mental health and psychiatric nursing to prevent PTSD. *J. Jpn. Assoc. Group Psychother.* **2017**, *33*, 18–22.
20. O'Sullivan, T.L.; Kuziemsky, C.E.; Corneil, W.; Lemyre, L.; Franco, Z. The EnRiCH community resilience framework for high-risk populations. *PLoS Curr.* **2014**. [CrossRef]
21. Généreux, M.; Petit, G.; Roy, M.; Maltais, D.; O'Sullivan, T. The "Lac-Mégantic tragedy" seen through the lens of the EnRiCH community resilience framework for high-risk populations. *Can. J. Public Health* **2018**, *109*, 261–267. [CrossRef]
22. Leadbeater, A. Community leadership in disaster recovery: A case study. *Aust. J. Emerg. Manag.* **2013**, *28*, 41–47.
23. Norris, F.H.; Friedman, M.J.; Watson, P.J.; Byrne, C.M.; Diaz, E.; Kaniasty, K. 60,000 disaster victims speak: Part I. An empirical review of the empirical literature, 1981–2001. *Psychiatry* **2002**, *65*, 207–239. [CrossRef]
24. Warsini, S.; West, C.; Dip, E.G.; Mills, J.; Usher, K. The psychosocial impact of natural disasters among adult survivors: An integrative review. *Issues Ment. Health Nurs.* **2014**, *35*, 420–436. [CrossRef]
25. Morgan, J.; Begg, A.; Beaven, S.; Schluter, P.; Jamieson, K.; Johal, S.; Johnston, D.; Sparrow, M. Monitoring wellbeing during recovery from the 2010–2011 Canterbury earthquakes: The CERA Wellbeing Survey. *Int. J. Disaster Risk Reduct.* **2015**, *14*, 96–103. [CrossRef]
26. Birnbaum, M.L.; Daily, E.K.; O'Rourke, A.P.; Kushner, J. Research and evaluations of the health aspects of disasters, part VI: Interventional research and the disaster logic model. *Prehosp. Disaster Med.* **2016**, *31*, 181–194. [CrossRef]
27. Tsutsumi, A.; Takashi, I.; Ito, A.; Thronicroft, G.; Patel, V.; Minas, H. Mental health mainstreamed in new UN disaster framework. *Lancet Psychiatry* **2015**, *2*, 679–680. [CrossRef]
28. Suzuki, Y.; Fukasawa, M.; Nakajima, S.; Narisawa, T.; Keiko, A.; Kim, Y. Developing a Consensus-Based Definition of "Kokoro-no Care" or Mental Health Services and Psychosocial Support: Drawing from Experiences of Mental Health Professionals Who Responded to the Great East Japan Earthquake. *PLoS Curr.* **2015**. [CrossRef]
29. Gamboa-Maldonado, T.; Marshak, H.H.; Sinclair, R.; Montgomery, S.; Dyjack, D.T. Building capacity for community disaster preparedness: A call for collaboration between public environmental health and emergency preparedness and response programs. *J. Environ. Health* **2012**, *75*, 24–29.
30. Jong, S.V.Z. Let's Talk Oil Spill Risk. Lessons Learned from Coastal Communities in British Columbia, Canada. Chapter 8. In *Responses to Disasters and Climate Change. Understanding Vulnerabilities and Fostering Resilience*; Taylor and Francis Group: Florida, FL, USA, 2016; pp. 83–92.
31. Svendsen, E.R.; Whittle, N.C.; Sanders, L.; McKeown, R.E.; Sprayberry, K.; Heim, M.; Caldwell, R.; Gibson, J.J.; Vena, J.E. GRACE: Public health recovery methods following an environmental disaster. *Arch. Environ. Occup. Health* **2010**, *65*, 77–85. [CrossRef]
32. Généreux, M.; Maltais, D.; Petit, G.; Roy, M. Monitoring adverse psychosocial outcomes one and two years after the Lac-Mégantic train derailment tragedy (Eastern Townships, Quebec, Canada). *Prehosp. Disaster Med.* **2019**. In press.
33. Schluter, P.J.; Hamilton, G.J.; Deely, J.M.; Ardagh, M.W. The impact of integrated health system changes, accelerated due to an earthquake, on emergency department attendances and acute admissions: A Bayesian change-point analysis. *BMJ Open* **2016**, *6*, e010709. [CrossRef]

34. Lichtveld, M.; Kennedy, S.; Krouse, R.Z.; Grimsley, F.; El-Dahr, J.; Bordelon, K.; Sterling, Y.; White, L.; Baelow, N.; DeGruy, S.; et al. From design to dissemination: Implementing community-based participatory research in postdisaster communities. *Am. J. Public Health* **2016**, *106*, 1235–1242. [CrossRef]
35. Aitsi-Selmi, A.; Murray, V. The Sendai framework: Disaster risk reduction through a health lens. *Bull. World Health Organ.* **2015**, *93*. [CrossRef]

10

Reducing the Future Risk of Trauma: On the Integration of Global Disaster Policy within Specific Health Domains and Established Fields of Practice

Lennart Reifels [1,2]

[1] Centre for Mental Health, Melbourne School of Population and Global Health, The University of Melbourne, Melbourne, VIC 3010, Australia; l.reifels@unimelb.edu.au

[2] Disaster Research Unit, Department of Political and Social Sciences, Free University of Berlin, 12165 Berlin, Germany

Abstract: The global increase in the frequency and severity of natural hazards and extreme climatic events necessitates more efficient global and national strategies to reduce the likelihood and impact of traumatic consequences for disaster-affected populations. The recent inclusion of mental health in the Sendai Framework for Disaster Risk Reduction marks a pivotal point in the recognition of the significant burden of disasters on mental health, and a global commitment to reducing its impacts. Nevertheless, effective agreement implementation and efforts to reduce disaster mental health risks are facing significant challenges. These include a lack of clarity about the conceptual interlinkages and place of disaster risk reduction principles within the field of disaster mental health, which is traditionally marked by a prevailing recovery orientation, and the need for effective translation into disaster mental health policy and practice. Therefore, this study drew on data from interviews with European disaster mental health and risk reduction experts in order to appraise the merit and implications of a global disaster risk reduction policy for advancing population mental health in the context of disaster. Study findings outline existing opportunities, challenges, and key strategies for the integration of disaster risk reduction within disaster mental health policy and practice.

Keywords: disaster; disaster risk reduction; Sendai framework; mental health

---

1. Introduction

At the global level, human mental health and wellbeing is being increasingly jeopardised through rising trends in population exposure to severe natural hazards and extreme climatic events [1,2]. Despite the often remarkable resilience of communities to the onslaught of such events, decades of disaster mental health research have demonstrated the significant burden that mass-traumatic events can inflict on the mental health of affected populations [3]. This mental health impact can vary in intensity, course, and duration, and find expression in temporary distress reactions among a large majority, ongoing mental health problems of mild to moderate severity, as well as more severe mental health issues (such as post-traumatic stress disorder or depression) among a significant minority of those affected by disaster [4]. Apart from constituting an important outcome domain in its own right, population mental health also plays a key role in facilitating effective rebuilding and recovery efforts and in terms of broader social, socio-economic, and societal functioning [5].

International recognition of the need to better manage the varied risks associated with disaster exposure has resulted in seminal intergovernmental agreements and policy frameworks to guide global and societal disaster risk reduction [6,7]. The Sendai Framework for Disaster Risk Reduction 2015–2030, which was adopted by 187 United Nations (UN) member states in March 2015, reflects an important conceptual shift in global disaster policy—away from managing disaster impacts and consequences, toward a proactive approach to managing and reducing disaster risks. Although this relatively subtle shift in global disaster policy may be unbeknownst to many outside of the field, it is likely to have important practical ramifications for concerted societal efforts to address disaster risks across varied sectors and practice domains over the next 15 years. It further requires a thorough understanding of both existing and newly emerging disaster risks facing societies today and the adoption of proactive and effective strategies to manage and reduce these risks in future.

The Sendai Framework is structured around the key elements of a global goal and expected outcome, operationalised through seven global targets primarily aimed at reducing: disaster mortality, the number of people affected, economic losses, damage to infrastructure, and disruption of basic (e.g., health) services. In addition, four cross-cutting priority areas for global action highlight the critical importance of: (1) understanding disaster risk, (2) strengthening disaster risk governance, (3) investing in disaster risk reduction, and (4) enhancing disaster preparedness for effective response and to 'build back better'. As part of a concerted implementation effort, the Sendai Framework also outlines local, national, and regional level stakeholder roles and responsibilities.

One of the cornerstones of the Sendai Framework is its strong emphasis on human health. This is particularly evident in 35 direct references to health, the explicit inclusion of health in the expected Sendai outcome ("the substantial reduction of disaster risk and losses in lives, livelihoods, and health and in the economic, physical, social, cultural, and environmental assets of persons, businesses, communities, and countries"), and direct links to health in four of the framework's seven global targets [8,9]. Within the context of this strong health emphasis, the explicit inclusion of mental health in the Sendai Framework marks a pivotal point in the recognition of the significant burden of disasters on the mental health of affected populations, and a simultaneous global commitment to reducing its impacts [10]. Mental health features, perhaps most prominently, as a national and local level responsibility under Sendai's priority action area (4) in terms of the aim to "enhance recovery schemes to provide psychosocial support and mental health services for all people in need" (paragraph 33o); whereas other key action areas underpin the critical importance of a better understanding of disaster risks across varied societal sectors and domains.

However, despite the formal inclusion and recognition of the importance of population mental health, significant challenges remain to the effective Sendai agreement implementation and associated efforts to reduce disaster mental health risks and consequences. These include a lack of clarity about the conceptual interlinkages and place of disaster risk reduction principles within the field of disaster mental health, which is traditionally marked by a prevailing recovery orientation, and the need for translation into disaster mental health policy and practice.

Conversely, key aspects relevant to disaster mental health have thus far received relatively little systematic attention in the context of disaster risk reduction frameworks. This, however, is in stark contrast to more general and public health domains, which are increasingly being considered in disaster risk reduction contexts [8,9,11,12]. As a direct consequence, the Sendai Framework currently provides little conceptual elaboration of the nature of disaster mental health risks or necessary guidance for future societal strategies to reduce and manage associated mental health risks and consequences of extreme climatic events and disasters. In view of the inevitable limits of global disaster treaties to provide health domain-specific guidance, there is therefore an urgent need to carefully consider the implications of the Sendai Framework for specific health domains, and to facilitate its integration within established fields of practice [13].

For brevity, this article adopts an inclusive definition of disaster mental health (DMH) as a scientific discipline and field of practice that is concerned with understanding, preventing, and addressing mental health problems and promoting psychosocial wellbeing and resilience in disaster and emergency contexts. Thus understood, DMH is not merely limited to efforts that seek to better understand or address psychiatric phenomena via therapeutic interventions, but rather includes recognition of the vital importance of a broader range of psycho-social factors, outcomes, and support strategies in disaster and emergency contexts. Emerging from traditions, such as trauma and stress studies, and incorporating related humanitarian practice fields, such as Mental Health and Psychosocial Support, DMH has amassed a considerable body of knowledge about the potential spectrum of disaster mental health outcomes and relevant intervention and support strategies over time [14,15]. Yet, traditionally, the primary focus of DMH strategies has been on facilitating recovery in the wake of disaster, whereas the field has remained fairly oblivious to broader developments in global disaster policy. In view of this circumstance, the current shift in disaster policy in the context of the Sendai Framework—from managing disaster impacts to reducing disaster risks—provides a pertinent and timely opportunity to examine the intersection of these two fields in more depth, and to explore the DMH field through a disaster risk reduction (DRR) lens.

This study therefore drew on data from interviews with European disaster mental health and risk reduction experts in order to appraise the merit and implications of global disaster risk reduction policy for advancing population mental health in the context of disaster. More specifically, this study examined the conceptual nature of disaster mental health risks, as well as concrete opportunities, current challenges, and key strategies for the integration of disaster risk reduction within disaster mental health policy and practice.

2. Materials and Methods

This study drew on data from interviews with 17 European key informants (including 14 DMH and 3 DRR experts), which were conducted between May and September 2016, as part of a larger research project that examined the early implementation of the Sendai Framework in Europe. In view of the relatively small pool of key informants in this area, this exploratory study adopted a purposive sampling frame informed by prior stakeholder mapping to recruit eminent DMH and DRR experts at the European regional and national levels (in the UK, the Netherlands, and Germany) for participation in semi-structured interviews. Participating DRR experts represented three of the 17 DRR experts recruited for the larger study who were both directly involved in the Sendai implementation and in a position to complete an interview schedule focused on disaster mental health. Key informants (10 men, 7 women) were typically affiliated with scientific institutions and national DMH or DRR advisory bodies across the UK, the Netherlands, and Germany, or European-based advisory bodies with a broader international mandate.

Semi-structured interviews were conducted on the basis of an interview schedule. The schedule included 15 questions that explored the intersection of DRR and DMH by eliciting information on: principal mental health risks in disaster contexts, DMH strategies to address these risks, and existing opportunities, current challenges, and key strategies for the integration of disaster risk reduction and disaster mental health. A copy of the full interview schedule is available from the author upon request. The interviews, which lasted between 40 and 95 minutes, were conducted either in person or remotely (via telephone or Skype), audio-recorded, and analysed thematically using NVivo11 (QSR International Pty Ltd., Melbourne, Australia). All key informants provided consent for study participation. The study protocol was approved by the Human Research Ethics Committee at the University of Melbourne (ID: 1646655.1).

3. Results

Key themes resulting from the expert interviews are summarised in the following, with the study's thematic coding framework and illustrative participant quotes outlined in Table S1.

3.1. Principal Disaster Mental Health Risks

Key informants were asked about what they would regard as the principal mental health risks in disaster contexts. The principal mental health risks identified by the experts fell into five broad thematic categories. The first two of these highlighted commonly established risk factors for adverse mental health outcomes, as well as newly emerging risks that were contextually bound to the unfolding European refugee/migration crisis. The three remaining categories were focused on risks associated with the conduct of appropriate disaster mental health responses and intervention strategies, e.g., in relation to the adequate recognition and detection of complex mental health impacts, the provision of appropriate mental health support, and overarching disaster response communication and coordination.

3.1.1. Common Risk Factors

Key informants frequently identified established risk factors for adverse mental health outcomes. These factors included, amongst others, the nature of the hazard, exposure level, peri-traumatic and post-event reactions, various forms of loss (of persons, resources, livelihoods), lack of (received or perceived) social support, distress impacting on normal functioning, the decay of the recovery environment, and secondary stressors in the disaster aftermath (related to damaged infrastructure, lacking health support, social conflict, and uncertainties about the future). Vulnerable population groups identified to be at particular risk and warranting special attention included those with pre-existing difficulties or severe mental illness, children, the elderly, socially isolated individuals, and people with disabilities.

3.1.2. Emerging Risks (European Migration Crisis)

A second set of emerging mental health risks revolved around the unfolding refugee and migration crisis in Europe, with many experts indicating involvement in this crisis either inside or outside of Europe. Principal mental health risks identified in this context were often reflective of underpinning social and physical determinants of health. These highlighted the role of displacement as a major mental health risk factor given the loss of continuity of care, the impact of family separation (on anxiety, depression, identity loss), as well as frequent occurrences of unresolved missing person situations (which provided no opportunity for closure or appropriate mourning). Mental health risks specific to younger generations were posed by: disrupted education and development paths for youth (during an already challenging and critical developmental stage); the impact of disrupted schooling and language barriers on cognitive development; as well as lacking access to normal peers, play, and structure for children; and the impacts of malnutrition on the mother-child bond, routine lactation, and cognitive/physical development of infants.

3.1.3. Recognition of Complex Mental Health Impacts

Failure to recognise the complexity and diversity of mental health impacts in disaster-affected populations was identified as a pivotal risk in the design and conduct of appropriate disaster mental health responses. Importantly, this included the risk of failing to detect those individuals who proceed to develop more persistent or severe mental health problems, distinct from those who initially experience common transitory distress responses. The shortcomings of a reductionist view were highlighted in terms of the failure to differentiate varying mental health risks of specific population groups (e.g., those affected directly or indirectly, or first responders), and in terms of a sole focus on specific signature disorders (such as post-traumatic stress disorder), rather than the relevant broader spectrum of disaster mental health outcomes and psychosocial consequences. Over-pathologisation on the part of disaster response planners further entails the risk of mismanaging normal human distress reactions to abnormal or disastrous circumstances. However, under-pathologisation may run the risk of failing to identify or reach those with significant mental health problems who may not otherwise readily access or seek support. Varied mental health risks posed by different disaster types and contexts, and interactions with pre-existing problems in disaster-affected communities, further compound the challenge of recognising complex disaster impacts in the design of appropriate mental health responses.

3.1.4. Provision of Appropriate Mental Health Support

Specific risks associated with the provision of appropriate mental health support to disaster-affected populations include the potential use of ineffective early interventions (such as debriefing), the lack of timely psychosocial care, the absence of clear and timely community information, and the lack of recognition of longer-term mental health provisions that needed to be put in place. In view of diverse emerging mental health problems and known barriers in the access to mental healthcare, the need was highlighted for a delicate balance between an emphasis on proactive support intervention and a stance of watchful waiting. This balance would help optimally align support efforts with the stage of recovery and nature of presenting problems, and not alienate affected individuals and communities in the process.

3.1.5. Disaster Response Communication and Coordination

Broader mental health risks were also identified in the context of disaster response communication and coordination. Non-consultative and top-down approaches of disaster response authorities can create mental health risks for affected communities further down the track. Politician behavior in disaster contexts can also be informed by and affecting public sentiment, whereas public perception of the way in which presenting health problems are handled or addressed by responsible authorities may pose a political risk for decision makers. Inherent risks of public disaster response communication included a general lack of communication, the uncertainty of (intended) outcomes, and possibility of unintended consequences. Moreover, disaster-poor countries can face challenges in communicating disaster risks to the wider public with a view to motivate self-protective action, which may lead to a stronger reliance on public authorities and experts in disaster contexts. Hierarchically organised civil protection systems, which are not traditionally citizen-centric, have therefore often failed to recognise existing community agency, resources, and self-help potential, or have struggled to translate a prevailing rhetoric of citizen engagement into effective practice. Conversely, the lack of public risk awareness, proper citizen engagement, and overarching stakeholder coordination and cooperation also increases the risk of adverse disaster outcomes and consequences.

3.2. Current DMH Strategies to Address Risks

When asked about key strategies through which the DMH field was addressing these principal disaster mental health risks, experts identified strategies within four main areas.

3.2.1. Development of Guidelines and Response Plans

The development of overarching psychosocial disaster guidelines and response plans was seen as pivotal to the design and conduct of effective disaster responses and to addressing mental health risks in disaster contexts. Specifically, organisations with routine involvement in disaster responses will need to have psychosocial disaster plans in place. Although generic plans may never be specific enough to capture unique disaster circumstances, these nevertheless provide an important planning framework that can be adapted to concrete scenarios.

3.2.2. Mechanisms to Identify and Direct People to Appropriate Support

Key mechanisms to detect and direct disaster-affected individuals to appropriate mental health support included the establishment of on-scene information and advice centres, the implementation of psychological screen and treat programs, and the establishment of disaster health registers. The role of public mental health awareness and wellbeing campaigns was raised in this context, as was the newly-developed concept of health passports for refugees and migrants, which may assist in providing greater continuity of care and access to vital medications across national boundaries.

3.2.3. Psychosocial and Mental Health Support Strategies

Designated mental health support strategies emphasised the need to provide screening, effective early intervention, and psychosocial support within the broader context of practical assistance. The need for basic psychosocial support strategies that could be provided by lay people and volunteer-based disaster relief agencies was highlighted. Specific psychosocial support strategies identified included the creation of safe spaces for vulnerable groups (in terms of child-friendly spaces, non-formal schooling, or breast-feeding tents), as well as the provision of parental support, livelihood skill building, general information, or legal advice. Awareness raising for the specific situation and issues affecting (and advocating the protection of) vulnerable groups was considered particularly critical in the context of violence against women and for residents of psychiatric institutions. The integration of mental health support within primary care and ceasing of opportunities to strengthen existing mental health systems and 'build back better' after disaster were equally highlighted as key avenues to address systemic mental health risks in disaster contexts.

3.2.4. Disaster Preparedness Planning

Other strategies and avenues to reduce disaster mental health risks were identified in the context of disaster preparedness planning. These included the provision of dedicated first responder training, the establishment of organisational support systems, mechanisms to facilitate multiagency networking, cooperation and joint planning, and the mapping of existing services. The importance of prior vulnerability and needs assessments (including geographical mapping of vulnerable groups) was highlighted, as was the need to involve these groups and the broader public in disaster preparedness planning. The resulting need to adapt existing alert systems, evacuation plans, and risk/crisis communication to the needs of vulnerable groups was emphasised, as was the potential to adopt a stronger focus on resilience-building activities throughout the whole cycle of disaster prevention, preparedness, response, and recovery planning.

3.3. Challenges to DMH/DRR Integration

Several questions explored the intersection of DMH and DRR in more depth, including existing challenges and opportunities for the integration of the two fields. Key integration challenges highlighted DMH and DRR as rather separate fields of practice, marked by practitioners from different professional backgrounds and a mutual lack of awareness. The use of technical jargon on either side was seen as an impediment to effective integration, as was the lack of DMH stakeholder involvement in the Sendai implementation process. The relative vagueness of the Sendai Framework, which does not specify key mental health risks to be addressed, along with its broad aims were seen to harbor the potential to lead to mental health initiatives that are not necessarily the most beneficial. Key challenges to greater recognition and use of existing DMH strategies within DRR included the lack of an empirical evidence base for specific psychosocial support strategies (which science requires to inform policy), and challenges in effective targeting of more preventative resilience-building initiatives before disaster strikes. Conversely, it was recognised that the Sendai implementation process did not necessarily follow a uniform international pattern but rather required unique integration within national systems and structures. Potential professional role and resource implications of the integration of the two fields were raised in terms of the necessary willingness of professionals to step outside of their brief, the perception that extra work or resources may be required, or that a stronger focus on community empowerment within DMH could result in less funding for traditional clinical or other core work. Other integration challenges included the limited sustainability of project-based initiatives, and lacking recognition of the vital role of DMH stakeholders in joint pre-disaster planning (beyond common ad-hoc involvement in response and recovery).

3.4. DMH/DRR Integration Opportunities

Notwithstanding these challenges, experts identified wide ranging opportunities for the stronger integration of the two fields. Key integration avenues involved the use of inter-sectoral platforms, joint stakeholder meetings, and preparedness summits, as well as disaster-related information and referral websites, and mobile phone applications. Joint DRR-DMH fact sheets and DRR primers for DMH staff may facilitate mutual practitioner understanding. Building on existing European projects and networks, the development of a shared European position was regarded as useful. In this context, major disaster events were also seen as progress catalysts that can provide opportunities to explore new solutions and trial different ways of operating.

DMH experts and practitioners can facilitate DMH/DRR integration by advocating the recognition of mental health issues in disaster prevention and response planning, integrating mental health knowledge at higher strategy and local planning levels, providing guidance on where mental health funding and efforts are best spent, and by continuing to build the underpinning DMH evidence base. Simultaneously, it was recognised that DMH must become better at providing clear and understandable messages and at marketing DMH knowledge, so that it can be more readily used by local authorities and stakeholders. Other DMH contributions to foster integration included psychosocial capacity analysis at the municipal level, prior vulnerability mapping, and knowledge and skill building in vulnerable groups to enhance self-help capacity and psychosocial stress management.

Integration can also be facilitated by expanding the prevailing DRR mandate to include mental health, such as by addressing psychological stressors in public crisis communication, including mental health messaging in non-formal education, as well as through professional selection and equipment of first responders with the vital skills to handle common stress reactions.

Promising conceptual interlinkages that facilitate future DMH/DRR integration efforts revolved around a shared focus on resilience building, the use of health promotion strategies, community-based and self-help approaches, and community mobilisation concepts that are already embedded in international guidelines for psychosocial emergency response. Other interlinkages exist between health and disaster literacy approaches, and between healthy cities and urban resilience frameworks.

Formal integration steps highlighted the benefits of incorporating DMH guidelines as an appendix to the Sendai Framework, the need to operationalise DMH/DRR linkages and interventions to support broader application and effectiveness testing, devote project funding to integration efforts, and mandate stronger interdisciplinary and interagency work, such as in joint disaster planning.

4. Discussion

The findings of this exploratory study provide a first look at the DMH field through a DRR lens, and a vital perspective on the intersection of these two fields that can facilitate future integration efforts. Study findings indicate that it is clearly early days in terms of the formal integration of the fields, and that Sendai disaster policy awareness within the mental health field may be limited. Yet, the impending application of DRR concepts and approaches across varied societal sectors and health domains in the context of the Sendai implementation provides a pertinent and timely opportunity to examine its conceptual and practical implications for DMH and other established fields of practice.

4.1. Conceptualising DMH Risks: The Place of Risk Within DMH

Application of the Sendai objective of understanding disaster risk within the context of a specific health domain and field of practice (such as DMH) inevitably involves the task of fleshing out an otherwise generic (or content-neutral) notion of disaster risk, with domain-specifically relevant content that is consistent with the broader Sendai notion. A better understanding of pre-existing notions of disaster risk held among practitioners within a given health domain therefore constitutes an important preliminary step in developing a shared conceptual understanding and joint future integration and work agenda.

In appraising the nature of principal DMH risks identified by the experts, and the place of risk within the DMH field more broadly, it is evident that DMH has developed an existing risk vocabulary (and associated evidence base) that is primarily centered on established risk factors for adverse disaster mental health outcomes. Such risk factors include a wide range of predisposing factors (such as age, gender, socio-economic status, or pre-existing difficulties), as well as factors related to disaster exposure and secondary stressors, all of which have been well established in the literature [3].

Nevertheless, beyond the primacy of this risk factor-driven understanding, the broad scope of identified principal DMH risks also spanned newly emerging mental health risks (contextually bound to the European migration crisis) and risks associated with the design and delivery of adequate support interventions (such as the recognition of complex disaster mental health impacts, the provision of appropriate mental health support, and broader disaster response communication and coordination). As a whole, these principal DMH risks are reflective of the developmental stage, existing sophistication, and key challenges of the field. Moreover, all these DMH risk notions (either directly or indirectly) have a shared concern with the potential for adverse disaster mental health outcomes.

Specific DMH risk factors identified in this study are structurally different from the broader (probabilistic) notion of disaster risk, elaborated and defined in the Sendai Framework as "The potential loss of life, injury, or destroyed or damaged assets which could occur to a system, society, or a community in a specific period of time, determined probabilistically as a function of hazard, exposure, vulnerability, and capacity" [16]. DMH risk factors are perhaps more akin to various elements of this definition, such as the key concepts of vulnerability, exposure, and (as in the case of the latter DMH risks) capacity.

When DMH risks are classified in terms of the specific nature of adverse disaster outcomes considered, it becomes possible to distinguish at least three different types of DMH risk, and to conceive of DMH risk more generally, as the likelihood and severity of:

(1) Newly emerging or exacerbated mental health issues among disaster-affected populations (Type A)
(2) Adverse impacts on existing mental health support systems (Type B), for example, in terms of client/staff safety and wellbeing, infrastructure damage, service disruption, surge capacity, evacuation, and business continuity
(3) Secondary effects of A and B on individual, community, business, and societal functioning (Type C)

Beyond these principal DMH risk types, it is also possible to identify more intermediate DMH risks, such as:

(4) Lack of DMH preparedness or capacity (Type D)
(5) Poor quality, lacking efficiency, efficacy, and coordination of DMH responses (Type E)

Nevertheless, although these latter intermediate risks may constitute ongoing key challenges of the field, these can also generally be regarded subordinate to principal DMH risks of Types A and B. In considering the nature of domain-specific DMH risks of Types A–C, it is again helpful to draw upon the broader Sendai notion of disaster risk. This notion calls us to move beyond the mere consideration of adverse outcomes, and to adopt a comprehensive understanding of disaster risk as determined by the key aspects of hazard, exposure, and existing vulnerabilities and capacities [16].

4.2. Current Focus of DMH (Risk Reduction) Strategies

In view of the nature of identified mental health risks in disaster contexts, much of the existing arsenal of DMH strategies has traditionally been focused on addressing these risks during disaster response and recovery phases. As such, these strategies could be seen to require the prior occurrence of disaster event exposure in order to become relevant or applicable. Yet, interview data also suggested an increasing trend toward the exploration of more proactive, preventative, and resilience building initiatives within DMH, which, while still fledging in terms of an empirical evidence base [17], would also be well aligned with broader developments in disaster policy and the move toward the promotion of disaster resilient communities, health systems, and societies [18,19].

4.3. Sendai's Dual Challenge for DMH

In this context, it is interesting to note that the principal reference to mental health in the Sendai Framework (Priority 4, paragraph 33o; see Introduction) encapsulates an implicit understanding of DMH that firmly locates the role of the field within disaster recovery and building back better phases. As such, this conceptual understanding also reinforces the traditional DMH focus and self-understanding. It is also in this narrow sense that the genuine conceptual challenge posed by the Sendai Framework for DMH policy may be considered comparatively negligible, notwithstanding substantial variability in the existing capacity of countries to effectively apply DMH policy and know-how in practice [20]. Put differently, the implications of this narrowly conceived Sendai challenge for DMH may be less about the aim of finding new and innovative ways of doing things, but rather about becoming more professional at those activities in which the field at large is already engaged; perhaps resulting in a greater need for capacity building or upscaling (particularly in resource-poor countries), rather than broader reorientation or reinvention.

Yet, while undoubtedly more work must be done in terms of strengthening the existing capacity, effectiveness, integration, and sustainability of DMH systems [21], Sendai's conceptual challenge for DMH policy and practice (in a broader sense) goes further. When Sendai's underpinning philosophy of understanding and reducing disaster risk is taken to heart, it becomes possible to look beyond DMH's established role as post-disaster savior, and to explore the potential role that the DMH field (via existing or future strategies) may be able to assume in reducing disaster risks and in averting adverse disaster mental health consequences, before these occur. The implications of this broader Sendai challenge for DMH may thus require a potential shift in conceptual emphasis—away from the current focus on downstream interventions and toward the exploration of more proactive upstream strategies that are effective at reducing DMH risks [13].

4.4. Sendai Implementation Requirements

Global Sendai Framework implementation between 2015 and 2030 will be monitored on the basis of national progress reporting across UN member states against agreed targets and indicators [16]. The ability of member states to demonstrate progress in terms of not only the existence but outcomes of effective DRR strategies has direct implications for societal sectors and health domains, and for the field of DMH. Key Sendai progress indicators of relevance to health include quantifiable reductions in the number of deaths (A-2), missing persons (A-3), injured or ill people (B-2), each per 100,000 population; as well as in the number of destroyed or damaged health facilities (D-2), and disruptions to health services (D-7) attributable to disasters [16,22].

When these health-related Sendai implementation requirements are viewed through the lens of the above DMH risk typology, these would primarily call for a better understanding and the reduction of principal DMH risks of Type A (in alignment with Sendai indicator B-2) and Type B (in alignment with indicators D-2 and D-7), whereas wider societal benefits of monitoring, enumerating, and reducing secondary, or more intermediate DMH risks of Types C–E, are also evident.

In this context, the Bangkok Principles, in support of the implementation of the health aspects of the Sendai Framework [23] and related UN guidance directives, also specifically highlight the importance of incorporating relevant (mental) health indicator data within comprehensive national disaster risk assessments [24], associated disaster loss databases [25], and multi-hazard early warning systems. Future monitoring of Sendai implementation progress in terms of the reduction of principal DMH risks is therefore critically dependent on the systematic identification, collection, and incorporation of mental health indicator data within these planning and reporting processes to ascertain reduced disaster impacts at population and service system levels over time.

4.5. Study Limitations

As the first study explicitly focussing on the nexus of DMH and DRR, this study adopted an open-exploratory and not theoretically-driven approach to examining DMH risks, strategies, and conceptual interlinkages of these fields from the perspective of European DMH and DRR experts. In view of the social construction of disaster risk [26], it is conceivable that exploration of these issues with other stakeholder groups (such as lay people or professionals from other regions) may have resulted in different conceptualisations of risk or priority strategies to address these. Specific DMH risks identified in this study may also, at least in part, be socio-historically contingent upon major events unfolding in the study region at the time. Although interview participants in this exploratory study represented eminent DMH and DRR experts at each of the targeted European regional and national levels, the purposive study sampling frame and relatively small sample size may have limited the representativeness and generalisability of study findings. The broader project policy focus on the Sendai Framework implementation across Europe placed restrictions on the extent to which its implications could be examined for more specific national or local DMH practice traditions.

4.6. Implications and Future Directions

DMH is in a favorable position to tackle the Sendai challenge to both inform DRR, and in turn, be informed by DRR. Expert identification of mental health risks and strategies does not necessarily imply that these risks are generally well understood or that such strategies are already widely in place across countries. The inclusion of mental health in the Sendai Framework is laudable, yet its general formulation does not reflect the existing key challenges and sophistication of the DMH field. DMH therefore needs to guide DRR on the relevant mental health risks and aspects of disasters and on the choice of effective strategies to address these. In turn, a shift in DMH orientation and further steps will be required to effectively translate DRR principles and concepts into DMH policy and practice.

This study outlined several strategies and conceptual interlinkages that can facilitate future DMH/DRR integration efforts and provided valuable insights and lessons for the integration of global disaster policy in other health domains and established fields of practice.

Future efforts to integrate global DRR policy within a given health domain need to address several interrelated levels. At a conceptual level, key DRR concepts and principles, such as disaster risk and risk reduction, need to be examined in terms of their compatibility with and implications for prevailing doctrines and practice approaches [27]. The application of a DRR approach within a given health domain, such as DMH, thus first and foremost requires completing a rather abstract notion of disaster risk with health domain-specifically relevant content and meaning. Whereas the Sendai Framework provides broad parameters and agreed-upon definitions of key DRR concepts, it is essential that we turn to practitioners and experts within these fields to better understand principal disaster risks and existing strengths and limitations of key strategies to address these risks at present.

At a policy level, integration can be facilitated through systematic mapping of the Sendai Framework against existing policies and practice guidelines to identify key areas of overlap, existing gaps, inform strategic future planning, and focus areas for further development. Insightful examples of comprehensive Sendai mapping exercises already exist in regard to EU policies [28], and the U.K.'s existing doctrine of integrated emergency management [29]. Future efforts to integrate DRR within DMH would thus benefit from systematically mapping the Sendai Framework against DMH policies and guidelines at varied entity levels including international, national, sub-national, and agency levels.

At a translational level, results of these foundational exercises can inform the shape and focus of key activities to operationalize existing linkages between these fields. These include the identification of promising bridging approaches or innovative case studies—at policy, service, or practical intervention levels—that can be applied more broadly and tested for effectiveness. Capitalizing upon and further developing existing avenues for joint cooperation between DMH and DRR sectors will become increasingly important, as is ensuring adequate DMH and health sector representation at all levels of the Sendai implementation process. In this respect, it is critical that mental health specific indicators be developed that align with broader Sendai indicators to facilitate ongoing monitoring and reporting of Sendai progress in terms of reduced mental health impacts at population and service system levels over time. One of the key strengths of the Sendai Framework is that it combines an ambitious and timely global policy program with broad multinational buy-in and clear guidance to facilitate its implementation at global, regional, national, and local levels.

Health domain-specific DRR integration efforts can complement broad-based, whole-society DRR approaches by highlighting the relevance of DRR policy and implications of key DRR concepts, addressing existing translation barriers, and helping to unlock the unique DRR potential within established fields of practice. Notably, designated DMH interventions constitute one key element in the broader arsenal of DRR strategies that can reduce future risk of disaster exposure, associated traumatic impacts, and adverse mental health consequences. Therefore, effective disaster mental health risk reduction requires the application and integration of effective DMH strategies in the context of broad-based DRR strategies [13]. To further strengthen its unique role and contribution in the Sendai implementation process, the DMH field needs to intensify its efforts to establish a sound evidence base to support the choice of effective interventions, to sustainably build its disaster preparedness and response capacity, and to actively explore the merit of more preventative upstream strategies. The recently established World Health Organization (WHO) Thematic Platform for Health Emergency and Disaster Risk Management Research [30,31] provides a promising overarching context in which to further examine principal disaster mental health risks (Types A–E) and more effective strategies to reduce these risks in future.

5. Conclusions

Successful Sendai Framework implementation and efforts to reduce disaster mental health risks critically hinge upon the application of both concerted broad-based DRR and effective DMH strategies, and on the effective integration of DRR principles within existing health domains and established fields of practice.

Acknowledgments: Some of the central ideas expressed in this paper were originally presented at the UNISDR Science and Technology Conference in Geneva, Switzerland in January 2016 and at the 32nd Annual Meeting of the International Society for Traumatic Stress Studies in Dallas, TX, USA in November 2016.

References

1. The Human Cost of Weather-related Disasters 1995–2015. Available online: https://www.unisdr.org/files/46796_cop21weatherdisastersreport2015.pdf (accessed on 4 September 2018).
2. Berry, H.L.; Bowen, K.; Kjellstrom, T. Climate change and mental health: A causal pathways framework. *Int. J. Public Health* **2010**, *55*, 123–132. [CrossRef] [PubMed]
3. Norris, F.H.; Friedman, M.J.; Watson, P.J.; Byrne, C.M.; Diaz, E.; Kaniasty, K. 60,000 disaster victims speak: Part I. An empirical review of the empirical literature, 1981–2001. *Psychiatry* **2002**, *65*, 207–239. [CrossRef] [PubMed]
4. Neria, Y.; Nandi, A.; Galea, S. Post-traumatic stress disorder following disasters: A systematic review. *Psychol. Med.* **2008**, *38*, 467–480. [CrossRef] [PubMed]
5. The Economic Cost of the Social Impact of Natural Disasters. Available online: http://australianbusinessroundtable.com.au/our-research/social-costs-report (accessed on 4 September 2018).
6. Sendai Framework for Disaster Risk Reduction 2015–2030. Available online: https://www.preventionweb.net/files/43291_sendaiframeworkfordrren.pdf (accessed on 4 September 2018).
7. Hyogo Framework for Action 2005–2015: Building the Resilience of Nations and Communities to Disasters. Available online: https://www.unisdr.org/files/1037_hyogoframeworkforactionenglish.pdf (accessed on 4 September 2018).
8. Murray, V.; Aitsi-Selmi, A.; Blanchard, K. The role of public health within the United Nations post-2015 framework for disaster risk reduction. *Int. J. Disaster Risk Sci.* **2015**, *6*, 28–37. [CrossRef]

9. Aitsi-Selmi, A.; Murray, V. The Sendai framework: Disaster risk reduction through a health lens. *Bull. World Health Organ.* **2015**, *93*, 362. [CrossRef] [PubMed]
10. Tsutsumi, A.; Izutsu, T.; Ito, A.; Thornicroft, G.; Patel, V.; Minas, H. Mental health mainstreamed in new UN disaster framework. *Lancet Psychiatry* **2015**, *2*, 679–680. [CrossRef]
11. Murray, V. Disaster Risk Reduction, Health, and the Post-2015 United Nations Landmark Agreements. *Disaster Med. Public Health Prep.* **2014**, *8*, 283–287. [CrossRef] [PubMed]
12. Dar, O.; Buckley, E.J.; Rokadiya, S.; Huda, Q.; Abrahams, J. Integrating health into disaster risk reduction strategies: Key considerations for success. *Am. J. Public Health* **2014**, *104*, 1811–1816. [CrossRef] [PubMed]
13. Reifels, L. Disaster Mental Health Risk Reduction: An Upstream Paradigm Shift for Disaster Mental Health. In Proceedings of the UNISDR Science and Technology Conference on the Implementation of the Sendai Framework for Disaster Risk Reduction 2015–2030, Geneva, Switzerland, 27–29 January 2016.
14. Halpern, J.; Tramontin, M. A history of disaster mental health. In *Disaster Mental Health: Theory and Practice*; Thomson: Belmont, CA, USA, 2007; pp. 46–79.
15. Watson, P.J.; Brymer, M.J.; Bonanno, G.A. Postdisaster psychological intervention since 9/11. *Am. Psychol.* **2011**, *66*, 482–494. [CrossRef] [PubMed]
16. Report of the Open-Ended Intergovernmental Expert Working Group on Indicators and Terminology Relating to Disaster Risk Reduction. Available online: https://www.preventionweb.net/files/50683_oiewgreportenglish.pdf (accessed on 4 September 2018).
17. Joyce, S.; Shand, F.; Tighe, J.; Laurent, S.J.; Bryant, R.A.; Harvey, S.B. Road to resilience: A systematic review and meta-analysis of resilience training programmes and interventions. *BMJ Open* **2018**, *8*, e017858. [CrossRef] [PubMed]
18. Beerlage, I. Community resilience. In *Atlas of Vulnerability and Resilience—Pilot Version for Germany, Austria, Liechtenstein and Switzerland*; Fekete, A., Hufschmidt, G., Eds.; Cologne: Bonn, Germany, 2016; pp. 32–33, ISBN 978-3-946573-12-8.
19. World Health Organization. *Operational Framework for Building Climate Resilient Health Systems*; World Health Organization: Geneva, Switzerland, 2015; ISBN 978 92 4 156507 3.
20. Te Brake, H.; Dückers, M. Early psychosocial interventions after disasters, terrorism and other shocking events: Is there a gap between norms and practice in Europe? *Eur. J. Psychotraumatol.* **2013**, *4*, 19093. [CrossRef] [PubMed]
21. Reifels, L.; Pietrantoni, L.; Prati, G.; Kim, Y.; Kilpatrick, D.G.; Dyb, G.; Halpern, J.; Olff, M.; Brewin, C.R.; O'Donnell, M. Lessons learned about psychosocial responses to disaster and mass trauma: An international perspective. *Eur. J. Psychotraumatol.* **2013**, *4*. [CrossRef] [PubMed]
22. Maini, R.; Clarke, L.; Blanchard, K.; Murray, V. The Sendai Framework for Disaster Risk Reduction and Its Indicators—Where Does Health Fit in? *Int. J. Disaster Risk Sci.* **2017**, *8*, 150–155. [CrossRef]
23. Bangkok Principles for the Implementation of the Health Aspects of the Sendai Framework for Disaster Risk Reduction 2015–2030. Available online: http://www.who.int/hac/events/2016/Bangkok_Principles.pdf (accessed on 4 September 2018).
24. Words into Action Guidelines: National Disaster Risk Assessment. Governance System, Methodologies, and Use of Results (Consultative Version). Available online: https://www.unisdr.org/files/52828_nationaldisasterriskassessmentwiagu.pdf (accessed on 4 September 2018).
25. Disaster Loss Data in Monitoring the Implementation of the Sendai Framework. Available online: https://council.science/cms/2017/05/DRR-policy-brief-2-data.pdf (accessed on 4 September 2018).
26. Chipangura, P.; Van Niekerk, D.; Van Der Waldt, G. An exploration of objectivism and social constructivism within the context of disaster risk. *Disaster Prev. Manag.* **2016**, *25*, 261–274. [CrossRef]
27. Phibbs, S.; Kenney, C.; Severinsen, C.; Mitchell, J.; Hughes, R. Synergising Public Health Concepts with the Sendai Framework for Disaster Risk Reduction: A Conceptual Glossary. *Int. J. Environ. Res. Public Health* **2016**, *13*, 1241. [CrossRef] [PubMed]
28. Action Plan on the Sendai Framework for Disaster Risk Reduction 2015–2030. A Disaster Risk-Informed Approach for All EU Policies. Available online: http://ec.europa.eu/echo/sites/echo-site/files/1_en_document_travail_service_part1_v2.pdf (accessed on 4 September 2018).

29. Disaster Risk Reduction and the Sendai Framework. What Does it Mean for UK resilience practitioners? Available online: https://www.epcresilience.com/EPC/media/Images/Knowledge%20Centre/Occasionals/OP21-Disaster-Risk-Reduction-Jun-2017.pdf (accessed on 4 September 2018).
30. Lo, S.T.T.; Chan, E.Y.Y.; Chan, G.K.W.; Murray, V.; Abrahams, J.; Ardalan, A.; Kayano, R.; Yau, J.C.W. Health Emergency and Disaster Risk Management (Health-EDRM): Developing the Research Field within the Sendai Framework Paradigm. *Int. J. Disaster Risk Sci.* **2017**, *8*, 145–149. [CrossRef]
31. Health Emergency and Disaster Risk Management: Mental Health and Psychosocial Support Factsheet. Available online: http://www.who.int/hac/techguidance/preparedness/risk-management-mental-health-december2017.pdf (accessed on 4 September 2018).

11

WHO Thematic Platform for Health Emergency and Disaster Risk Management Research Network (TPRN): Report of the Kobe Expert Meeting

Ryoma Kayano [1,*], Emily YY Chan [2], Virginia Murray [3], Jonathan Abrahams [4] and Sarah Louise Barber [1]

1 World Health Organization Centre for Health Development, Kobe 651-0073, Japan; barbers@who.int
2 Collaborating Centre for Oxford University and Chinese University of Hong Kong for Disaster and Medical Humanitarian Response (CCOUC), School of Public Health and Primary Care, The Chinese University of Hong Kong, HongKong, China; Emily.chan@cuhk.edu.hk
3 Public Health England, London SE1 8UG, UK; Virginia.Murray@phe.gov.uk
4 Country Health Emergency Preparedness and International Regulations Department, WHO Health Emergencies Programme, World Health Organization, CH-1211 Geneva, Switzerland; abrahamsj@who.int
* Correspondence: kayanor@who.int

Abstract: The WHO Thematic Platform for Health Emergency and Disaster Risk Management Research Network (TPRN) was established in 2016 in response to the Sendai Framework for Disaster Risk Reduction 2015–2030. The TPRN facilitates global collaborative action for improving the scientific evidence base in health emergency and disaster risk management (Health EDRM). In 2018, the WHO convened a meeting to identify key research questions, bringing together leading experts from WHO, TPRN, World Association for Disaster and Emergency Medicine (WADEM), and the Japan International Cooperation Agency, and delegates to the Asia Pacific Conference on Disaster Medicine (APCDM). The meeting identified research questions in five major areas for Health EDRM: health data management, psychosocial management, community risk management, health workforce development, and research methods and ethics. Funding these key research questions is essential to accelerate evidence-based actions during emergencies and disasters.

Keywords: health emergency and disaster risk management (Health EDRM); Sendai Framework for Disaster Risk Reduction 2015–2030; WHO Thematic Platform for Health EDRM; health data; psychosocial; risk communication; capacity building; research methods; ethics

---

1. Introduction

Over the past few decades, the frequency of disasters has increased as a result of a number of risk drivers including unplanned urbanization and unmitigated climate change. The impact of many of these disasters on human health has also become more severe, due in part to increasing numbers of vulnerable populations, including older persons. The 2015 Third UN World Conference on Disaster Risk Reduction (WCDRR) established the Sendai Framework on Disaster Risk Reduction 2015–2030 (SFDRR), which introduced a framework for action across the disaster risk management (DRM) continuum (prevention, preparedness, response, and recovery) and sought to enhance the resilience of communities and health and social systems. With more than 30 references to health issues specifically, the framework includes health in its goal as "the substantial reduction of disaster risk and losses in lives, livelihoods and health . . . ." [1]. It also emphasizes the importance of improving the scientific evidence base to advance health emergency and disaster risk management (Health EDRM).

In response, World Health Organization (WHO) established the WHO Thematic Platform for Health EDRM Research Network (TPRN) to promote global collaboration among academia [2,3], government officials and other stakeholders to generate better scientific evidence to inform policy and practice for managing health risks associated with emergencies and disaster. In 2017, leaders of this research network published a review paper on the Sendai Framework implementation and recommendations on Health EDRM research [4,5]. The paper highlighted the critical importance of research before, during and after disasters (not only the acute phase) and gave consideration to the following: a holistic approach, including physical, mental and psychosocial health and well-being; identifying populations at risk with specific health needs; standardization of needs assessments, standardization of evaluation methodologies and reporting systems for countries, communities and individual cases; multidisciplinary and multi-sectoral approaches; and a review of research for informing better policy development and implementation.

To accelerate research in Health EDRM, the WHO organized a meeting to identify key research gaps and questions by convening the leading experts from WHO, World Association for Disaster and Emergency Medicine (WADEM), and Japan International Cooperation Agency (JICA), and delegates to the Asia Pacific Conference on Disaster Medicine (APCDM). The WHO Kobe Center (WKC) organized the meeting as one of the programs during APCDM 2018 on 17 October 2018, in Kobe, Japan [6].

2. Materials and Methods

The purpose of the meeting was to identify concrete research questions based on the established overarching priorities in line with the published reviews of research needs conducted by the coordinators of the WHO Thematic Platform for Health EDRM Research Network (TPRN) [4,5]. The selection of the research themes, meeting participants and research questions were conducted as below.

As a first step, an open-ended consultation was conducted with the ten TPRN coordinators. Background information from the above-mentioned references [4,5] was shared for the consultation. Through this process, the first draft of the expert meeting agenda with potential discussion themes and background information was developed. Based on the potential discussion themes, 25 participants from 10 countries for the expert meeting were selected based on their global expertise in responding to health emergencies and natural disasters in consultation with the TPRN coordinators and APCDM organizers. They included the WHO Health-EDRM responsible officers in headquarters and regional offices in the Asia Pacific Region (Western Pacific Region and Southeast Asia Region), the TPRN co-chairs and representatives from international, regional or national organizations and societies involved in Health-EDRM (Public Health England, the Chinese University of Hong Kong, WADEM, Association of South-East Asian Nations (ASEAN) Secretariat, JICA, Government of Thailand, Japan Disaster Medical Assistance Team Secretariat; and leading researchers selected based on their previous academic works and Health-EDRM related activities.

As a second step, another consultation to finalize the major research themes was conducted with all of the potential 25 participants to obtain their feedback, and five major discussion themes were selected (Table 1). Based on the final confirmed meeting themes, participants were then selected to cover all the five research themes through consultation with stakeholders. Through this process, 32 experts from 12 countries (Australia, Canada, Hong Kong, India, Indonesia, Japan, Myanmar, New Zealand, Philippines, Thailand, UK, USA) were selected for the expert meeting. The meeting agenda with the five major discussion themes and their background information was shared with all the participants.

As a third step, the expert meeting was conducted as a session of APCDM. Two rounds of group discussions were conducted. The discussion on each theme was facilitated by a lead discussant selected based on their expertise and previous research under each area in Health-EDRM (Table 1). After the group discussions, a plenary discussion was conducted to integrate the results of the group discussions and reach consensus among the participants.

3. Key Research Gaps and Questions in Five Key Research Areas

The process resulted in a series of questions listed in Table 1.

Table 1. Key research questions in five major areas.

Area	Research Questions
Area 1 Health data management before, during and after emergencies and disasters Lead discussant: Tatsuhiko Kubo, University of Occupational and Environmental Health, Japan	(a) What are the national and regional challenges inhibiting implementation of the WHO standardized medical data collection systems after emergencies and disasters? (b) What is the broader health-related data needed to inform effective Health emergency and disaster risk management (EDRM), i.e., community vulnerabilities, hospital functional status, infrastructure, lifelines and health workforce?
Area 2 Psychosocial management before, during and after emergencies and disasters, and other medium and long-term effects on the public health and health system Lead discussant: Yoshiharu Kim, National Center for Neurology and Psychiatry, Japan	(a) How can mental health and psychosocial risk be classified using longitudinal and multi-centric studies? (b) How can methods for screening, diagnosis and treatment for affected people be standardized across different settings? (c) How can assets associated with greater community resilience be identified before, during, and after disaster?
Area 3 Community emergency and disaster risk management, including risk literacy and addressing needs of sub-populations Lead discussant: Emily Y.Y. Chan, The Chinese University of Hong Kong	(a) What architecture is needed to support research in Health EDRM including consensus among disciplines and ethics? (b) How can research be better translated to policy and practice across different backgrounds and contexts? (c) What kind of technology for information and data management and communication is needed for risk communication, emergency response and research design?
Area 4 Health workforce development for health emergency and disaster risk management Lead discussant: Jonathan Abrahams, World Health Organization	(a) How can different countries strengthen Health EDRM through disaster risk management training programs, and what strategies will support retention, motivation and deployment of trained people? (b) What are the best practices for sustaining the development of the local health workforce for Health EDRM, fostering positive interactions between external support workers and the local workforce, and enabling the transition to recovery and post-event Health EDRM? (c) What is the common knowledge or competencies required for Health EDRM?
Area 5 Research methods and ethics Lead discussant: Virginia Murray, Public Health England	(a) What are the definitions of research methods and technical terms for Health EDRM? (b) How can impact evaluation methods for intervention and qualitative–quantitative mixed methods be standardized? (c) How can the publication process for Health EDRM research become more systematic and effective? (d) What are the challenges and best practices in addressing national health system, cultural and religious issues before, during and after interventions?

The first research area was health data management before, during and after emergencies and disasters. Experts highlighted the significant progress made through the development of the WHO Emergency Medical Team (EMT) Minimum Data Set (MDS) in 2017 [7], enabling standardized data collection and reporting by EMTs dispatched to emergency areas. However, it was noted that implementation was not optimal. Further research is needed on reducing the implementation barriers in national and regional contexts, and the supplementary data required for broader public health action.

The second area was psychosocial management. Experts identified research priorities in the classification of mental health and psychosocial risk, standardization of methods for screening, diagnosis and treatment, and the identification of characteristics of risk and resilience among affected individuals and communities.

The third research area was community risk management and risk literacy. Experts identified the need to strengthen the components of research architecture to support research for Health EDRM, the means to translate research to policy and practice, and research to advance the technology of information and data management and communication for risk communication for Health EDRM, with the focus on an effective and localized risk communication approach to meet the requirements of the local community.

The fourth area was health workforce development. Experts identified knowledge gaps in a common understanding of relevant knowledge and competencies required for the Health EDRM workforce as well as the contents for in-house training/professional development and their interaction with stakeholders, and in understanding how to sustain the development of the local health workforce for Health EDRM, foster positive interactions between external support workers and the local workforce and the effective transition to recovery, integrating measures to reduce risks of future events and build stronger systems. More understanding is needed about how countries can strengthen Health EDRM through disaster risk management training programs, and how they are able to retain, motivate and utilize trained personnel, including for deployment.

The fifth area was research methods and ethics. To move beyond case studies, key research priorities including the basic definitions of research methods and technical terms in the field of Health EDRM setting, standardizing impact evaluation methodologies, and promoting publication of result in a systematic way. Lastly, the group identified the need for best practices in addressing national health systems, and cultural and religious issues. A research methods resource and book were thought to be important additions to the TPRN tools.

4. Follow-Up Actions

The expert meeting focused on identifying the key research needs in five major areas through formulating research questions. Specific approaches in responding to each research question should be discussed and implemented with additional studies and literature reviews conducted in a systematic way. These include: (a) conducting more implementation research using currently available health data collection tools (Area 1); (b) standardization of monitoring of long-term psychological consequences, and validation of individual-level and community-level interventions for better psychological consequences (Area 2); (c) identifying the existing challenges for better translation of research findings to policy and programs (Area 3); (d) conducting an inventory of the existing workforce development programs and identifying essential components of training programs (Area 4); and (e) integrating existing knowledge about research methods for Health-EDRM by developing guidance by global experts (Area 5). These follow-up actions are addressed in greater detail in the later theme-based articles.

Given this background, the meeting concluded with the commitment to organize an annual TPRN meeting and utilize other forums in collaboration with partner organizations to promote and update knowledge and experience in Health EDRM research. The meetings will update progress in the key research areas, and further expert consultations will be held to identify further research gaps and possible sources of funding. In 2019, the WKC will function as the secretariat of TPRN in collaboration with WHO HQ. The WHO will establish an information sharing platform to facilitate interactions among TPRN participants about Health EDRM research and science, as well as opportunities for funding, conferences and collaborative research.

5. Conclusions

The expert meeting contributed to setting forth some key research gaps to be addressed for the advancement of Health EDRM research. Successful implementation will require further research collaborations through the TPRN initiative, partnerships and resource mobilization.

The expert meeting did not reach consensus through blind rating, voting or a structured questionnaire-based approach, which are recommended by Delphi Method. This limitation will be addressed during the next follow-up expert meeting.

Author Contributions: Conceptualization, R.K. and E.Y.Y.C.; Writing-Original Draft Preparation, R.K.; Writing-Review & Editing, E.Y.Y.C., V.M., S.L.B. and J.A.; Project Administration, R.K., J.A.

Acknowledgments: The opinions contained in the paper are those of its authors and, except where specifically stated, are not intended to represent the official policies or positions of the WHO. The expert meeting was organized under the collaboration among WHO, APCDM 2018, and JICA. The authors express their gratitude to the following individuals who contributed substantially to meeting organization: Shinichi Nakayama (APCDM) and Masako Tani (Project for Strengthening the ASEAN Regional Capacity on Disaster Health Management (ARCH Project), JICA). The authors thank all the meeting participants who contributed to achieving the results (in alphabetical order of their last name): Myo Nyein Aung (Chiang Mai Rajabhat University, Thailand), Nilesh Buddh (WHO Regional Office for South East Asia), Cheuk Pong Chiu (The Chinese University of Hong Kong, China), Shinichi Egawa (Tohoku University, Japan), Paul Farrell (WADEM), Ferdinal Moreno Fernando (ASEAN Secretariat), Sayaka Gomei (Dokkyo Medical University, Japan), Mélissa Généreux (University of Sherbrooke, Canada), Teodoro Herbosa (University of the Philippines, Philippines), Shuichi Ikeda (ARCH Project, JICA), Tatruro Kai (Saiseikai Senri Hospital, Japan), Hiroshi Kato (Hyogo Institute for Traumatic Stress), Yoshiharu Kim (National Center for Neurology and Psychiatry, Japan), Yuichi Koido (Japan Disaster Medical Assistance Team (DMAT) Secretariat, Ministry of Health, Labor and Welfare, Japan), Tomoko Komagata (Tokyo Medical and Dental University, Japan), Tatsuhiko Kubo (University of Occupational and Environmental Health, Japan), Sonoe Mashino (University of Hyogo, Japan), Yasushi Nakajima (ARCH Project, JICA), Toshiyuki Ojima (Hamamatsu University School of Medicine, Japan), Yasuhiro Otomo (Tokyo Medical and Dental University, Japan), Heather Papowitz (WHO Regional Office for the Western Pacific), Philip Schluter (University of Canterbury, New Zealand), Phumin Silapunt (Chulabhorn Hospital, Thailand), Yosuke Takada (Okayama University, Japan), Sho Takahashi (University of Tsukuba, Japan), Nobuyo Tsuboyama-Kasaoka (National Institute of Health and Nutrition, Japan), Shiori Usami (Kumamoto University, Japan).

References

1. Sendai Framework for Disaster Risk Reduction 2015–2030. Available online: https://www.unisdr.org/we/inform/publications/43291 (accessed on 02 April 2019).
2. WHO Thematic Platform for Health Emergency and Disaster Risk Management. Available online: http://www.who.int/hac/techguidance/preparedness/WHO-Thematic-Platform-Health-EDRM-Terms-Reference-2018.pdf?ua=1 (accessed on 02 April 2019).
3. WHO Thematic Platform for Health Emergency and Disaster Risk Management Research Network. Available online: http://www.who.int/hac/techguidance/preparedness/WHO-Thematic-Platform-Health-EDRM-Research-Network-2018.pdf?ua=1 (accessed on 02 April 2019).
4. Chan, E.Y.Y.; Murray, V. What are the health research needs for the Sendai Framework. *Lancet* **2017**, *390*, e35–e36. [CrossRef]
5. Lo, S.T.T.; Chan, E.Y.Y.; Chan, G.K.W.; Murray, V.; Abrahams, J.; Ardalan, A.; Kayano, R.; Yau, J.C.W. Health Emergency and Disaster Risk Management (Health-EDRM): Developing the Research Field within the Sendai Framework Paradigm. *Int. J. Disaster Risk Sci.* **2017**, *8*, 145–149. [CrossRef]
6. Asian Pacific Conference for Disaster Medicine. 2018. Available online: http://www.apcdm2018.org/index.html (accessed on 02 April 2019).
7. Benin-Goren, O.; Kubo, T.; Norton, I. Emergency Medical Team Working Group for Minimum Data Set. *Prehosp. Disaster Med.* **2017**, *32* (Suppl. S1), S96. [CrossRef]

12

Outcomes of Establishing an Urgent Care Centre in the Same Location as an Emergency Department

Annelie Raidla [1,2], Katrin Darro [1,2], Tobias Carlson [2,3], Amir Khorram-Manesh [2,4], Johan Berlin [5] and Eric Carlström [2,6,7,*]

1 Emergency Department at Östra Hospital, Sahlgrenska University Hospital, 413 90 Gothenburg, Sweden; annelie.raidla@vgregion.se (A.R.); katrin.darro@vgregion.se (K.D.)
2 Gothenburg Emergency Research Group (GEMREG), Sahlgrenska University Hospital, 413 90 Gothenburg, Sweden; tobias.carlson@vgregion.se (T.C.); amir.khorram-manesh@surgery.gu.se (A.K.-M.)
3 Center of Emergency Department Development, Sahlgrenska University Hospital, 413 90 Gothenburg, Sweden
4 Institute of Clinical Sciences, Sahlgrenska Academy, Gothenburg University, 405 30 Gothenburg, Sweden
5 Department of Social and Behavioral Studies, University West, 461 86 Trollhättan, Sweden; johan.berlin@hv.se
6 Institute of Health and Care Sciences, Sahlgrenska Academy, University of Gothenburg, 405 30 Gothenburg, Sweden
7 USN School of Business, Campus Vestfold, University of South-Eastern Norway, 3603 Kongsberg, Norway
* Correspondence: eric.carlstrom@gu.se

Abstract: The emergency department (ED) is one of the busiest facilities in a hospital, and it is frequently described as a bottleneck that limits space and structures, jeopardising surge capacity during Major Incidents and Disasters (MIDs) and pandemics such as the COVID 19 outbreak. One remedy to facilitate surge capacity is to establish an Urgent Care Centre (UCC), i.e., a secondary ED, co-located and in close collaboration with an ED. This study investigates the outcome of treatment in an ED versus a UCC in terms of length of stay (LOS), time to physician (TTP) and use of medical services. If it was possible to make these parameters equal to or even less than the ED, UCCs could be used as supplementary units to the ED, improving sustainability. The results show reduced waiting times at the UCC, both in terms of TTP and LOS. In conclusion, creating a primary care-like facility in close proximity to the hospitals may not only relieve overcrowding of the hospital's ED in peacetime, but it may also provide an opportunity for use during MIDs and pandemics to facilitate the victims of the incident and society as a whole.

Keywords: urgent care centre; emergency department; length of stay; surge capacity; Sweden

---

1. Introduction

The increasing number of Major Incidents and Disasters (MIDs), either natural or man-made, necessitates preparedness in both human and material resources. This has become evident during the COVID 19 pandemic, which has caused tremendous pressure on Emergency Departments (EDs) in several countries. The concept of surge capacity initiated within the immediate period after an MID or the outbreak of a pandemic has the aim of increasing the number of staff and material, as well as creating spaces and structures based on validated and tested systems and procedures. However, an expanding incident necessitates an additional surge, a so-called secondary surge capacity with the intention of utilizing other possible resources. All these measures are implemented in accordance with the contingency plans for each organization, including healthcare, in order to create a more flexible surge capacity [1].

Most of the hospitals call in their staff and create operational spaces. The first stage entails sending home patients who are already admitted but do not need emergency care, or those who have already been treated and who can continue their recovery at home. This stage creates new beds and spaces for incoming patients. In the second phase, extra space should be created for the admission of emergency cases. Besides the ordinary ED, another admission unit is normally set up to handle either urgent patients or ordinary, non-emergency cases. An outpatient department is usually used. Whilst adequate, this approach needs to be planned as there is a clear need for staff who are familiar with the locales, equipment that has to be adjusted to emergency requirements, and procedures that can be put in place as quickly as possible based on disaster medicine principles [2].

Previous studies have shown that staff who lack such familiarity can cause more harm than save lives, and unfavourable spaces can cause more challenges than facilitating the process. In particular, EDs should have staff qualified in emergency medicine, areas for triage and sorting, and proper devices for the care of the severely injured. The optimum suggestion is actually an existing unit that already handles emergency cases, i.e., a secondary ED [3–6].

The emergency department is one of the hospital's busiest facilities and is frequently described as a bottleneck that limits space and structures, jeopardising surge capacity [7,8]. In recent decades, overcrowding in emergency departments (EDs) has been reported as an increasingly worrying occurrence [9,10]. It has been associated with longer waiting times prior to treatment for severely ill patients, risk of in-hospital mortality and a higher probability of leaving the ED against medical advice or without being seen [11]. During the height of the COVID 19 epidemic in Europe and the US in spring 2020, EDs experienced a tremendous peak in the number of patient presentations. Preparedness for disasters became a significant concern in relation to health-care sustainability, and several city-based hospitals throughout the world were operating at or near to capacity limits [12].

The issue of everyday overcrowding of EDs and the impact on preparedness to handle peaks such as that during COVID 19 appeared to be complex, with several factors including physical distancing, use of personal protective equipment and hygienic measures needing to be considered along with remedies required [13].

In the early 1980s, an increasing number of emergency cases led to the establishment of Urgent Care Centres (UCCs) [14]. They function as a healthcare provider staffed by primary care physicians, registered nurses and nurse practitioners, with the ability to handle emergency conditions that do not need ED amenities. UCCs are often managed by a hosting hospital and share mutual support systems such as laboratory, radiation and medical services. It has been reported that UCCs reduce the overuse of EDs by up to 48% [15]. Doran showed that patients treated by UCCs, sited together with and in close collaboration with an ED, received swift service and better follow-up than the control group in the study [16]. UCCs and EDs have also proven to be horizontally integrated and collaborative and function informally between ED and UCC staff [17].

This paper suggests that UCCs may be suitable units for beneficial use both in peacetime and during an MID. They fulfil the function as a supportive unit in peacetime, and by using the same staff and resources can easily be converted to an extra ED or a pandemic admission unit as evidenced by the current need during the COVID 19 epidemic. With the first UCC having been set up in Sweden, the aim of this study was to investigate the outcome of treatment in the ED versus the UCC in terms of quality, LOS, time to physician (TTP), use of medical services, referrals, revisits, hospitalisation, mortality and costs. If it was the case that these parameters were equal to the ED, the UCC could be used as a complementary unit to the ED, improving sustainability not only in peacetime but also during MIDs.

2. Methods

The ED and UCC studied were situated in a hospital in Gothenburg in western Sweden. The ED was part of a University Hospital, distributed over three main hospital complexes in different districts, with one ED each. Each of the EDs received approximately one-third of the 150,000 presentations annually in the city. The ED included was typical, i.e., treating diseases and injuries from age 16, excluding orthopaedic and psychiatric diseases. It received 53,840 visits during 2018, an increase of 4.8% over the year before (2017). The trend of more visits had been apparent during the last few decades. The ED served the part of the county characterised by the weakest socioeconomic status and highest proportion of immigrants. A UCC was established in spring 2018, staffed with primary care physicians and registered nurses. The UCC shared the triage line with the ED, with attendees being assessed post-triage as either ED or UCC patients. The UCC was expected to optimise shared resources and provide improved services for low-urgency patients. The study was approved by the Regional Ethical Review Board in Gothenburg with approval number: D 374-18.

2.1. Sample

The study was based on 200 patients fulfilling the inclusion criteria for visiting the UCC. The exclusion criteria were patients triaged red, patients with a preliminary diagnosis in most cases referred from the primary care centre to the ED (e.g., potential distal deep vein thrombosis, emergent vertigo etc.) and patients with a preliminary diagnosis potentially developing from non-red triage to a state of emergency (e.g., suspected ectopic pregnancy, dyspnoea, suspected urosepsis, etc.). A list of exclusion criteria based on a literature review was developed and implemented as a selective tool used in the triage at the ED. The STROBE checklist (strengthening the communication of observational studies in epidemiology) was used to guide the study process [18].

The first half (n = 100) of the 200 patients were selected retrospectively on a consecutive basis just prior to the UCC being established. Consequently, the first half were treated by the ED. The second half of the patients (n = 100) were selected consecutively from patients triaged to the UCC six months after it was established. No other substantial changes in organization or methods occurred at the ED during the study period.

The 200 patients were distributed over 104 men and 96 women, with an average age of 45 (SD = 20.24). The study size was based on a power estimation of a standardized statistical power of 0.80 and medium effect size of 0.3 premeditated the appropriate sample size to 93 participants in each population. The α significance level was 0.05 [19]. The two populations were compared in order to concur in terms of emergency and severity. They were triaged on a five-level scale from red (highest degree of emergency) to blue (non-urgent). The distribution was red = 0, orange = 3, yellow = 107, green = 89 and blue = 13 patients. The patients were all triaged according to the Rapid Emergency Triage Treatment Scale [20]. The most common symptoms were wounds/burns, headache/dizziness, fever/infection and chest pain/vascular symptoms (Table 1).

Table 1. Symptoms distributed over the two samples, before (ED population) and after (UCC population). (n = 200).

	Before (ED)	After (UCC)	Total
Headache/Dizziness	20	8	28
Infection/Fever	15	11	26
Wound/Burn	14	16	30
Dyspnoea	8	1	9
Abdominal	7	8	15
Colorectal	7	7	14
Urology	7	8	15
Extremities	7	9	16
Chest pain/Vascular	5	14	19
Unspecific	10	18	28
All	100	100	200

2.2. Analysis

We produced a before (n = 100 ED patients) and after (N = 100 UCC patients) design, i.e., prior and after the UCC being established. Focus was on dimensions concerning the outcome of treatment at the ED in comparison to the UCC. Aspects studied were LOS, TTP, use of medical services (radiology, laboratory analysis), revisits, hospitalisations, mortality and cost. Descriptive statistics included central tendency and dispersion. LOS was defined as the time spent from admission to discharge from the UCC or the ED or admission to a ward. TTP was defined as the time spent from admission to seeing a physician. Paired-sample calculations of LOS, TTP and laboratory analysis showed a statistical difference of means. However, the results of normality measured by the Kolmogorov Smirnov test did indicate LOS, TTP and laboratory analysis to be significantly skewed (LOS sig. 0.00, TTP sig. 0.00, and laboratory analysis sig. 0.00). The samples could consequently not be regarded as normally distributed due to outliers. A complementary non-parametric test was therefore conducted using a Wilcoxon signed-rank test.

3. Results

The results include aspects (mainly LOS, TTP and laboratory analysis) of patients visiting the UCC versus visiting the ED, a Wilcoxon signed-rank test of LOS, TTP and laboratory analysis and the cost in Euros/average attendee at the UCC versus the ED.

Several differences appeared when comparing the first and second half of the sample (treated by the ED versus treated by the UCC). From arrival to discharge, the UCC patients spent an average of 2.11 h less at the hospital than the ED patients. TTP was thus 1.57 h less at the UCC than at the ED. There was also a reduction in terms of laboratory analysis at the UCC compared to the ED. Even though the numbers of radiology, findings, referrals, revisits and hospitalisations were minor (26 and below), the sample visiting the UCC appeared to be almost similar to the one visiting the ED (Table 2).

Table 2. Aspects studied of patients visiting the UCC versus patients visiting the ED (N = 200).

	ED	UCC	All
n	100	100	200
LOS (SD)	3.21 (2.32)	1.10 (0.63)	2.15 (2.00)
TTP (SD)	2.14 (2.28)	0.57 (0.46)	1.36 (1.82)
Laboratory analysis (SD)	449 (5.15)	31 (0.66)	480 (4.22)
Radiology	9	4	13
Radiology findings	1	3	4
Referrals	26	21	47
Revisits 72 Hours	3	1	4
Hospitalisation	1	0	1
5-day Mortality	0	0	0

LOS, TTP and laboratory analyses were selected for the Wilcoxon rank test, confirming both LOS and TTP to be significantly more time consuming at the ED than at the UCC. A similar result emerged with regard to laboratory analysis.

Total cost of attendees at the UCC and the ED differed. The cost of UCC attendees was less than the cost of ED attendees (Table 4). (Table 3).

On average, an UCC attendee was 67–210 Euros cheaper. One reason for the difference was fewer medical services, i.e., radiology and laboratory than at the ED. The total cost of medical services at the UCC for the population studied was an average of 37.28 Euros less than at the ED (radiology = 16.62, laboratory = 20.66) (Table 4).

Table 3. Ranks and statistics of LOS, TTP and laboratory analysis of attendees at UCC versus ED (N = 200).

	Ranks	n	Mean Rank	Sum of Ranks
Z based on positive ranks = −7.547 Assympt Sig. (2-tailed) = 0.00	Negative Ranks	82 (UCC LOS < ED LOS)	55.23	4474.00
	Positive Ranks	16 (UCC LOS > ED LOS)	17.44	279.00
	Ties	2 (UCC LOS = ED LOS)		
	Total	100		
	Ranks	**n**	**Mean Rank**	**Sum of Ranks**
Z based on positive ranks = −6.928 Assympt Sig. (2-tailed) = 0.00	Negative Ranks	80 (UCC TTP < ED TTP)	56.75	4540.00
	Positive Ranks	20 (UCC TTP > ED TTP)	25.50	510.00
	Ties	0 (UCC TTP = ED TTP)		
	Total	100		
	Ranks	**n**	**Mean Rank**	**Sum of Ranks**
Z based on positive ranks = −6.723 Assympt Sig. (2-tailed) = 0.00	Negative Ranks	63 (UCC lab. < ED lab.)	36.05	2271.00
	Positive Ranks	5 (UCC lab. > ED lab.)	15.00	75.00
	Ties	32 (UCC lab. = ED lab.)		
	Total	100		

Table 4. Cost in Euros/average attendee at the UCC and the ED distributed in total cost, radiology cost and laboratory cost.

	Total Cost/Average Attendee	Radiology Cost/Average Attendee in the Population Studied (N = 200)	Laboratory Cost/Average Attendee in the Population Studied (N = 200)
ED (n = 100)	362 E (Physician) 219 E (Nurse)	18.11 E	22.19 E
UCC (n = 100)	152 E (Physician and Nurse)	1.49 E	1.53 E

4. Discussion

This study shows that waiting times for the patients studied who were referred to the UCC were reduced, both in terms of TTP and LOS. There was also a reduction in the number of blood tests performed at the UCC. Accordingly, there was a substantial cost reduction for UCC visits compared to the ED on the studied population. These components contribute to cost-effective and sustainable care. However, the sample was too small to draw any conclusions regarding the outcome in terms of assessment and treatment accuracy, though it was not possible to register any increase in revisits.

The most important effect was probably the reduced LOS. The UCC relieved the ED of low-urgency patients and, in the long run, potential crowding. This might consequently have contributed to fewer complex and diversified assignments at the ED. Extrapolating the results, a consequence of establishing a UCC might contribute to EDs maintaining their focus on emergencies and avoid time-consuming challenges such as maintaining continuity and follow-up routines [21]. The UCC studied cut the LOS by two-thirds in relation to the population studied, which may improve disaster preparedness [22]. An integrated UCC/ED may also be used as a fast track and flexible area of care during pandemic peaks and emergencies [23,24].

It can tentatively be suggested that one more important function of UCC in crisis is its networking capacity as part of the primary care system. Non-urgent and non-MID patients can easily be referred to other primary care centres for follow-up [1]. Patients who have access to continuous primary care are known to have an improved health status and lower rates of unnecessary hospitalisation compared to those which do not have such access [25]. In contrast, crowding in the emergency room not only contributes to patient dissatisfaction, but it also increases the risk of spread of infection, misdiagnosis and delayed administration of drugs and, in the long run, prolongs hospitalisation [22].

The proximity of the UCC used in this study seems to be an advantage, not only for peacetime use but also for a future MID, when immediate staff and material and structures are essential factors in successful MID management. The close distance between the UCC and the ED may not only alleviate the ED's burdens but also improve close interprofessional collaboration between colleagues from both units. A study four months after the establishment of an integrated ED/UCC reported inter-organizational and inter-professional collaboration. The staff, physicians and nurses crossed a stairwell and a corridor to discuss common challenges. Questions about the parties' capacity for diagnosing and treating patients were sorted out, and non-conventional solutions were occasionally invented to handle strenuous situations and tricky cases. Mistakes in assessments and patients whose health conditions rapidly changed could easily be handled by swift re-referrals from the UCC back to the ED [17].

The differences observed in this study regarding the utilization of medical services by UCC and ED on a similar population may simply reflect the ability of UCC to adjust to new conditions, procedures and perspectives when assessing patients. The ED staff may be more focused on recent symptoms and a rapidly emerging illness. The UCC staff, on the other hand, may be focused on long-term medical history [26]. While the ED assesses and reassesses the patient in a broad manner, the UCC may use anamnesis and bedside information to construct a picture of the status of the patient [16]. However, when comparing the strengths of the two units, the UCC has the potential to optimize care for both urgent and non-urgent patients. The difference in working methods can be considered an asset when providing sustainable care to the mix of needs in the population of attendees, and during pandemics and disaster management [27]. Despite fewer blood tests and X-rays at the UCC, the results obtained did not indicate any incorrect assessments or treatments at UCC. However, generalising the results of this study will require studies of larger populations. Placing a UCC close to an ED may, however, become a promising establishment in terms of reduction in costs, LOS, TTP and the use of medical services, which is beneficial in the management of an MID.

The pressure on EDs during COVID 19 underscores the need for further studies on interventions aiming to relieve and facilitate ED capacity. Even though a silver bullet for the issue of ED crowding has not yet been found, different methods may be combined to improve preparedness. UCCs are one promising method when it comes to preparedness, along with cost-reductions and improved continuity.

5. Limitations

As already mentioned, this is a study of a limited population from a single UCC. If the results are to be generalised, a substantial study population from several UCCs will be desirable.

This study did not include a follow-up on patient satisfaction. The next study on the outcome of the UCC established should include such a study. Even though there are reasons to believe that patients perceive the UCC as a favourable alternative to the ED, based on the shorter TTP and LOS, other factors such as treatment, follow-up and expectations may impact on patient satisfaction. Such satisfaction is also important for non-MID patients seeking help during a major emergency. It is important that the public feel secure and that patient safety for non-MID patients can be guaranteed by using ordinary staff, material and structures. Another limitation is the scarcity of research related to hospital-based UCCs, especially in a European context. Hopefully, this limited study might inspire other researchers to conduct new research on UCCs in order to improve the sustainability of healthcare.

6. Conclusions

In conclusion, Major Incidents and Disasters (MIDs) and pandemics such as COVID 19 are inevitable and demand hospital and prehospital preparedness in order to guarantee and enhance the capability of healthcare to save lives. Hospitals need to surge capacity by obtaining the necessary staff, material and structure, as well as valid and tested systems. Professional, trained staffs are an important factor in successful MID management; however, their familiarity with the facility in which they work and the devices they need to use is also essential. In this perspective, creating a primary care-like facility in close proximity to the hospitals may not only relieve overcrowding in hospital EDs in peacetime, but it also provides an opportunity for such units to be used to facilitate care of the victims of MIDs and pandemics.

Author Contributions: Conceptualization, A.R., K.D., T.C., A.K.-M, J.B., E.C.; methodology, E.C., A.R. and K.D.; Writing—original draft, E.C., A.R., K.D., A.K.-M.; Writing—review and editing, A.R., K.D., T.C., A.K.-M., J.B., E.C.; supervision, E.C. All authors have read and agreed to the published version of the manuscript.

References

1. Khorram-Manesh, A. Flexible surge capacity—Public health, public education, and disaster Management. *Health Promot. Perspect.* **2020**, *10*, 175–179. [CrossRef] [PubMed]
2. Khorram-Manesh, A.; Lönroth, H.; Rotter, P.; Wilhelmsson, M.; Aremyr, J.; Berner, A.; Nero Andersson, A.; Carlström, E. Non-medical aspects of civilian–military collaboration in management of major incidents. *Eur. J. Trauma Emerg. Surg.* **2017**, *43*, 595–603. [CrossRef] [PubMed]
3. Khorram-Manesh, A.; Yttermyr, J.; Sörensson, J.; Carlström, E. The impact of disaster and major incidents on vulnerable groups: Risk and medical assessment of patients with advanced care at home. *Home Health Care Manag. Pract.* **2017**, *29*, 183–190. [CrossRef]
4. Ablah, E.; Konda, K.S.; Konda, K.; Melbourne, M.; Ingoglia, J.N.; Gebbie, K.M. Emergency preparedness training and response among community health centers and local health departments: Results from a multi-state survey. *J. Community Health* **2010**, *35*, 285–293. [CrossRef] [PubMed]
5. Jacobs, L.M.; McSwain, N.E.; Rotondo, M.F.; Wade, D.; Fabbri, W.; Eastman, A.L.; Butler, F.K.; Sinclair, J. Improving survival from active shooter events: The Hartford Consensus. *J. Trauma Acute Care Surg.* **2013**, *74*, 1399–1400. [CrossRef] [PubMed]
6. Shoaf, K.I.; Rottman, S.J. The role of public health in disaster preparedness, mitigation, response, and recovery. *Prehospital Disaster Med.* **2000**, *15*, 144–146. [CrossRef]
7. Berlin, J.; Carlström, E. The 20-minutes Team.—A critical study from the emergency room. *J. Eval. Clin. Pract.* **2008**, *14*, 569–576. [CrossRef]
8. Berlin, J.; Carlström, E. From Artefact to Effect.—The organising effect of artefacts on teams. *J. Health Organ. Manag.* **2010**, *24*, 412–427. [CrossRef]
9. Carter, E.; Pouch, S.M.; Larson, E.L. The Relationship between Emergency Department Crowding and Patient Outcomes: A Systematic Review. *J. Nurs. Scholarsh.* **2014**, *46*, 106–115. [CrossRef]
10. Kellerman, A.L. Crisis in the emergency department. *N. Engl. J. Med.* **2006**, *355*, 1300–1303. [CrossRef]
11. Bernstein, S.L.; Aronsky, D.; Duseja, R.; Epstein, S.; Handel, D.; Hwang, U.; McCarthy, M.; McConnell, K.J.; Pines, J.M.; Rathlev, N.; et al. The Effect of Emergency Department Crowding on Clinically Oriented Outcomes. *Acad. Emerg. Med.* **2009**, *16*, 1–10. [CrossRef] [PubMed]
12. Rosovski, R.P.; Andonian, J.S.; Hayes, B.D. The impending storm: COVID-19, pandemics and our overwhelmed emergency departments. *Am. J. Emerg. Med.* **2019**, *38*, 1270–1294.
13. Khorram-Manesh, A.; Carlström, E.; Hertelendy, A.J.; Goniewicz, K.; Casady, C.B.; Burkle, F.M. Does the prosperity of a country play a role in COVID 19 outcomes? *Disaster Med. Public Health Prep.* **2020**, *12*, 1–10. [CrossRef] [PubMed]
14. Weinick, R.M.; Bristol, S.J.; DesRoches, C.M. Urgent care centers in the US: Findings from a national survey. *BMC Health Serv. Res.* **2009**, *9*, 79. [CrossRef]
15. Yee, T.; Lechner, A.E.; Boukus, E.R. The surge in urgent care centers: Emergency department alternative or costly convenience. *Res. Brief* **2013**, *26*, 1–6.
16. Doran, K.M.; Raven, M.C.; Rosenheck, R.A. What drives frequent emergency department use in an integrated health system? National data from the veterans' health administration. *Annu. Emerg. Med.* **2013**, *62*, 151–159. [CrossRef]
17. Wennman, I.; Wittholt, M.; Carlström, E.; Carlsson, T.; Khorram-Manesh, A. Urgent care centre in Sweden—The integration of teams and perceived effects. *Int. J. Health Plan. Manag.* **2019**, *34*, 1–12. [CrossRef]
18. Vandenbroucke, J.; von Elm, E.; Altman, D.G.; Gøtzsche, P.C.; Mulrow, C.D.; Pocock, S.J. Strengthening the Reporting of Observational Studies in Epidemiology (STROBE): Explanation and Elaboration. *PLoS Med.* **2007**, *4*, 1628–1654. [CrossRef]

19. Cohen, J. *Statistical Power Analysis for the Behavioral Sciences*; Academic Press: Cambridge, MA, USA, 2013.
20. Wireklint, S.C.; Elmqvist, C.; Parenti, N.; Göransson, K.E. A descriptive study of registered nurses' application of the triage scale RETTS©; a Swedish reliability study. *Int. Emerg. Nurs.* **2018**, *38*, 21–28. [CrossRef]
21. Raidla, A.; Dárro, K.; Carlson, T.; Carlström, E. Characterising double frequent users in an emergency department. *J. Hosp. Adm.* **2018**, *7*, 35–39. [CrossRef]
22. Wickman, L.; Svensson, P.; Djärv, T. Effect of crowding on length of stay for common chief complaints in the emergency department: A STROBE cohort study. *Medicine* **2017**, *96*, e8457. [CrossRef] [PubMed]
23. Wennman, I.; Nordling, P.; Herlitz, J.; Lernfelt, B.; Kihlgren, M.; Gustafsson, C.; Hansson, P.-O. The clinical consequences of a prehospital diagnosis of stroke by the emergency medical services. A pilot study. *Scand. J. Trauma Resusc. Emerg. Med.* **2012**, *20*, 48. [CrossRef] [PubMed]
24. Morley, C.; Unwin, M.; Peterson, G.M.; Stankovich, J.; Kinsman, L. Emergency department crowding: A systematic review of causes, consequences and solutions. *PLoS ONE* **2018**, *13*, e0203316. [CrossRef] [PubMed]
25. O'Malley, A.S.; Forrest, C.B.; Politzer, R.M.; Wulu, J.T.; Shi, L. Health center trends, 1994–2001: What do they portend for the federal growth initiative? *Health Aff.* **2005**, *24*, 465–472. [CrossRef]
26. Tricco, A.C.; Antony, J.; Ivers, N.M. Effectiveness of quality improvement strategies for coordination of care to reduce use of healthcare services: A systematic review and meta-analysis. *Can. Med. Assoc. J.* **2014**, *186*, E568–E578. [CrossRef]
27. Wertheimer, B.; Jacobs, R.E.A.; Baily, M. Discharge before noon: An achievable hospital goal. *J. Hosp. Med.* **2014**, *9*, 210–214. [CrossRef]

13

Increased Medical Visits and Mortality among Adults with Cardiovascular Diseases in Severely Affected Areas After Typhoon Morakot

Hsin-I Shih [1,2,3], Tzu-Yuan Chao [4], Yi-Ting Huang [2], Yi-Fang Tu [2,5], Tzu-Ching Sung [6], Jung-Der Wang [3] and Chia-Ming Chang [2,7,*]

1 Department of Emergency Medicine, National Cheng Kung University Hospital, College of Medicine, National Cheng Kung University, Tainan 70403, Taiwan; hshihnckutw@gmail.com
2 School of Medicine, College of Medicine, National Cheng Kung University, Tainan 70101, Taiwan; alage@gs.ncku.edu.tw (Y.-T.H.); nckutu@gmail.com (Y.-F.T.)
3 Department of Public Health, College of Medicine, National Cheng Kung University, Tainan 70101, Taiwan; jdwang121@gmail.com
4 Department of Urban Planning, National Cheng Kung University, Tainan 70101, Taiwan; tychao@mail.ncku.edu.tw
5 Department of Paediatrics, National Cheng Kung University Hospital, College of Medicine, National Cheng Kung University, Tainan 70403, Taiwan
6 School of Medicine for International Students, I-Shou University, Kaohsiung 82445, Taiwan; vivian1223@isu.edu.tw
7 Division of Geriatrics & Gerontology, Department of Internal Medicine, National Cheng Kung University Hospital, Tainan 70403, Taiwan
* Correspondence: 10108040@gs.ncku.edu.tw

Abstract: Natural disasters have negative health impacts on chronic diseases in affected populations. Severely affected areas are usually rural areas with limited basic infrastructure and a population have that has limited access to optimal healthcare after a disaster. Patients with cardiovascular diseases are required to maintain quality care, especially after disasters. A population-based case-control study enrolled adults from the National Health Insurance Registry who had ischemic heart disease and cerebrovascular disease histories and lived in the area affected by Typhoon Morakot in 2009. Monthly medical visits for acute cerebrovascular and ischemic heart diseases markedly increased at approximately 1–2 months after the typhoon. Survival analysis during the two years following the typhoon indicated a significant increase in mortality in adults with an acute ischemic heart disease history who lived in the severely affected area. Mortality hazard analysis showed that among affected adults with previous cerebrovascular diseases and acute ischemic heart diseases, patients with diabetes (adjusted hazard ratio [HR]: 1.3–1.7), Chronic Kidney Disease (CKD) (adjusted HR: 2.0–2.7), chronic obstructive pulmonary diseases (COPD) and asthma (adjusted HR: 1.7–2.1), liver cirrhosis (adjusted HR: 2.3–3.3) and neoplasms (adjusted HR: 1.1–2.1) had significantly increased mortality rates. Consequently, high-quality and accessible primary healthcare plans should be made available to maintain and support affected populations after disasters.

Keywords: disaster; typhoon; flood; elderly; cardiovascular diseases; cerebrovascular diseases

1. Introduction

The number of reported weather-related natural disasters has been increasing since the 1960s. These disasters result in over 60,000 deaths each year worldwide [1,2]. Increasingly variable rainfall patterns have increased the frequency and intensity of flooding, which has had great impacts on human health. People may be forced to move, which heightens the risk of health effects on mental disorders, communicable diseases, and chronic comorbidities. Heavy floods cause substantial infrastructure damage and lead to massive economic and personal losses for communities [3,4]. These disasters require large-scale, multinational coordination to provide urgent humanitarian aid and continuous relief [5] to the affected areas.

Severely affected areas are usually rural and coastal areas with limited basic infrastructure and a small population. Rural and coastal areas are more likely than urban areas to have an inequitably high burden due to healthcare disparities. These disparities contribute to the inadequate provision of basic healthcare services that arise from few medical facilities, a minimal number of providers, few specialty practices, and a lack of accompanying technical innovations and health promotion programs [6–8]. In medically underserved rural settings, people experiencing barriers to primary healthcare tend to have a low income, low education level and high rate of unemployment [9]. Patients with chronic comorbidities need to maintain a delicate balance of care to decrease complications during and after disasters. A previous study found that 24.3% of visits to emergency treatment facilities after Hurricane Katrina were for chronic diseases or related conditions [10]. Following the March 2011 earthquake and tsunami in Japan, increased mortality was observed in some patients with chronic comorbidities [11]. Increased numbers of visits for acute ischemic heart disease and stroke following natural disasters have been identified after natural disasters. Survivors also have to cope with stressors such as searching for food and shelter, relocating, crowding, financial hardship, and navigating social services [12]. Stressors from hurricanes and other natural disasters can cause chronic and acute mental stress, which can trigger cardiovascular events. Affected communities, especially those who are severely affected and in a rural area, are faced with a myriad of disparities, each posing a barrier to timely response and complete recovery from a disaster.

The Asia-Pacific region has been recognized as the region with the highest risk of major disasters [13]. Moreover, Taiwan may be the location most vulnerable to natural hazards, with 73% of its land and population exposed to three or more hazards [14]. Typhoon Morakot affected the West Pacific Region from August 6 to 11 August 2009. On August 7, it caused copious amounts of rainfall in Taiwan, peaking at 2777 mm (109.3 in). This extreme amount of rain triggered massive mudflows and severe flooding throughout southern Taiwan, causing 702 deaths and roughly US$6.76 billion in financial losses [15,16]. Almost all southern Taiwan experienced record-breaking heavy rain, and the associated flood damage required people to relocate to temporary shelters for approximately six months to one year. After Typhoon Morakot, multidisciplinary, large-scale reconstruction and relief actions were initiated. Residents who lived in the affected areas before the disaster were identified by the Ministry of Health and Welfare and received partial medical expense reimbursement for 3 months. Medical teams and clinics were established in the temporary shelters to provide primary basic healthcare in the severely affected areas for at least 6 months. A series of recovery and relief measures were implemented and initiated in the following years. To evaluate the parameters affecting health outcomes of cardiovascular and cerebrovascular diseases among different levels of affected areas (Appendix A Table A1), we conducted a longitudinal follow-up study to assess health parameters among adult residents in different areas affected by Typhoon Morakot, a major disaster.

2. Materials and Methods

2.1. Data Source

Data from the Taiwan National Health Insurance (NHI) Database from the National Health Research Institute (NHRI) was analyzed. All claims submitted by physicians to the National Health Insurance Registry must include a diagnostic code based on the International Classification of Diseases, Ninth Revision, Clinical Modification (ICD-9-CM) developed by the World Health Organization which allows the NHI Registry to verify claims and generate statistics about causes of illness and death [17].

The NHRI recorded data included residents' demographic data, medications, treatments (including operations), and disease diagnoses at four different levels of healthcare facilities. After Typhoon Morakot, the NHI Bureau identified residents who had lived in the affected areas before the disaster and provided partial reimbursement of their medical expenses based on the Regulation "National Health Insurance Reimbursement for Medical Expenses after Typhoon Morakot". Adult residents living in the affected area were enrolled for further analysis.

2.2. Study Design

A population-based longitudinal case-control study was conducted. In total, historical data of 715,244 adults who had lived in the affected areas were obtained for this study. Adult patients with healthcare facility visit records were analyzed. The index date was 8 August 2009, the date that Typhoon Morakot struck Taiwan. The adults were separated into non-elderly and elderly groups (18–64 years and 65 years and older, respectively). Patients with chronic medical conditions requiring long-term follow-up, such as diabetes mellitus (DM), hypertension, chronic kidney disease (CKD), heart disease, hyperlipidemia, chronic obstructive pulmonary disease (COPD), liver cirrhosis and neoplasms, were identified from long-term medical records, and records of their most recent follow-up visit for their chronic medical conditions were reviewed to assess their comorbidities after the disaster. The observation period of the study was from January 2008 to December 2011.

Patients with underlying medical comorbidities, including hypertension (ICD-9-CM: 401–405), DM (ICD-9-CM: 250), asthma (ICD-9-CM: 493), chronic heart failure (ICD-9-CM: 428, 410–414), COPD (ICD-9-CM: 491–496, excluding 493, 495), liver cirrhosis (ICD-9-CM: 571.5), neoplasms (ICD-9-CM: 140–239) and CKD (ICD-9-CM: 585, 582, 583.9), that were recorded before the index date were selected and noted. All medical service utilization records after the index date were reviewed. The calculated Charlson Comorbidity Index (CCI) values indicated the severity of these patients' comorbidities. The patients' socioeconomic statuses were based on their income records, as reported to the NHI bureau.

The rates of acute ischemic heart diseases and cerebrovascular diseases in adults who lived in the affected areas were analyzed. The study analyzed patients with acute ischemic heart disease (ICD-9-CM: 410–414), intracranial hemorrhage (ICH) (ICD-9-CM: 430–432) and ischemic stroke (ICD-9-CM: 433–437) before and after Typhoon Morakot. The above diseases that occurred after the index date were evaluated to determine patients' health outcomes before and after Typhoon Morakot. The monthly visits of acute illnesses were measured from the patients' medical records. For each person, the occurrence of the same event within the same one-month period was counted only once. Hospitalization records after Typhoon Morakot were also analyzed to evaluate the health hazards, heart failure (ICD-9-CM: 428); common infections such as lower respiratory tract infection (ICD-9-CM: 480–488), urinary tract infection (ICD-9-CM: 590, 595, 597, 599), and skin and soft tissue infections (ICD-9-CM: 680–686); and trauma and injury (ICD-9-CM: 850–959).

The validated definition of mortality was adapted from the NHI database and was based on the insurance status among those affected adults enrolled in our study. Mortality cases were defined as enrolled adults withdrawn due to death or critical discharge with the diagnosis of one of the most common twenty causes of death (ICD-9-CM) of National Statistics in Taiwan, and without any medical records after withdrawal date, missing for more than six months, and were disqualified as an insurance applicant of the NHI program such as immigration and the expiration of the duration of stay of aliens [18]. All causes of death for the affected adults enrolled in this study between August 2009 and December 2011 were enrolled for further survival and hazard ratio analysis.

2.3. Spatial-Temporal Analysis

The classification of township and metropolitan areas in Taiwan was adapted from the 2005 Taiwan Social Change Survey, which tracks and provides insights into long-term societal trends and developments in each town or metropolitan area in six prospective areas through nationally representative survey data obtained through cluster sampling; data obtained included the proportion of the working population employed in the service sector, the proportion of the industrial population, the proportion of the population 15–64 years old, the proportion of the elderly population, the proportion of the population that attained at least a bachelor's degree, and the population density of the area. In total, three different town or metropolitan areas (urban, suburban, and rural) were included [19].

2.4. Covariates

In addition to age and sex, area of residence was incorporated into the study design as a demographic variable. Comorbidities considered in this study included hypertension, DM, hypertension, COPD and asthma, liver cirrhosis, and neoplasms, which were defined by major diagnosis codes with at least three months' long-term prescriptions before the index date with relevant ICD-9-CM codes mentioned above.

2.5. Statistical Analysis

The distribution of the study population, which was based on demographic and disease history data such as sex, age, diabetes, chronic kidney, pulmonary, and liver diseases, living place, social economic status, cardiovascular, cerebrovascular diseases, and mortality was analyzed. Besides A case control study to evaluate time-to-event outcomes was applied. To evaluate differences among different study groups, the chi-square test was used for categorical variables, and the Student's t test was used for continuous variables. The control group was matched for age and sex using propensity scoring methods. Major underlying diseases and living locations were selected from the univariate and multi-variate Cox proportional hazard regression models with backward eliminations to estimate hazard ratios of mortality among affected adults with a history of cardiovascular and cerebrovascular events. All tests of significance were 2-tailed, and a p value of 0.05 or less was considered statistically significant. Robust Cox models using robust sandwich variance estimators were applied considering clustering within matched sets. Moreover, stratified Cox models using stratification of the propensity scores were also adopted to treat the matched sets. The former approach resulted in an unbiased estimation of marginal hazard ratios that were compared with a biased estimation of marginal hazard ratios resulting from the latter approach. Each comparison value and its 95% confidence interval (95% CI) were also analyzed. All data management and statistical analyses were performed with SAS 9.4 software (SAS Institute, Cary, NC, USA). All statistical tests were 2-sided, and p values less than 0.05 were considered statistically significant.

2.6. Ethical Issues

All provisions of the study were performed in accordance with the principles of the Declaration of Helsinki and the Declaration of Taipei [20]. Patients' personal information was encrypted to protect their privacy, and the electronic databases were decoded for research; therefore, the requirement for informed consent was waived by the institutional review board (IRB). This study was approved by the IRB of the study hospital (IRB No: A-ER-103-176).

3. Results

A total of 715,244 adult patient files were identified; 199,991 patients (28%) were in the elderly group. Female patients were predominant (398,819, 56%). The study diagram is shown in the Appendix A Figure A1. The demographic characteristics of the study population between different severity of affected areas are presented in Table 1. Compared to the adults living in the moderately affected area, those in the severely affected area before Typhoon Morakot were older, lived more in rural areas, had a higher rate of multiple underlying diseases (CCI $\geq$ 1: 45% vs. 41%) and cardiovascular disease history (18% vs. 15%). Besides, the adults living in the severely affected area also had higher rates of underlying chronic diseases, such as DM (16% vs. 14%), hypertension (33% vs. 26%), heart disease (12% vs. 10%), COPD and asthma (6% vs. 4%).

Table 1. Demographic and clinical characteristics of adults living between different severity of affected areas before Typhoon Morakot.

Characteristics	Adults Living in the Affected Area			Chi^2-Test p Value
	Moderately Affected (n = 574,089) No. (%)	Severely Affected (n = 141,155) No. (%)	Total (n = 715,244) No. (%)	
Sex				
Female	321,697 (56)	77,122 (55)	398,819 (56)	<0.0001
Age (years)				
Mean ± SD *	51.69 ± 17.87	55.29 ± 17.64	52.40 ± 17.88	
Age Group				
Elderly	151,801 (26)	48,190 (34)	199,991 (28)	<0.0001
Related Cardiovascular History (January 2008–July 2009)				
Either of the following	86,198 (15)	24,969 (18)	111,167 (16)	<0.0001
Ischemic heart diseases	59,226 (10)	17,093 (12)	76,319 (11)	<0.0001
Acute cerebrovascular diseases	36,559 (6)	11,003 (8)	47,562 (7)	<0.0001
Socioeconomic Status (USD/month)				
Low < $750 USD	301,416 (53)	93,431 (66)	394,847 (55)	
Location				
Urban	150,232 (26)	0 (0)	150,232 (21)	<0.0001
Suburban	276,951 (48)	47,890 (34)	324,841 (45)	
Rural	146,906 (26)	93,265 (66)	240,171 (34)	
CCI †				
0	338,653 (59)	77,717 (55)	416,370 (58)	<0.0001
1–2	183,175 (32)	49,034 (35)	232,209 (32)	
>2	52,261 (9)	14,404 (10)	66,665 (9)	
Underlying diseases				
DM	79,653 (14)	21,886 (16)	101,539 (14)	<0.0001
Hypertension	143,332 (26)	45,940 (33)	189,272 (26)	<0.0001
CKD	12,959 (2)	3058 (2)	16,017 (2)	0.04
Heart disease	57,835 (10)	17,171 (12)	75,006 (10)	<0.0001
COPD & asthma	25,612 (4)	8116 (6)	33,728 (6)	<0.0001
Liver cirrhosis	9570 (2)	2007 (1)	11,577 (1)	0.02
Neoplasms	32,304 (6)	7341 (5)	39,645 (6)	0.01

* Standard deviation; † Charlson Comorbidity Index. DM: Diabetes mellitus; CKD: Chronic kidney disease; COPD: Chronic obstructive pulmonary diseases.

Figure 1 shows the number of monthly visits for acute ischemic heart disease and cerebrovascular events by affected adults before and after Typhoon Morakot, i.e., from 2008 to 2010. There was a markedly increased peak in visits in the same month Typhoon Morakot occurred in both the severely and moderately affected areas and in both elderly and non-elderly adults. Compared to that for acute ischemic heart disease, the difference in the number of monthly visits for acute cerebrovascular diseases was more prominent in the moderately affected areas, particularly in the elderly group.

The demographic data before and after matching are summarized in Table 2. After matching for age and sex, the proportions of adults living in the severely affected area with a history of cerebrovascular diseases (44% vs. 42%, $p < 0.001$), hypertension (62% vs. 58%, $p < 0.0001$), hypertension (62% vs. 58%, $p < 0.0001$), COPD and asthma (12% vs. 11%, $p = 0.0001$) was higher than those in the moderately affected area. Adults living in the severely affected area had a higher proportion of living in rural area (71% vs. 32%, $p < 0.0001$) and low-income status than those living in the moderately affected area (monthly income < 750 USD: 73% vs. 60%, $p < 0.0001$). However, there was no significant difference in the CCI score between adults living in the moderately and severely affected areas.

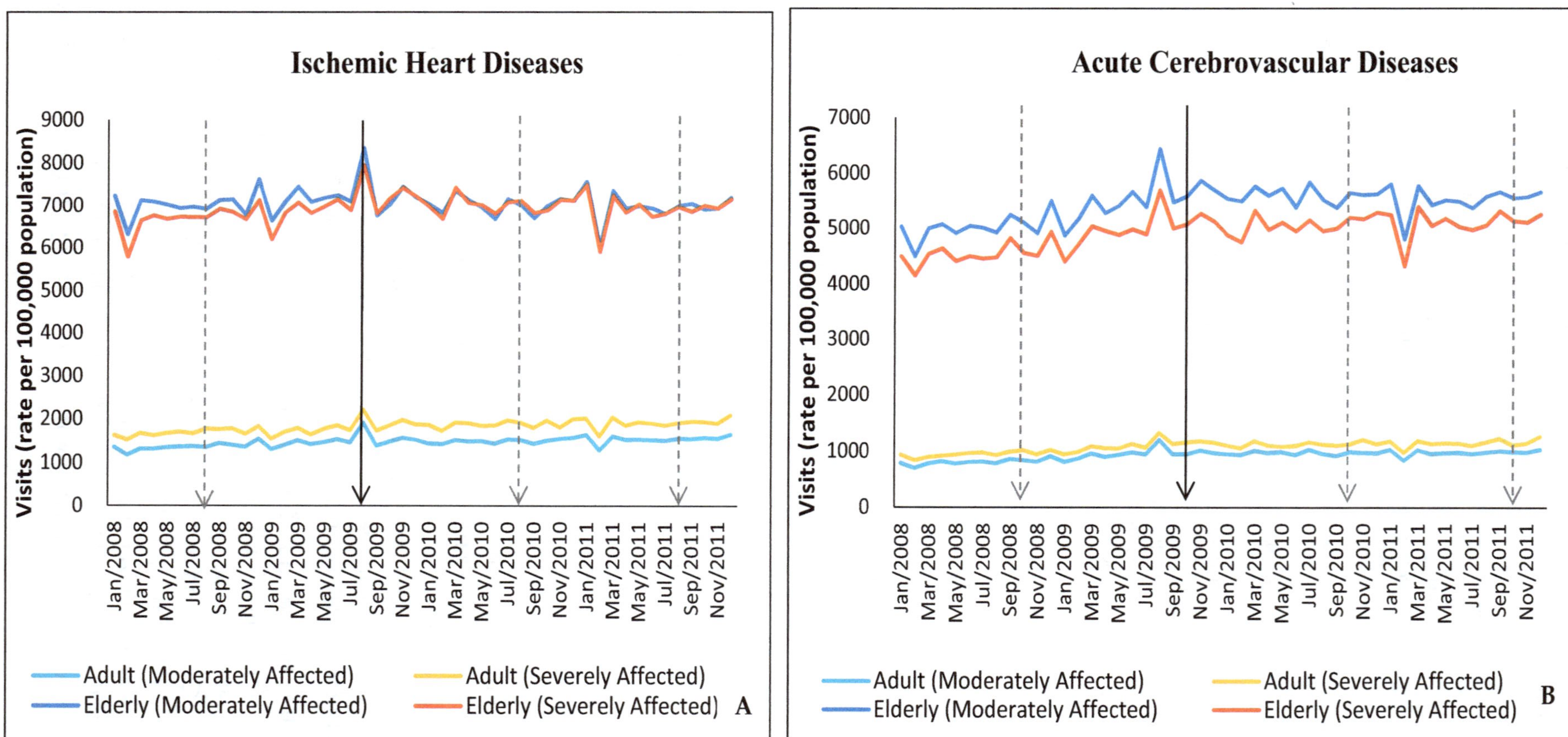

Figure 1. Monthly visits for acute cardiovascular and cerebrovascular events by affected adults before and after Typhoon Morakot. (**A**): Ischemic Heart Diseases; (**B**): Acute Cerebrovascular Diseases. Vertical solid lines: Index Month (August/2009); vertical dotted lines: August/2008, August/2010 and August/2011.

Table 2. Demographics of affected adults before and after matching.

Characteristics	Adult Patients with a Related Cardiovascular History (January 2008–July 2009)					
	Pre-Match			Post-Match		
	Moderately Affected (n = 86,198) No. (%)	Severely Affected (n = 24,969) No. (%)	Chi[2] Test p Value	Moderately Affected (n = 24,969) No. (%)	Severely Affected (n = 24,969) No. (%)	Chi[2] Test p Value
Sex						
Female	45,030 (52)	13,257 (53)	0.02	13,257 (53)	13,257 (53)	1.00
Age (years)						
Mean ± SD *	66.84 ± 12.76	67.72 ± 12.37		67.52 ± 12.63	67.72 ± 12.37	
Age Group						
Elderly	51,724 (60)	15,814 (63)	<0.0001	15,814 (63)	15,814 (63)	1.00
Related Cardiovascular History (January 2008–July 2009)						
Ischemic heart disease	59,226 (69)	17,093(68)	0.45	17,158 (69)	17,093 (68)	0.53
Acute cerebrovascular diseases	36,559 (42)	11,003 (44)	<0.0001	10,568 (42)	11,003 (44)	<0.0001
Socioeconomic Status (USD/month)						
Low < $750 USD	51,230 (59)	18,169 (73)	<0.0001	14,985 (60)	18,169 (73)	<0.0001
Location						
Urban	21,279 (25)	0 (0)		6213 (25)	0 (0)	<0.0001
Suburban	36,826 (42)	7267 (29)	<0.0001	10,650 (43)	7267 (29)	
Rural	28,093 (33)	17,702 (71)		8106 (32)	17,702 (71)	
CCI †						
0	17,928 (21)	4918 (20)	0.0007	5102 (20)	4918 (20)	0.11
1–2	44,003 (51)	12,911 (52)		12,744 (51)	12,911 (52)	
> 2	24,267 (28)	7140 (29)		7123 (29)	7140 (29)	
Underlying diseases						
DM	24,863 (29)	7063 (28)	0.09	7225 (29)	7063 (28)	0.11
Hypertension	49,642 (58)	15,468 (62)	<0.0001	14,430 (58)	15,468 (62)	<0.0001
CKD	4613 (5.4)	1195 (4.8)	0.0004	1372 (5.5)	1195 (4.8)	0.0003
Heart disease	41,546 (48)	12,326 (49)	0.0012	12,111 (48)	12326 (49)	0.05
COPD & asthma	8891 (10)	2933 (12)	<0.0001	2662 (11)	2933 (12)	0.0001
Liver cirrhosis	1946 (2.3)	424 (1.6)	<0.0001	553 (2.2)	424 (1.7)	<0.0001
Neoplasms	6520 (7.6)	1748 (7.0)	0.0028	1933 (7.7)	1748 (7.0)	0.0015

* Standard deviation; † Charlson Comorbidity Index. DM: Diabetes mellitus; CKD: Chronic kidney disease; COPD: Chronic obstructive pulmonary diseases.

A mortality analysis of adults with cardiovascular and cerebrovascular disease histories was performed. Robust Cox models using robust sandwich variance estimators for clustering within matched sets were used to analyze survival after Typhoon Morakot in affected adults with cardiovascular and cerebrovascular disease histories in the moderately and severely affected areas. Before Typhoon Morakot, the robust sandwich estimation for three-year survival between moderately and severely affected areas revealed a significant difference in the survival rate of affected adults with a cardiovascular events history ($p = 0.0047$) but did not reveal a significant difference in the survival rate of affected adults with a cerebrovascular event history.

Hospitalizations after Typhoon Morakot in affected adults with cardiovascular and cerebrovascular histories before Typhoon Morakot were analyzed (Table 3). Compared to the hospitalization rate in affected adults in the moderately affected area, a slightly increased hospitalization rate was noted among affected adults living in the severely affected area after Typhoon Morakot in terms of acute ischemic heart diseases, acute cerebrovascular diseases, heart failure, infection-related diseases, trauma- and injury-related diseases ($p < 0.0001$).

Table 3. Hospitalizations after Typhoon Morakot in affected adults with preexisting histories of cardiovascular and cerebrovascular diseases before Typhoon Morakot.

Characteristics	Adult Patients with a Related Cardiovascular History (January 2008–July 2009/)			
	Post-Match			
	Moderately Affected (n = 24,969) No. (%)	Severely Affected (n = 24,969) No. (%)	OR 95% CI	Chi²-Test p Value
Acute ischemic heart diseases	2607 (10)	2896 (12)	1.096 * (1.037–1.16)	<0.0001
Acute cerebrovascular diseases	1852 (7.4)	2118 (8.4)	1.129 * (1.058–1.205)	<0.0001
Heart failure	1399 (5.6)	1633 (6.5)	1.152 * (1.07–1.24)	<0.0001
Infection	4661 (19)	5301 (21)	1.123 * (1.075–1.173)	<0.0001
Trauma and injury	1238 (4.9)	1456 (5.8)	1.161 * (1.074–1.255)	<0.0001

* $p < 0.05$.

To determine the important risk factors for mortality among affected adults with cardiovascular and cerebrovascular disease histories and to eliminate confounding factors, a multivariate stratified Cox proportional hazards regression model was estimated (Table 4). Among affected adults with a cerebrovascular disease history, patients with diabetes (adjusted HR: 1.40, 95% CI: 1.29–1.52, $p < 0.0001$), CKD (adjusted HR: 2.05, 95% CI: 1.81–2.33), COPD and asthma (adjusted HR: 1.89, 95% CI: 1.72–2.08, $p < 0.0001$), liver cirrhosis (adjusted HR: 2.25 95% CI: 1.79–2.79, $p < 0.0001$) and neoplasms (adjusted HR: 1.51, 95% CI: 1.33–1.71, $p < 0.0001$) had significantly increased mortality rates. Additionally, among affected adults with acute ischemic heart disease histories, patients with diabetes (adjusted HR: 1.55, 95% CI: 1.43–1.68, $p < 0.0001$), CKD (adjusted HR: 2.40, 95% CI: 2.15–2.69), COPD and asthma (adjusted HR: 1.69, 95% CI: 1.54–1.86, $p < 0.0001$), liver cirrhosis (adjusted HR: 2.76, 95% CI: 2.29–3.32, $p < 0.0001$) and neoplasms (adjusted HR: 1.87, 95% CI: 1.67–2.09, $p < 0.0001$) had higher mortality.

Table 4. Hazard ratio of all-cause mortality in affected adults with previous histories of cerebrovascular and ischemic heart diseases before Typhoon Morakot.

	Cerebrovascular Disease History † (n = 21,571)				Ischemic Heart Disease History † (n = 34,251)			
	Univariate Analysis		Multivariate Analysis		Univariate Analysis		Multivariate Analysis	
	HR	95% CI	aHR	95% CI	HR	95% CI	aHR	95% CI
Location (Ref = Nonrural)								
Rural	0.93	0.86–1.00			1.01	0.93–1.09		
DM (Ref = No)								
Yes	1.43 *	1.32–1.56	1.40 *	1.29–1.52	1.58 *	1.46–1.71	1.55 *	1.43–1.68
Hypertension (Ref = No)								
Yes	0.96	0.88–1.04			0.85 *	0.79–0.92	0.84 *	0.77–0.91
CKD (Ref = No)								
Yes	2.24 *	1.97–2.54	2.05 *	1.81–2.33	2.60 *	2.32–2.91	2.40 *	2.15–2.69
COPD & asthma (Ref = No)								
Yes	1.88 *	1.71–2.07	1.89 *	1.72–2.08	1.69 *	1.54–1.86	1.69 *	1.54–1.85
Liver cirrhosis (Ref = No)								
	2.35 *	1.88–2.93	2.23 *	1.79–2.79	3.18 *	2.64–3.82	2.76 *	2.29–3.32
Neoplasms (Ref = No)								
	1.61 *	1.42–1.82	1.51 *	1.33–1.71	2.07 *	1.85–2.31	1.87 *	1.67–2.09

† Enrolled variables in Cox model for cerebrovascular disease history and cerebrovascular disease history: Location, DM, Hypertension, CKD, COPD and asthma, liver cirrhosis, Neoplasm. DM: Diabetes mellitus; CKD: Chronic kidney disease, COPD: Chronic obstructive pulmonary diseases. * $p < 0.05$.

4. Discussion

This study suggested that affected adults with acute ischemic heart diseases and acute cerebrovascular disease histories before Typhoon Morakot had an increased numbers of visits healthcare facilities for acute ischemic heart disease and acute cerebrovascular diseases two months after Typhoon Morakot in both the moderately and severely affected areas. The survival analysis suggested that affected adults with acute ischemic heart disease history before Typhoon Morakot living in the severely affected area had significantly higher mortality than those living in the moderately affected area. Compared with those of affected adults in the moderately affected area, slightly more hospitalizations were noted among affected adults living in the severely affected area after Typhoon Morakot. Increased mortality rates were observed in affected adults with cerebrovascular disease and ischemic heart disease histories who had comorbidities such as diabetes, CKD, COPD and asthma, liver cirrhosis, and neoplasms.

Increases in the numbers of hospital visits for acute ischemic heart disease and stroke following natural disasters have been reported. A medical records analysis after the Great Hanshin-Awaji Earthquake in 1995 found that acute coronary syndrome and stroke rates rapidly increased and then decreased within 7 weeks, similar to rates after the Great East Japan Earthquake in 2011 [21,22]. After Hurricane Sandy in 2012, researchers detected increases in hospitalizations and deaths due to myocardial infarction and stroke during the 2 weeks following the hurricane compared to the same 2 weeks from 5 years previously [23]. In Taiwan, the rate of hospitalization due to acute myocardial infarction increased during the 6 weeks after the Ji-Ji Earthquake in 1999, and a significantly higher number of patients were hospitalized with acute myocardial infarction during that period than during the same 6-week period in the previous year [24]. Our study revealed similar results. Increased numbers of visits for acute cardiovascular and cerebrovascular events were observed in the first two months after Typhoon Morakot. The survival analysis also indicated a significant increase in mortality in the two years following the typhoon in those with previous acute ischemic heart disease who had lived in the severely affected area. Typhoon Morakot has had significantly short- and long-term health impacts on affected adults with acute ischemic heart diseases and cerebrovascular disease histories, especially those with chronic comorbidities such as DM, CKD or end-stage renal disease (ESRD), COPD, liver cirrhosis and neoplasms.

The abrupt increase in cardiovascular diseases (CVDs) in the acute phase was likely due to psychosocial and posttraumatic stress caused by the disaster and inadequate response after the disaster, especially in the severely affected areas [25–27]. Early morbidity from some cardiovascular events was likely predominantly attributable to the psychological stress of the event2 and corresponding physiologic derangements; psychosocial factors such as missed medications, changed diet, poor living conditions, and the stress of disorders following a disaster have been noted as well [26,28,29]. Psychosocial stressors and lack of medication and a proper support system likely play a key role. After Hurricane Katrina, multiple reports indicated high rates of psychosocial stress and posttraumatic stress [30]. Survivors had to cope with stressors such as searching for food and shelter, relocating, crowding, financial hardship, and navigating social services. Events such as hurricanes and other natural disasters can cause chronic and acute mental stress, which can trigger cardiovascular events [31]. Traditional cardiac risk factors account for only half of the incidence of CVDs, with most of the remaining risk explained by psychosocial factors [31]. Our study revealed similar results and indicated a short-term increase in the numbers of visits for acute ischemic heart and cerebrovascular diseases by affected adults with cardiovascular and cerebrovascular disease histories after Typhoon Morakot. After matching, increased two-year mortality was observed in severely affected adults with an acute ischemic heart disease history, highlighting the importance of the care of high-risk populations with cardiovascular diseases, especially those residing in severely affected rural areas. However, our study also suggested that affected populations with more co-morbidities (i.e., liver cirrhosis, CKD, COPD, asthma and neoplasms other than cardiovascular disease) have higher all-cause mortality hazards. The increased all-cause mortality occurred when patients with multimorbidity and pre-existing cardiovascular diseases such as stroke and ischemic heart diseases had increased risk of complications from either underlying diseases or comorbidities [32–37].

Health disparities are differences in the health statuses of specific populations and the general population. Health disparities are usually defined as "a particular type of health difference that is closely linked with social, economic, and/or environmental disadvantages" [8,38]. Although medical teams and acute social and financial relief programs are provided to affected populations in affected areas, affected populations with chronic comorbidities in severely affected areas still have an increased risk of mortality. Specialty and subspecialty healthcare services are usually less likely to be available in rural areas, and rural areas are less likely to offer specialized and highly sophisticated or high-intensity care than suburban or urban areas. Reliable transportation to healthcare facilities might also be a barrier for rural residents due to long distances, poor road conditions, and the limited availability of public transportation options in rural areas. These exacerbate problems for rural patients seeking specialized care who are required to travel significant distances for treatment [39]. Following a disaster, medical infrastructure usually becomes overwhelmed with acute injury and illness patients [40,41]. If chronic diseases controlled, preexisting chronic health problems can quickly become acute in nature, and these diseases have been linked to increased mortality in vulnerable populations in the wake of a disaster [40]. Chronic disease within the context of a disaster might have a bidirectional effect, whereby initial acute disorders may advance to long-term illnesses if insufficiently treated. This effect creates a "secondary surge" in required medical treatment long after the event and amplifies health disparities among medically underserved populations. The secondary surge of chronic diseases after a disaster coupled with inherent healthcare disparities, such as those commonly found in medically deprived rural areas, makes access to routine healthcare very difficult during the recovery phase [7]. Our data revealed similar results. Severely affected areas were more likely to comprise households with low socioeconomic levels. Patients with underlying comorbidities had higher mortality rates and morbidities after Typhoon Morakot that those without underlying comorbidities. Affected adults with an acute ischemic heart disease history before Typhoon Morakot living in severely affected areas had substantially increased hospitalization and mortality rates, highlighting the importance of medical accessibility. Most of the acute medical teams departed the severely affected areas approximately 6 months after Typhoon Morakot. Although relocation villages with permanent houses and healthcare centers were established within one year after Typhoon Morakot in the severely affected area, the accessibility of public transportation from these relocation villages to advanced cardiovascular care centers was limited. Accessibility limitations have great negative impacts on affected adults with cardiovascular risks, resulting in negative health outcomes.

The effects of spatial disparities after a disaster could be improved by the adoption of an improved universal healthcare system. Previous studies have suggested that universal healthcare systems substantially reduce socioeconomic inequalities in primary care access and quality but lead to only modest reductions in disparities in healthcare outcomes [42–44]. The Sendai framework for disaster risk reduction 2015–2030 aims to achieve substantial reductions in disaster risks and losses by enhancing the resilience of national health systems; corresponding efforts include strengthening the development and implementation of inclusive policies and social safety-net mechanisms and ensuring access to basic healthcare services, with the ultimate aim of eradicating poverty [45]. High-quality and accessible universal healthcare systems could maintain and support affected populations after disasters and are regarded as an important aspect of community resilience [46]. In order to be well-prepared for the foreseeable catastrophic natural events caused by the climate change, after Typhoon Morakot, a series of laws have been enacted including the most important "Spatial Planning Act 2016" [47] (state of the new climate-adaptive and environmental-oriented land use policy). In 2018, the Ministry of the Interior announced the implementation of the National Spatial Plan in accordance with the law and further emphasized on prioritizing the conservation of environmentally sensitive areas as well as important public facilities including medical services in rural and coastal areas. In addition, the United Nations Sustainable Development Goals (SDGs) [48] (United Nations, 2015) form the basis of spatial plans at all levels to ensure the health inequality and urban-rural gaps are taken into account in future land use policies. At the same time, more comprehensive affected area response plans including early evacuation of vulnerable groups and more medical and mental resources deployments before and after the heavy rainfall in susceptible areas were implemented to decrease the vulnerabilities and increase the resilience of the communities [49].

This study has several strengths. First, the large sample of population-based data covering almost the entire population affected by this disaster provided a large enough sample size for matching. Second, in addition to the use of traditional analyses, stratified Cox models and robust Cox models using robust sandwich variance estimators considering clustering within matched sets were employed. The latter approach resulted in unbiased estimations of marginal hazard ratios that could be compared with biased estimations of marginal hazard ratios resulting from the former approach.

Some limitations also need to be mentioned. The limitations of this study include the fact that the clinical data were collected from a registry; thus, completely verifying the data was impossible. Additionally, the registry does not include non-affected adults as reference group and provide detailed cardiovascular risk information regarding smoking habits, alcohol consumption, body mass index, physical activity, and family history, which are potential confounding factors in the analysis of chronic diseases and populations affected by disasters. The estimates of mortality among patients in this study were not verified with death certificates; however, the missing for more than 6 months is closely related to death and the proportion of disqualifications as an insurance applicant is negligible given the fact that foreigners only constitute around 2% of all insured individuals of Taiwan's NHI from the insurance service database. The misclassification rate of the estimated mortality method was <2.37%, and the method we used has been adapted from some previous studies [50,51]. Sex and age were chosen to match in these two groups to minimize the effects of comorbidities in the elderly. Although the underlying diseases between the two groups were still different, the CCI between the two groups after matching was similar and revealed similar comorbidities between groups. Hypertension is known as an important risk factor for cardiovascular death during the acute phase of a disaster. In most patients, the increases in clinic blood pressure and self-measured blood pressure are transient, and the blood pressure levels return to the pre-disaster baseline levels within 4 weeks. The blood pressure levels should be monitored and the dose of antihypertensive medication should be reconsidered every 2 weeks during the disaster situation [52]. An inverse relationship between diastolic pressure and adverse cardiac ischemic events (i.e., the lower the diastolic pressure the greater the risk of coronary heart disease and adverse outcomes) has been observed in numerous studies. This effect is even more pronounced in patients with underlying coronary artery disease (CAD) [53]. Previous studies also indicated uncontrolled hypertension increased risk of all-cause and cardiovascular disease mortality but no significant differences were identified between normotensives, and treated and controlled hypertensives [54]. Non-adherence to antihypertensive medication increased the risk of all adverse health outcomes, including all-cause mortality and hospitalization for cardiovascular diseases such as myocardial infarction, heart failure and stroke [55,56]. The hypertension-mortality risk would be significant reduced if good adherence to anti-hypertension agents is achieved [57,58]. Our study suggested that hypertension did not increase all-cause mortality within two years among affected adults with an ischemic heart disease history after Typhoon Morakot; patients with hypertension have lower mortality hazard might be because patients marked as hypertension received regular anti-hypertensive agent treatment with relative good adherence and blood pressure levels. Further longer follow-up studies should be considered to observe the effects. The monthly visits and mortality rates after this disaster might be underestimated if affected adults were not enrolled in the national healthcare system or did not have medical records during the study period. Furthermore, the areas covered in the spatial-temporal analysis were based on the primary medical facilities that were most commonly used by the residents of the affected areas after the disaster. It was difficult to locate all the affected individuals because some patients visiting these medical facilities might not have been residing in the same area they did before the disaster. The database did not include the unaffected population as the reference group in evaluating the baseline status of mental health before and after Typhoon Morakot. The effects of Typhoon Morakot are difficult to evaluate precisely. Moreover, classifications of township development and the proportions of elderly individuals in the populations were based on the 2005 Taiwan Social Change Survey (Round 5), which primarily considered socioeconomic change and township development in Taiwan; thus, these results may not apply to other spatiotemporal analyses of the relationships between socioeconomic factors and diseases. However, data from the national census, such as the proportion of elderly individuals in the population and household income, were acquired to achieve optimal validity. Finally, nondifferential misclassification of diseases in the registry at baseline might lead to bias toward the null.

In conclusion, the health status of patients with histories of acute cerebrovascular and cardiovascular diseases before Typhoon Morakot was negative effected in both the short term and long term after Typhoon Morakot. The increase in mortality was predominant among the elderly population and was associated with comorbidities and living in the severely affected area. High-quality and accessible universal healthcare systems are important to maintain and support affected populations after disasters. Further long-term spatial and socioeconomic analyses of the health of affected populations with chronic diseases are warranted to build community resilience with optimal deployment, beneficial healthcare strategies and a collaborative framework.

Author Contributions: Conceived and designed the study: H.-I.S., C.-M.C. Provided study materials and assembled the data: H.-I.S., T.-Y.C., C.-M.C., Y.-F.T. Analysed and interpreted the data: H.-I.S., C.-M.C., Y.-T.H., T.-C.S. and J.-D.W. Wrote the paper: H.-I.S., C.-M.C., T.-C.S. and Y.-T.H. Final approval of the manuscript: H.-I.S. and C.-M.C. All authors have read and agreed to the published version of the manuscript.

Appendix A

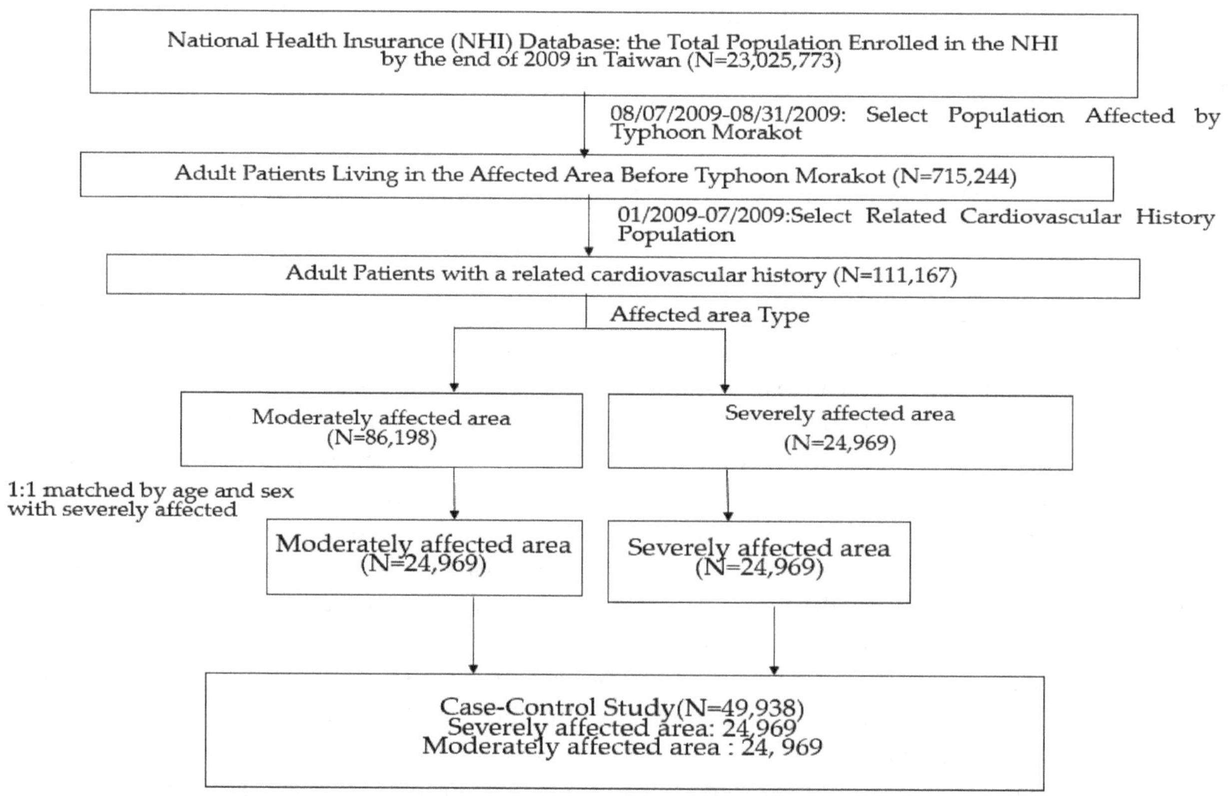

Figure A1. Flow diagram for patients enrolled in this study.

Table A1. Affected Townships of Typhoon Morakot.

County	Severely Affected Townships
Kaohsiung County *	Jiaxian, Taoyuan, Namaxia, Maolin, Neimen, Liugui, Qishan, Dashu, Shanlin, Meinong
Pingtung County *	Jiadong, Linbian, Neipu, Sandimen, Gaoshu, Taiwu, Shizi, Chunri, Wutai, Laiyi, Mudan, Donggang Majia
Chiayi County *	Dongshi, Alishan, Meishan, Zhuqi, Fanlu, Dapu
Taitung County	Taimali, Jinfeng, Dawu, Daren, Haiduan
Tainan County *	Nanhua, Danei, Yujing, Madou, Xuejia
Nantou County	Xinyi, Ren'ai, Shuili, Guoxing
Yulin County	Gukeng, Kouhu, Yuanchang

* All townships were severely affected.

References

1. Costello, A.; Abbas, M.; Allen, A.; Ball, S.; Bellamy, R.; Friel, S.; Groce, N.; Johnson, A.; Kett, M.; Lee, M.; et al. Managing the health effects of climate change. *Lancet* **2009**, *373*, 1693–1733. [CrossRef]
2. Smith, K.R.; Woodward, A.; Campbell-Lendrum, D.; Chadee, D.D.; Honda, Y.; Liu, Q.; Olwoch, J.M.; Revich, B.; Sauerborn, R. Human health: Impacts, adaptation, and co-benefits. In *Climate Change 2014: Impacts, Adaptation, and Vulnerability*; Field, C.B., Barros, V.R., Dokken, D.J., Mach, K.J., Mastrandrea, M.D., Bilir, T.E., Chatterjee, M., Ebi, K.L., Estrada, Y.O., Genova, R.C., et al., Eds.; Cambridge University Press: Cambridge, UK, 2014; pp. 709–754.
3. World Health Organization. Climate Change and Health. Available online: https://www.who.int/news-room/fact-sheets/detail/climate-change-and-health (accessed on 15 March 2020).
4. Regional Office for the Western Pacific World Health Organization. *Emergencies and Disasters*; Regional Office for the Western Pacific, World Health Organization: Manila, Philippines, 2005.
5. Bui, T.; Cho, S.; Sovereign, M. Negotiation issues in multinational humanitarian assistance/disaster relief. In *Proceedings of the 32nd Annual Hawaii International Conference on Systems Sciences, Maui, HI, USA, 5–8 January 1999*; HICSS-32. [CD-ROM]; Institute of Electrical and Electronics Engineers (IEEE): Piscataway Township, NJ, USA, 2003; p. 10.
6. Bathi, J.R.; Das, H.S. Vulnerability of Coastal Communities from Storm Surge and Flood Disasters. *Int. J. Environ. Res. Public Health* **2016**, *13*, 239. [CrossRef] [PubMed]
7. Davis, J.R.; Wilson, S.; Brock-Martin, A.; Glover, S.; Svendsen, E.R. The Impact of Disasters on Populations With Health and Health Care Disparities. *Disaster Med. Public Health Prep.* **2010**, *4*, 30–38. [CrossRef] [PubMed]
8. Braveman, P. What Are Health Disparities and Health Equity? We Need to Be Clear. *Public Health Rep.* **2014**, *129*, 5–8. [CrossRef] [PubMed]
9. Hsu, C.E.; Mas, F.S.; Jacobson, H.E.; Harris, A.M.; Hunt, V.I.; Nkhoma, E.T. Public health preparedness of health providers: Meeting the needs of diverse, rural communities. *J. Natl. Med. Assoc.* **2006**, *98*, 1784–1791.
10. Sharma, A.J.; Weiss, E.C.; Young, S.L.; Stephens, K.; Ratard, R.; Straif-Bourgeois, S.; Sokol, T.M.; Vranken, P.; Rubin, C.H. Chronic Disease and Related Conditions at Emergency Treatment Facilities in the New Orleans Area After Hurricane Katrina. *Disaster Med. Public Health Prep.* **2008**, *2*, 27–32. [CrossRef]
11. Hasegawa, A.; Ohira, T.; Maeda, M.; Yasumura, S.; Tanigawa, K. Emergency Responses and Health Consequences after the Fukushima Accident. *Clin. Oncol.* **2016**, *28*, 237–244. [CrossRef]
12. McCann, D.G. A Review of Hurricane Disaster Planning for the Elderly. *World Med. Health Policy* **2011**, *3*, 5–30. [CrossRef]
13. Pelling, M.; Uitto, J.I. Small Island developing states: Natural disaster vulnerability and global change. *Environ. Hazards* **2001**, *3*, 49–62.
14. Lamont-Doherty Earth Observatory Risk Analysis Reports over Half of World's Population Exposed to One or More Major Natural Hazards. Available online: http://www.earth.columbia.edu/news/2005/story03-29-05.html (accessed on 11 December 2019).
15. Kaohsiung County Office The Official List of survivors in Kaohsiung during the Typhoon Morakot. Available online: http://88taiwan.blogspot.tw/2009/08/0815.html (accessed on 11 April 2020).

16. National Science and Technology Center for Disaster Reduction, Disaster Survey and Analysis of Morakot Typhoon. *National Science and Technology Center for Disaster Reduction Anual Report, 2010*; National Science and Technology Center for Disaster Reduction: Taipei, Taiwan, 2010.
17. Hsieh, C.-Y.; Su, C.-C.; Shao, S.-C.; Sung, S.-F.; Lin, S.-J.; Yang, Y.-H.K.; Lai, E.C.-C. Taiwan's National Health Insurance Research Database: Past and future. *Clin. Epidemiol.* **2019**, *11*, 349–358. [CrossRef]
18. Lee, T.C.; Yang, C.L.; Wang, T.M. Population Aging and NHI Expenditures in Taiwan. *J. Popul. Stud.* **2011**, *43*, 1–35.
19. Center for Survey Research Academia Sinica Taiwan Social Change Survey. Available online: https://www2.ios.sinica.edu.tw/sc/en/home2.php (accessed on 10 January 2018).
20. The World Medical Association Annexe 2. WMA Declaration of Taipei on ethical considerations regarding health databases and biobanks. *J. Int. Bioethique Ethique Sci.* **2017**, *28*, 113–117. [CrossRef]
21. Aoki, T.; Fukumoto, Y.; Yasuda, S.; Sakata, Y.; Ito, K.; Takahashi, J.; Miyata, S.; Tsuji, I.; Shimokawa, H. The Great East Japan Earthquake Disaster and cardiovascular diseases. *Eur. Hear. J.* **2012**, *33*, 2796–2803. [CrossRef] [PubMed]
22. Aoki, T.; Takahashi, J.; Fukumoto, Y.; Yasuda, S.; Ito, K.; Miyata, S.; Shinozaki, T.; Inoue, K.; Yagi, T.; Komaru, T.; et al. Effect of the Great East Japan Earthquake on cardiovascular diseases—Report from the 10 hospitals in the disaster area. *Circ. J.* **2013**, *77*, 490–493. [CrossRef] [PubMed]
23. Swerdel, J.N.; Janevic, T.M.; Cosgrove, N.M.; Kostis, J.B. The Myocardial Infarction Data Acquisition System (MIDAS 24) Study Group the Effect of Hurricane Sandy on Cardiovascular Events in New Jersey. *J. Am. Hear. Assoc.* **2014**, *3*, 001354. [CrossRef]
24. Tsai, C.-H.; Lung, F.-W.; Wang, S.-Y. The 1999 Ji-Ji (Taiwan) Earthquake as a Trigger for Acute Myocardial Infarction. *J. Psychosom. Res.* **2004**, *45*, 477–482. [CrossRef]
25. Dedert, E.A.; Calhoun, P.S.; Watkins, L.L.; Sherwood, A.; Beckham, J.C. Posttraumatic Stress Disorder, Cardiovascular, and Metabolic Disease: A Review of the Evidence. *Ann. Behav. Med.* **2010**, *39*, 61–78. [CrossRef]
26. Edmondson, D.; Cohen, B.E. Posttraumatic stress disorder and cardiovascular disease. *Prog. Cardiovasc. Dis.* **2013**, *55*, 548–556. [CrossRef]
27. Onose, T.; Nochioka, K.; Sakata, Y.; Miura, M.; Tadaki, S.; Ushigome, R.; Yamauchi, T.; Sato, K.; Tsuji, K.; Abe, R.; et al. Predictors and Prognostic Impact of Post-Traumatic Stress Disorder After the Great East Japan Earthquake in Patients With Cardiovascular Disease. *Circ. J.* **2015**, *79*, 664–667. [CrossRef]
28. Lavie, C.J.; Gerber, T.C.; Lanier, W.L. Hurricane Katrina: The Infarcts beyond the Storm. *Disaster Med. Public Health Prep.* **2009**, *3*, 131–135. [CrossRef]
29. Kivimäki, M.; Steptoe, A. Effects of stress on the development and progression of cardiovascular disease. *Nat. Rev. Cardiol.* **2017**, *15*, 215–229. [CrossRef] [PubMed]
30. Peters, M.N.; Moscona, J.C.; Katz, M.J.; DeAndrade, K.B.; Quevedo, H.C.; Tiwari, S.; Burchett, A.R.; Turnage, T.A.; Singh, K.Y.; Fomunung, E.N.; et al. Natural Disasters and Myocardial Infarction: The Six Years After Hurricane Katrina. *Mayo Clin. Proc.* **2014**, *89*, 472–477. [CrossRef] [PubMed]
31. Epel, E.; Lin, J.; Wilhelm, F.H.; Wolkowitz, O.; Cawthon, R.; Adler, N.; Dolbier, C.; Mendes, W.; Blackburn, E. Cell aging in relation to stress arousal and cardiovascular disease risk factors. *Psychoneuroendocrinology* **2006**, *31*, 277–287. [CrossRef] [PubMed]
32. Glynn, L.; Buckley, B.; Reddan, N.; Newell, J.; Hinde, J.; Dinneen, S.F.; Murphy, A.W. Multimorbidity and risk among patients with established cardiovascular disease: A cohort study. *Br. J. Gen. Pr.* **2008**, *58*, 488–494. [CrossRef] [PubMed]
33. Lekoubou, A.; Ovbiagele, B. Prevalence and influence of chronic obstructive pulmonary disease on stroke outcomes in hospitalized stroke patients. *eNeurologicalSci* **2017**, *6*, 21–24. [CrossRef]
34. Yen, Y.-S.; Harnod, D.; Lin, C.-L.; Harnod, T.; Lin, C.-L. Long-Term Mortality and Medical Burden of Patients with Chronic Obstructive Pulmonary Disease with and without Subsequent Stroke Episodes. *Int. J. Environ. Res. Public Health* **2020**, *17*, 2550. [CrossRef]
35. Strand, L.B.; Tsai, M.K.; Wen, C.P.; Chang, S.-S.; Brumpton, B.M. Is having asthma associated with an increased risk of dying from cardiovascular disease? A prospective cohort study of 446 346 Taiwanese adults. *BMJ Open* **2018**, *8*, e019992. [CrossRef]

36. Sturgeon, K.M.; Deng, L.; Bluethmann, S.M.; Zhou, S.; Trifiletti, D.M.; Jiang, C.; Kelly, S.P.; Zaorsky, N.G. A population-based study of cardiovascular disease mortality risk in US cancer patients. *Eur. Heart J.* **2019**, *40*, 3889–3897. [CrossRef]
37. Kim, D.; Adejumo, A.C.; Yoo, E.R.; Iqbal, U.; Li, A.A.; Pham, E.A.; Cholankeril, G.; Glenn, J.S.; Ahmed, A. Trends in Mortality From Extrahepatic Complications in Patients with Chronic Liver Disease, From 2007 Through 2017. *Gastroenterology* **2019**, *157*, 1055–1066. [CrossRef]
38. Healthy People 2020. Disparities. Available online: https://www.healthypeople.gov/2020/about/foundation-health-measures/Disparities (accessed on 15 August 2020).
39. Basu, S.; Berkowitz, S.A.; Phillips, R.L.; Bitton, A.; Landon, B.E.; Phillips, R.S. Association of Primary Care Physician Supply With Population Mortality in the United States, 2005–2015. *JAMA Intern. Med.* **2019**, *179*, 506. [CrossRef]
40. Ford, E.S.; Mokdad, A.H.; Link, M.W.; Garvin, W.S.; McGuire, L.C.; Jiles, R.B.; Balluz, L.S.; B., J.R. Chronic disease in health emergencies: In the eye of the hurricane. *Prev. Chronic Dis.* **2006**, *3*, A46. [PubMed]
41. Cunningham, P.J.; Felland, L.E. Falling behind: Americans' access to medical care deteriorates, 2003–2007. *Track. Rep.* **2008**, *19*, 1–5.
42. Asaria, M.; Ali, S.; Doran, T.; Ferguson, B.; Fleetcroft, R.; Goddard, M.; Goldblatt, P.; Laudicella, M.; Raine, R.; Cookson, R. How a universal health system reduces inequalities: Lessons from England. *J. Epidemiol. Community Health* **2016**, *70*, 637–643. [CrossRef] [PubMed]
43. Marmot, M.; Friel, S.; Bell, R.; Houweling, T.A.J.; Taylor, S. Closing the gap in a generation: Health equity through action on the social determinants of health. *Lancet* **2008**, *372*, 1661–1669. [CrossRef]
44. Veugelers, P.; Yip, A.M. Socioeconomic disparities in health care use: Does universal coverage reduce inequalities in health? *J. Epidemiol. Community Health* **2003**, *57*, 424–428. [CrossRef]
45. Aitsi-Selmi, A.; Murray, V. The Sendai framework: Disaster risk reduction through a health lens. *Bull. World Health Organ.* **2015**, *93*, 362. [CrossRef]
46. Plough, A.; Fielding, J.E.; Chandra, A.; Williams, M.; Eisenman, D.; Wells, K.B.; Law, G.Y.; Fogleman, S.; Magana, A. Building community disaster resilience: Perspectives from a large urban county department of public health. *Am. J. Public Health* **2013**, *103*, 1190–1197. [CrossRef]
47. Ministry of the Interior. Toward a Sustainable Taiwan: Summary National Spatial Plan. Taiwan. Available online: https://www.cpami.gov.tw/filesys/file/rp6/rp1081203e.pdf (accessed on 15 August 2020).
48. United Nations. United Nations Sustainable Development Goals. Available online: https://sdgs.un.org/goals (accessed on 15 August 2020).
49. Ministry of the Interior. Disaster Prevention and Protection Act. Available online: https://law.moj.gov.tw/ENG/LawClass/LawAll.aspx?pcode=D0120014 (accessed on 15 August 2020).
50. Pan, Y.-J.; Yeh, L.-L.; Chan, H.-Y.; Chang, C.-K. Transformation of excess mortality in people with schizophrenia and bipolar disorder in Taiwan. *Psychol. Med.* **2017**, *47*, 2483–2493. [CrossRef]
51. Chiu, Y.-W.; Wu, C.-S.; Chen, P.-C.; Wei, Y.-C.; Hsu, L.-Y.; Wang, S.-H. Risk of acute mesenteric ischemia in patients with diabetes: A population-based cohort study in Taiwan. *Atherosclerosis* **2020**, *296*, 18–24. [CrossRef]
52. Kario, K. Disaster hypertension—Its characteristics, mechanism, and management. *Circ. J.* **2012**, *76*, 553–562. [CrossRef]
53. Messerli, F.H.; Panjrath, G.S. The J-Curve between Blood Pressure and Coronary Artery Disease or Essential Hypertension. *J. Am. Coll. Cardiol.* **2009**, *54*, 1827–1834. [CrossRef] [PubMed]
54. Zhou, N.; Xi, B.; Zhao, M.; Wang, L.; Veeranki, S.P. Uncontrolled hypertension increases risk of all-cause and cardiovascular disease mortality in US adults: The NHANES III Linked Mortality Study. *Sci. Rep.* **2018**, *8*, 9418. [CrossRef]
55. Shin, S.; Song, H.; Oh, S.-K.; Choi, K.E.; Kim, H.; Jang, S. Effect of antihypertensive medication adherence on hospitalization for cardiovascular disease and mortality in hypertensive patients. *Hypertens. Res.* **2013**, *36*, 1000–1005. [CrossRef]
56. Kim, S.; Shin, D.W.; Yun, J.M.; Hwang, Y.; Park, S.K.; Ko, Y.-J.; Cho, B.L. Medication Adherence and the Risk of Cardiovascular Mortality and Hospitalization Among Patients With Newly Prescribed Antihypertensive Medications. *Hypertension* **2016**, *67*, 506–512. [CrossRef] [PubMed]

57. Yang, Q.; Chang, A.; Ritchey, M.D.; Loustalot, F. Antihypertensive Medication Adherence and Risk of Cardiovascular Disease among Older Adults: A Population-Based Cohort Study. *J. Am. Hear. Assoc.* **2017**, *6*, 6. [CrossRef] [PubMed]
58. Bowling, C.B.; Davis, B.R.; Luciano, A.; Simpson, L.M.; Sloane, R.; Pieper, C.F.; Einhorn, P.T.; Oparil, S.; Muntner, P. Sustained blood pressure control and coronary heart disease, stroke, heart failure, and mortality: An observational analysis of ALLHAT. *J. Clin. Hypertens.* **2019**, *21*, 451–459. [CrossRef] [PubMed]

14

Spatio-Temporal Distribution of Negative Emotions in New York City After a Natural Disaster as Seen in Social Media

Oliver Gruebner [1,2,*], Sarah R. Lowe [3], Martin Sykora [4], Ketan Shankardass [5], SV Subramanian [6] and Sandro Galea [7]

1 Department of Geography, Humboldt-Universität zu Berlin, Berlin 10099, Germany
2 Epidemiology, Biostatistics, and Prevention Institute (EBPI), University of Zurich, 8001 Zurich, Switzerland
3 Department of Psychology, Montclair State University, Montclair, NJ 07043, USA; lowes@mail.montclair.edu
4 Centre for Information Management (CIM), School of Business and Economics (SBE), Loughborough University, Loughborough LE11 3TU, UK; M.D.Sykora@lboro.ac.uk
5 Department of Health Sciences, Wilfrid Laurier University, Waterloo, ON M5B 1W8, Canada; ketan.shankardass@gmail.com
6 Department of Social and Behavioral Sciences, Harvard T.H. Chan School of Public Health, Boston, MA 02115, USA; svsubram@hsph.harvard.edu
7 School of Public Health, Boston University, Boston, MA 02118, USA; sgalea@bu.edu
* Correspondence: oliver.gruebner@geo.hu-berlin.de

Abstract: Disasters have substantial consequences for population mental health. We used Twitter to (1) extract negative emotions indicating discomfort in New York City (NYC) before, during, and after Superstorm Sandy in 2012. We further aimed to (2) identify whether pre- or peri-disaster discomfort were associated with peri- or post-disaster discomfort, respectively, and to (3) assess geographic variation in discomfort across NYC census tracts over time. Our sample consisted of 1,018,140 geo-located tweets that were analyzed with an advanced sentiment analysis called "Extracting the Meaning Of Terse Information in a Visualization of Emotion" (EMOTIVE). We calculated discomfort rates for 2137 NYC census tracts, applied spatial regimes regression to find associations of discomfort, and used Moran's I for spatial cluster detection across NYC boroughs over time. We found increased discomfort, that is, bundled negative emotions after the storm as compared to during the storm. Furthermore, pre- and peri-disaster discomfort was positively associated with post-disaster discomfort; however, this association was different across boroughs, with significant associations only in Manhattan, the Bronx, and Queens. In addition, rates were most prominently spatially clustered in Staten Island lasting pre- to post-disaster. This is the first study that determined significant associations of negative emotional responses found in social media posts over space and time in the context of a natural disaster, which may guide us in identifying those areas and populations mostly in need for care.

Keywords: advanced sentiment analysis; digital epidemiology; geographic information system; geo-social media; hotspots; post-disaster mental health; psychogeography; spatial epidemiology; spatial regimes regression; Twitter data

---

1. Introduction

Large-scale natural disasters are observed worldwide [1–3] and can have substantial consequences for population mental health [4–7]. Although research to date has documented a great deal of mental health resilience in the aftermath of disasters, elevated rates of mental health consequences, including depression and post-traumatic stress, have been observed [7–10]. One of the key risk factors for adverse post-disaster mental health outcomes is experiencing overwhelming emotions in the context of disaster, which may be caused by the event itself, such as by exposure to trauma (i.e., actual or threatened death, serious injury, or sexual violence) [9]. These emotions may also be influenced by non-traumatic *stressors* either in the short or long term, such as loss of financial property, personal belongings, and/or one's home [4,7,9–11]. For example, emotions may convey information about how people evaluate what is happening and how they cope with it when they experience stress [11]. Sadness is usually related to experiencing an irreversible loss, and fright related to perception of immediate, concrete, and overwhelming physical danger [11]. Many studies have shown such negative emotional responses during a disaster being predictive of mental health problems in the aftermath of disaster [4], which may reflect the impact of disaster in terms of experienced stress. It is, however, important to differentiate "normal responses to abnormal events" from a lack of mental health resilience because the majority of people who report negative emotional reactions during a disaster do not develop mental health problems in the aftermath [7,10]. Nevertheless, we might expect the spatial and temporal distribution of emotional responses to follow the location and timing of disaster impacts, with implications for the burden of related adverse mental health problems.

The majority of studies on disaster mental health to date have relied solely on post-disaster data. Post-disaster studies are prone to possible recall bias, with the consequence that we are potentially missing important information on the time before the event. Some notable studies to date have included pre-event data [12–14]. Although these studies have brought a much better understanding of changes in mental health from pre- to post-disaster, research on this topic would further benefit from information that is gathered both prior to and during the event. Such information could, for example, demonstrate multiple dimensions of emotional reactions over time in the context of a disaster that could increase the precision of data relevant to mental health responses. Specifically, investigating multiple specific emotions, as defined by Ekman [15], such as fear, anger or disgust, or a combination thereof, could inform about the quality and strength of emotions as they are experienced during the disaster and could inform about risk for possible post-disaster mental health outcomes [16–23].

Research to date has provided little insight into geographic variability in where emotions are excessively expressed during or in the aftermath of large-scale disasters. Geographic concentrations of emotional expression would be indicative of some form of stress that is jointly experienced in specific populations within areas at specific times. Information on the concentration of specific emotional responses may exhibit people's alertness, and geographically mapping those places could reveal the spatial extent of areas in which possible issues arise guiding early intervention to minimize adverse mental health consequences. Better knowledge about the location and timing of specific emotional concentrations could provide important information about how to more efficiently roll out emergency public health interventions in the aftermath of disasters and other mass traumatic events.

Social media data, such as from Twitter, may help to fill these gaps, as they are largely and publicly available, have been successfully applied to disaster research, and provide pre-, peri-, and post-disaster information [23–25]. For example, specific emotions, such as fear or sadness, can be detected from Twitter streams through advanced sentiment analysis [26,27] and can be related to periods before, during, and after disasters. Furthermore, such data provide the opportunity for the geographic assessment of single posts. Hence, ecological momentary assessment of emotional reactions—that is, ongoing evaluation of in-the-moment experiences—becomes possible [26]. For example, in a study on emotional responses in the greater New York City area during Superstorm Sandy, Gruebner et al. [21] used Twitter data and found specific negative emotions clustered over space and time. However, this previous study used a relatively narrow time frame during the disaster.

We set out to explore the spatial distribution of *discomfort* in the population before, during, and after Superstorm Sandy that formed over the Caribbean on 22 October, hit the New York City (NYC) area on 29 October, and disappeared on 2 November 2012 [28]. The storm caused 43 deaths and about US$ 19 billion in damages within NYC alone making it the most costly and destructive disaster to impact public housing in the history of this city [29]. Specifically, we aimed to (1) identify a composite of negative emotions (i.e., discomfort) as expressed by the population that posted geo-located Twitter tweets in NYC over three time periods, each of approximately two weeks, representative of the pre-disaster period, the peri-disaster period, and the post-disaster period. We further aimed to (2) assess whether pre- or peri-disaster discomfort were associated with peri- or post-disaster discomfort, and to (3) investigate whether there was geographic variation in discomfort risk across NYC boroughs over time.

2. Materials and Methods

We used Twitter for this study because it is a publicly available resource that can be widely used for research purposes. Furthermore, tweets were geo-referenced facilitating spatial analysis informing our research questions. In addition, Twitter has already been used in other studies in that context [21,30–32].

About 45 million social media users that were mostly under the age of 50 in the United States were monthly active on Twitter by the end of 2012 [33–35]. Approximately three percent of them potentially used geolocation services producing geo-located Twitter data [36]. We used geo-located Twitter data published within NYC for the time frame of 10 October to 18 November 2012. Our sample was composed of 1,018,140 tweets that were suitable for our analysis, i.e., had information about geographic locations from where the tweets had been issued and were in English (see Table 1). We used tweets that were geo-located within those NYC census tracts that shared a border in order to facilitate spatial analyses at the census tract level. Thereby, 399,089 tweets were within the pre-disaster period (8 October to 21 October), 235,423 tweets were within the peri-disaster period (22 October to 4 November), and 383,628 tweets were within the post-disaster period (5 November to 18 November). Our level of analysis was the census tract (N = 2137). The dataset was available from the Harvard Center for Geographic Analysis Geo-tweet Archive (CGA) [37], the institution that collected the data. For transparency in research, the Tweet IDs used in this study can be made available for interested researchers, according to Twitter's sharing policy. Harvard provides a rehydration app to facilitate conversions of TweetIDs back to full tweets [38].

Table 1. Descriptive figures for aggregated Tweets at the census tract level over the entire study period in New York City from 10 October–18 November 2012. For example, the range of tweet population (or individual emotions) indicates the minimum and maximum number of all tweets, or of tweets with a specific emotion, found in census tracts. Note that discomfort is a combination of the negative emotions anger, confusion, disgust, fear, sadness, and shame. Tweets were coded as discomfort when they were indicative of any of these emotions at the individual level. Therefore, the numbers do not sum up at the census tract level when single emotions are compared to discomfort at that level.

Variable	Range	1st/3rd Quintile	Median	Mean	Sum
Tweet population	1–6507	24/149	59	158.8	1,018,140
Discomfort	0–158	0/5	2	5.03	32,254
Anger	0–119	0/1	0	0.77	4918
Confusion	0–8	0/0	0	0.25	1620
Disgust	0–45	0/1	0	1.11	7126
Fear	0–34	0/1	0	0.59	3841
Sadness	0–77	0/3	1	2.24	14,333
Shame	0–23	0/0	0	0.17	1079

We first analyzed the raw data with the advanced sentiment detection program "Extracting the Meaning Of Terse Information in a Visualization of Emotion" (EMOTIVE) [25,39]. While standard sentiment analysis tools only separate the mood as identified from social media texts into negative, positive, or neutral, EMOTIVE is able to detect basic emotions as defined by Ekman [40], such as *anger, disgust, fear, happiness, sadness, surprise*, and also *shame* and *confusion*, thereby preserving the original tweet texts and timestamps. We combined six of these emotions that are typically considered as negative emotions, i.e., *anger, confusion, disgust, fear, sadness,* and *shame* into one single emotion which we named *discomfort* to maximize statistical power. We coded each tweet dichotomously for the presence (case = 1) or absence (no case = 0) of discomfort. We then separated the dataset into three sets of two weeks each, representative of the pre-disaster period (8 October to 21 October), the peri-disaster period (22 October to 4 November), and the post-disaster period (5 November to 18 November). We then noted all discomfort cases at the census tract level and calculated smoothed spatial empirical Bayes (SEB) rates using the percentage of tweets that were indicative of discomfort out of all tweets (tweet population) for each census tract during each time period. This method was used to adjust for heterogeneity of variances of the rates [41] that evolved due to varying population sizes in the total tweets across NYC's census tracts. Empirical Bayes rates were calculated in GeoDa (Center for Spatial Data Science, Chicago, IL, USA) [41]. In addition, we checked whether SEB rates were significantly different across pre-, peri-, and post-disaster with paired t-tests in R (The R Foundation, Vienna, Austria) [42].

Second, we assessed associations between pre- and peri-disaster discomfort and between pre- as well as peri- and post-disaster discomfort rates at the census tract level initially with Ordinary Least Squares (OLS) regression models. Because OLS residuals exhibited spatial autocorrelation indicated by a Lagrange multiplier test, with the lag model performing well over the spatial error model, we chose a spatial lag model (Spatial Two Stage Least Squares regression (S2SLS)) as suggested in Anselin and Rey [43]. This model explicitly included a spatial lag variable on the right-hand side of the regression equation to account for the spatial structure found in the data stemming from non-independence of discomfort SEB rates in neighboring census tracts.

Third, we investigated spatial clusters of above average SEB (discomfort) across the census tracts at each time period by applying spatial autocorrelation analyses (Global and local Moran's I) in GeoDa [41]. We then ran a series of spatial regimes regression models (S2SLS) to further account for structural instability [43], that is, geographic variation in the associations between pre- and peri-disaster discomfort and post-disaster discomfort across NYC boroughs, i.e., the regimes. Furthermore, a Chow test [44] was applied for regime diagnostics. Regression analysis was applied in GeoDaSpace (Center for Spatial Data Science, Chicago, IL, USA) [45].

3. Results

3.1. Rates of Discomfort in Twitter Data

We extracted and combined six negative emotions from the Twitter activity of users in the given area and time frames in a single index that we termed *discomfort*. We identified 2649 cases (i.e., tweets) (0.66%) indicative of discomfort pre-disaster, 1641 cases (0.70%) peri-disaster, and 2845 cases (0.74%) post-disaster. We noted that compared to pre-disaster, overall discomfort rates were significantly different peri-disaster with $t(2136) = -6.65$, $p < 0.001$ and a mean of difference of -0.003. Post-disaster rates were also significantly different from pre-disaster rates $t(2136) = -3.06$, $p = 0.002$ (mean of difference = -0.001) and from peri-disaster rates $t(2136) = 4.76$, $p < 0.001$ (mean of difference -0.002). In addition, we noted that median rates of discomfort were different across boroughs and time periods, with the highest rates across all time periods in Staten Island as compared to the other boroughs, and Brooklyn having the lowest rates across all time periods compared to the other boroughs (Figure 1).

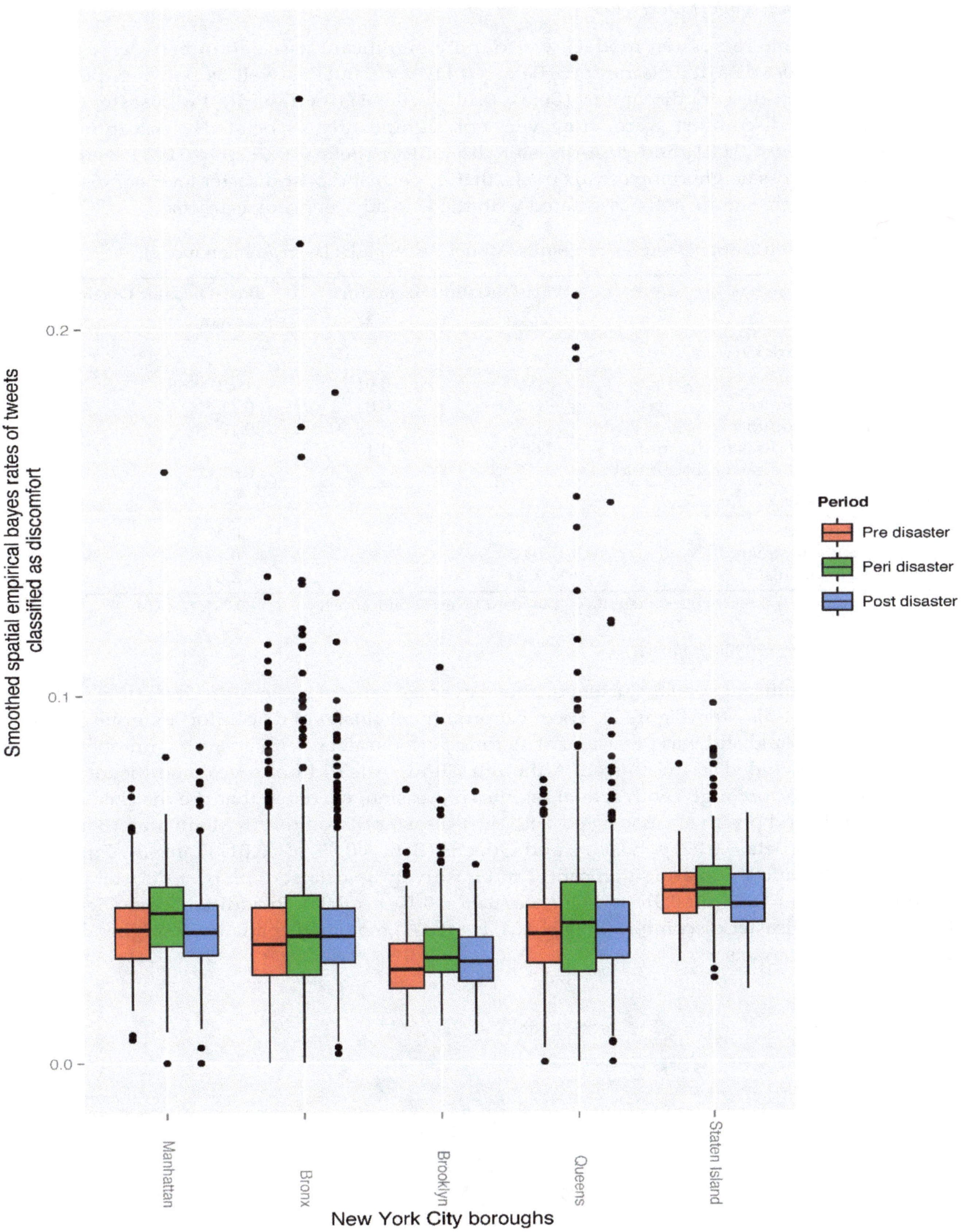

Figure 1. Spatial Empirical Bayes smoothed rates of tweets classified as discomfort for each NYC borough across time periods.

3.2. Associations of Discomfort Over Time

In multivariable regression models, we found a significant association between pre-disaster discomfort and post-disaster discomfort (Beta = 0.11, $p < 0.001$) as well as between peri-disaster discomfort and post-disaster discomfort (Beta = 0.10, $p < 0.001$) (see Table 2). Pre-disaster discomfort and peri-disaster discomfort were, however, not significantly associated. Additionally, both peri- (Beta = 0.68, $p < 0.001$) and post-disaster discomfort (Beta = 0.61, $p < 0.001$) were spatially interdependent across neighboring census tracts, that is, peri- and post-disaster levels of discomfort in one census tract were significantly associated with those in adjacent census tracts.

Table 2. Spatial regression results. Model 1 is a spatial lag regression model.

Variable	Peri-Disaster Discomfort		Post-Disaster Discomfort	
	Coef.	S.E.	Coef.	S.E.
Model 1: New York City				
NYC Intercept	0.00	0.01	0.01 **	0.00
Pre-disaster discomfort	0.03	0.04	0.11 ***	0.02
Peri-disaster discomfort	/		0.10 ***	0.01
Spatial lag of peri-disaster discomfort	0.68 ***	0.18	/	
Spatial lag of post-disaster discomfort	/		0.61 ***	0.07
Model diagnostic				
Pseudo R-squared	0.33		0.47	
Spatial Pseudo R-squared	0.03		0.13	
Anselin-Kelejian Test	1.99		2.67	

Coef. = Coefficient estimate; S.E. = Standard Error; Significance level: *** <0.001, ** <0.01.

3.3. Spatial Variation in Discomfort Risk

We found significant spatial clusters of above average rates of discomfort in all time frames, i.e., pre-, peri-, and post-disaster (Figure 2). The most prominent cluster of discomfort in terms of size was located in Staten Island and was persistent at all time periods, albeit with a varying number of census tracts that were included in the cluster. Although Chow tests did not reveal significant structural instability across the boroughs with spatial regimes regression, we noted that pre-disaster discomfort was significantly and positively associated with post-disaster discomfort in Manhattan (Beta = 0.18, $p < 0.01$), the Bronx (Beta = 0.22, $p < 0.001$), and Queens (Beta = 0.09, $p < 0.01$) (Table 3). Furthermore, peri-disaster discomfort was also significantly and positively associated with post-disaster discomfort in Manhattan (Beta = 0.13, $p < 0.01$) and Queens (Beta = 0.10, $p < 0.05$). In addition, peri- (Beta = 0.91, $p < 0.001$) and post-disaster discomfort (Beta = 0.64, $p < 0.001$) remained spatially interdependent across neighboring census tracts.

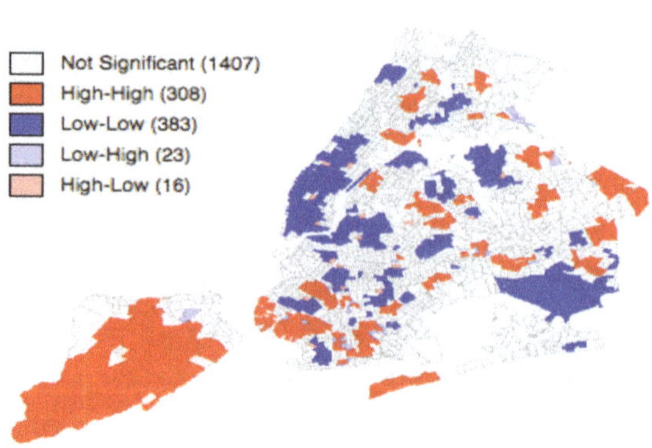

(A)

Figure 2. *Cont.*

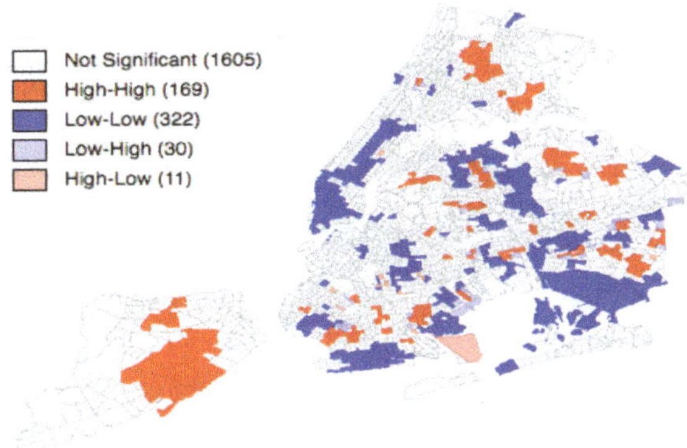

(B)

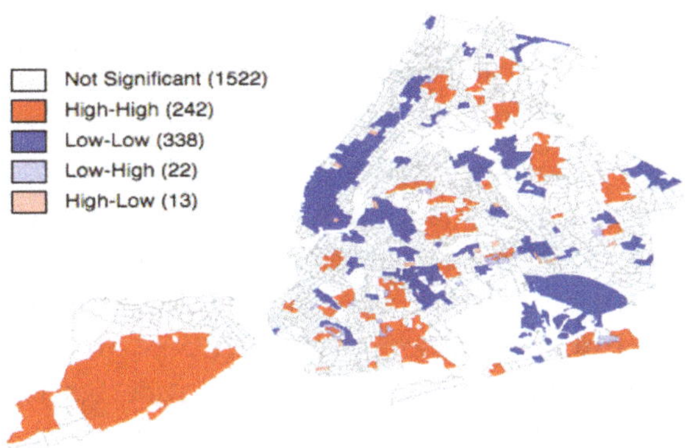

(C)

Figure 2. Local clusters of above average discomfort rates (shaded in red) in NYC geo-located Twitter tweets for the three periods before (**A**), during (**B**) and after (**C**) Superstorm Sandy, indicating that high rates were found next to other high rates (High-High). Rates were smoothed with the spatial empirical Bayes smoother prior to the cluster analysis. Notably, the statistic also calculates below average rates (low rates next to other low rates) and outliers (high rates next to low rates and vice versa) that are not considered in this study.

Table 3. Spatial regression results. Model 2 is a spatial lag regression model with regimes, i.e., the boroughs.

Variable	Peri-Disaster Discomfort		Post-Disaster Discomfort	
	Coef.	S.E.	Coef.	S.E.
Model 2: New York City boroughs				
Manhattan Intercept	0.00	0.01	0.00	0.00
Pre-disaster discomfort	0.09	0.12	0.18 **	0.06
Peri-disaster discomfort	/		0.13 **	0.04
Bronx Intercept	0.00	0.01	0.00	0.00
Pre-disaster discomfort	0.07	0.07	0.22 ***	0.07
Peri-disaster discomfort	/		0.05	0.04
Brooklyn Intercept	0.00	0.01	0.01	0.00
Pre-disaster discomfort	0.01	0.06	0.07.	0.04
Peri-disaster discomfort	/		0.10	0.06
Queens Intercept	0.00	0.01	0.01	0.00
Pre-disaster discomfort	0.03	0.08	0.09 **	0.04
Peri-disaster discomfort	/		0.10 *	0.05
Staten Island Intercept	0.01	0.01	0.01 *	0.01
Pre-disaster discomfort	−0.03	0.09	0.07	0.09
Peri-disaster discomfort	/		0.04	0.04

Table 3. *Cont.*

Variable	Peri-Disaster Discomfort		Post-Disaster Discomfort	
	Coef.	S.E.	Coef.	S.E.
Global spatial lag of peri-disaster discomfort	0.91 ***	0.25	/	
Global spatial lag of post-disaster discomfort	/		0.64 ***	0.14
Model diagnostic				
Pseudo R-squared	0.33		0.47	
Spatial Pseudo R-squared	0.03		0.14	
Chow test for intercept	1.84		9.09	
Chow test for pre-disaster discomfort	1.97		6.99	
Chow test for peri-disaster discomfort	/		4.01	
Global Chow test	2.36		18.06	
Anselin-Kelejian Test	1.93		1.04	

Coef. = Coefficient estimate, S.E. = Standard Error, Significance level: *** <0.001, ** <0.01, * <0.1.

4. Discussion

We found negative emotional reactions that we combined in one variable, which we called discomfort. Overall, discomfort rates were significantly different after the disaster as compared to before or during the pre-disaster period across boroughs. Further, we showed that pre- and peri-disaster discomfort were significantly associated with post-disaster discomfort rates. Moreover, discomfort rates were spatially clustered across NYC census tracts and associations of discomfort rates over time were different across boroughs with significant associations only in Manhattan, the Bronx, and Queens.

The Twitter activity of users can exhibit perceived and real risk as experienced by users [21,31]. Our results show that there were higher rates of discomfort expressed in Tweets during the post-disaster period as compared to during the peri-disaster period, likely corresponding to the time period in which residents had to deal with the greatest stressors (e.g., losses) after the storm. Staten Island had the highest median rates of discomfort among all boroughs and across all time frames, which was consistent with what one might expect based on the variability of Sandy's impact across NYC. Staten Island was one of the boroughs that was hit the hardest by Superstorm Sandy due to a combination of the storm's arrival and high tide leading to high levels of inundations and crucial service outage after the storm [46]. All the above might explain why we see highest rates of discomfort in Staten Island.

Taking into account all census tracts in a global regression model, we found that higher volumes of specific negative emotions at pre- or during the disaster were associated with negative emotions also after the disaster. From studies that compared mental health symptoms from before with after the disaster we know that pre-disaster conditions are one of the strongest predictors for post-disaster conditions [12–14]. This may also be true for emotional responses as expressed on Twitter and other social media platforms.

We further investigated geographic concentrations in discomfort rates across NYC regions (i.e., census tracts) within and across the boroughs and found significant spatial clustering of above average discomfort rates in all boroughs except Manhattan, with biggest clusters across census tracts in Staten Island. Spatial clusters may occur due to spatial dependence of rates across census tracts. Our analysis did not investigate the possible causes of small-area variation in discomfort over time; however, we have at least three possible explanations for spatial dependence causing the clusters. First, there were environmental issues, such as flooding and houses affected by the storm with some of them being totally destroyed [47]. Further, reported power shortages, falling trees, or strong winds spanning across census tracts may have affected a wider population in several neighboring census tracts simultaneously. This might have been particularly true across several neighboring census tracts in Staten Island, where considerable flooding and destroyed houses have been reported by the Federal Emergency and Management Agency (FEMA) [47,48]. While people collectively experienced these environmental issues, they may have processed feelings in the affected areas leading to these spatial patterns of negative emotions. There has also been more localized environmental damage, such as floods and affected houses in parts of other boroughs, for example in the Queens areas spanning from Averne to the Far Rockaway, where we found clusters, too [47,48].

Second, daily interaction of, for example, residents of one census tract with facilities of other census tracts (e.g., coffee shop, work place, shelter, drop-off location for receiving aid and goods) while tweeting might have produced spatial patterns of emotions spanning across several adjacent census tracts.

Third, people may have perceived environmental issues differently depending on their socio-demographic characteristics or socio-ecological context in which they live, for example with people living in better structural quality of housing worrying less about strong winds. Socio-demographic characteristics or socio-ecological contexts vary substantially across NYC boroughs (with some neighborhoods being highly segregated across census tracts), which may have further contributed to the clusters. Future studies should include neighborhood level socio-demographic and socio-ecologic variables to further understand these patterns.

We also found that clusters of above average discomfort rates in several census tracts were persistent over time from peri- to post-disaster. The most prominent clusters at all time periods spanning across the largest number of census tracts were also located in Staten Island. These clusters and those elsewhere may exhibit areas of increased risk for mental health needs due to, e.g., increased environmental issues, mobility (or displacement) of tweeters, different perceptions among tweeters, or a combination of the three.

In addition, we investigated the spatial variability of associations of discomfort rates over time. We found that pre-disaster discomfort was significantly associated with post-disaster discomfort only in Manhattan, the Bronx, and Queens, while peri-disaster discomfort was significantly associated with post-disaster discomfort only in Manhattan and Queens. We may expect other factors being more important predictors for post-disaster discomfort in the other boroughs, such as neighborhood-level socio-ecological factors (e.g., socio-economic status, physical exposure to the storm). With regard to the boroughs in which we found significant positive associations of discomfort rates across the time periods, our results may indicate that the associations were place dependent with socio-ecological factors specific to local census tracts and boroughs. Our results may also indicate that those areas with higher discomfort rates during the storm—presumably due to issues such as service outfalls or strong winds—may be more likely to exhibit discomfort also after the storm, when neighborhoods were flooded or houses seriously affected by the storm. Since early emotional reactions predict post-disaster mental health problems [4], this should be investigated in more depth in future studies.

Our study had several limitations. First, we used geo-located English tweets from Twitter. Future studies may also include non-geo referenced data including further languages or data sources. Second, due to likely service shortages during and in the immediate aftermath of the storm, the three time frames under investigation had different number of tweets with the lowest number of tweets during the disaster, which should be kept in mind when interpreting the findings. For example, it is possible that Twitter users were unable to charge their phones, that they were trying to conserve battery life, or that they were restricted in their cell phone usage due to interrupted cell phone services, hence limiting the activity of Twitter users during that time. Third, we only used tweets from NYC census tracts that shared a border with another NYC census tract to facilitate spatial analysis. This excluded tweets that were published in census tracts not directly connected to other census tracts (e.g., Ellis Island) or that were posted while travelling on water. Fourth, since tweeters were assumingly using mobile devices while tweeting, it is possible that tweets were not always sent from the same location but rather while on the daily commute, at home, at work, or in a shelter before or during the storm. After the storm, some of the Twitter population may have been displaced and would be tweeting from other locations as before or during the storm. Finally, we have worked at the ecological level, that is, census tracts in which tweets have been posted rather than at the individual Twitter user level. Use of individual Twitter identifiers would permit the application and testing of more traditional paradigms of stress response variation during a trauma as predicting post-trauma distress.

5. Conclusions

This is the first study that identified emotions representative of discomfort in social media along with their concentration in space and time. Discomfort, i.e., negative emotional responses including amongst others fear, anger, and sadness, were concentrated in some neighborhoods across NYC and were persistent over time, most prominently so in Staten Island. These concentrations may provide knowledge about areas and communities with mental health need.

High discomfort rates pre-disaster were associated with high rates during and after the disaster. The association of pre-, peri-, and post-disaster discomfort over time was place dependent, suggesting different socio-ecological factors responsible for discomfort across the five boroughs.

Since early emotional reactions may predict longer-term mental health needs, this approach could further assist in the long-term allocation of services. EMOTIVE is currently being extended to also evaluate stress responses that in conjunction with a spatially explicit approach, as it has been applied here may help to estimate the development of symptoms indicative of depression and PTSD [49,50]. Given that social media use has dramatically increased worldwide since 2012, these data provide enormous potential for mental health research to study e.g., the functional relationship between socio-ecological factors and mental health. For example, working at the individual social media user level might inform about individual people's exposure in addition to weather-related damage and flooding, such as loss of resources and restricted access to services in real time. In addition, this level of analysis could also capture other community-level risk factors such as geographic variation in pre-existing mental health conditions or social support. In countries with limited formal surveillance infrastructure, the approach may also have potential for the identification of areas and populations in need for care.

Author Contributions: Conceptualization, O.G. and S.R.L.; Methodology, M.S. and O.G.; Software, M.S.; Formal Analysis, M.S. and O.G. Data Curation, M.S. and O.G. Writing-Original Draft Preparation, O.G. and S.R.L.; Writing-Review & Editing, O.G., S.R.L. and K.S.; Visualization, O.G.; Supervision, S.G. and S.V.S.

Acknowledgments: We thank Suzanne Elayan for her help with data preparation for EMOTIVE. We acknowledge support by the German Research Foundation (DFG) and the Open Access Publication Fund of Humboldt-Universität zu Berlin.

References

1. International Federation of Red Cross and Red Crescent Societies World disasters report: Focus on Culture and Risk. Available online: http://www.ifrc.org/Global/Documents/Secretariat/201410/WDR%2014.pdf (accessed on 12 October 2018).
2. Hoeppe, P. Trends in weather related disasters—Consequences for insurers and society. *Weather Clim. Extrem.* **2015**. [CrossRef]
3. NOAA National Centers for Environmental Information, N. O. and A. A. Billion-Dollar Weather and Climate Disasters: Summary Stats. Available online: http://www.ncdc.noaa.gov/billions/summary-stats (accessed on 12 October 2018).
4. Norris, F.H.; Friedman, M.J.; Watson, P.J.; Byrne, C.M.; Diaz, E.; Kaniasty, K. 60,000 disaster victims speak: Part I. An empirical review of the empirical literature, 1981–2001. *Psychiatry-Interpers. Biol. Process.* **2002**, *65*, 207–239. [CrossRef]
5. Neria, Y.; Galea, S. *Mental Health and Disasters*; Cambridge University Press: Cambridge, UK, 2009; ISBN 0521883873.
6. Neria, Y.; Nandi, A.; Galea, S. Post-traumatic stress disorder following disasters: A systematic review. *Psychol. Med.* **2008**, *38*, 467–480. [CrossRef] [PubMed]

7. Goldmann, E.; Galea, S. Mental health consequences of disasters. *Annu. Rev. Public Health* **2014**, *35*, 169–183. [CrossRef] [PubMed]
8. Dückers, M.L.A. A multilayered psychosocial resilience framework and its implications for community-focused crisis management. *J. Contingencies Crisis Manag.* **2017**, *25*, 182–187. [CrossRef]
9. North, C.S.; Pfefferbaum, B. Mental health response to community disasters. *JAMA* **2013**, *310*, 507. [CrossRef] [PubMed]
10. North, C.S. Disaster mental health epidemiology: Methodological review and interpretation of research findings. *Psychiatry* **2016**, *79*, 130–146. [CrossRef] [PubMed]
11. Lazarus, R.S. *Stress and Emotion A New Synthesis*; SPRINGER: New York, NY, USA, 2006; ISBN 9780826102614.
12. Lowe, S.R.; Chan, C.S.; Rhodes, J.E. Pre-hurricane perceived social support protects against psychological distress: A longitudinal analysis of low-income mothers. *J. Consult. Clin. Psychol.* **2010**, *78*, 551–560. [CrossRef] [PubMed]
13. Weems, C.F.; Pina, A.A.; Costa, N.M.; Watts, S.E.; Taylor, L.K.; Cannon, M.F. Predisaster trait anxiety and negative affect predict posttraumatic stress in youths after Hurricane Katrina. *J. Consult. Clin. Psychol.* **2007**, *75*, 154–159. [CrossRef] [PubMed]
14. La Greca, A.M.; Silverman, W.K.; Wasserstein, S.B. Children's predisaster functioning as a predictor of posttraumatic stress following Hurricane Andrew. *J. Consult. Clin. Psychol.* **1998**, *66*, 883–892. [CrossRef] [PubMed]
15. Ekman, P. Basic emotions. In *Handbook of Cognition and Emotion*; John Wiley&Sons, Ltd.: Chichester, UK, 2005; pp. 45–60. ISBN 9780471978367.
16. Sutton, J.; Gibson, C.B.; Phillips, N.E.; Spiro, E.S.; League, C.; Johnson, B.; Fitzhugh, S.M.; Butts, C.T. A cross-hazard analysis of terse message retransmission on Twitter. *Proc. Natl. Acad. Sci. USA* **2015**, *112*, 14793–14798. [CrossRef] [PubMed]
17. Houston, J.B.; Hawthorne, J.; Perreault, M.F.; Park, E.H.; Goldstein Hode, M.; Halliwell, M.R.; Turner McGowen, S.E.; Davis, R.; Vaid, S.; McElderry, J.A.; et al. Social media and disasters: A functional framework for social media use in disaster planning, response, and research. *Disasters* **2015**, *39*, 1–22. [CrossRef] [PubMed]
18. Glass, K.; Colbaugh, R. Estimating the sentiment of social media content for security informatics applications. *Secur. Inform.* **2012**, *1*, 3. [CrossRef]
19. Johansson, F.; Brynielsson, J.; Quijano, M.N. Estimating Citizen Alertness in Crises Using Social Media Monitoring and Analysis. In Proceedings of the 2012 European Intelligence and Security Informatics Conference, Odense, Denmark, 22–24 August 2012. [CrossRef]
20. Kumar, S.; Barbier, G.; Abbasi, M.A.; Liu, H. Tweet Tracker: An Analysis Tool for Humanitarian and Disaster Relief. In Proceedings of the Fifth International AAAI Conference on Weblogs and Social Media, Barcelona, Spain, 17–21 July 2011.
21. Gruebner, O.; Lowe, S.R.; Sykora, M.; Shankardass, K.; Subramanian, S.V.; Galea, S. A novel surveillance approach for disaster mental health. *PLoS ONE* **2017**, *12*, e0181233. [CrossRef] [PubMed]
22. Gruebner, O.; Sykora, M.; Lowe, S.R.; Shankardass, K.; Trinquart, L.; Jackson, T.; Subramanian, S.V.; Galea, S. Mental health surveillance after the terrorist attacks in Paris. *Lancet* **2016**, *387*, 2195–2196. [CrossRef]
23. Gruebner, O.; Sykora, M.; Lowe, S.R.; Shankardass, K.; Galea, S.; Subramanian, S.V. Big data opportunities for social behavioral and mental health research. *Soc. Sci. Med.* **2017**, *2012*, 2016–2018. [CrossRef] [PubMed]
24. Hirschberg, J.; Manning, C.D. Advances in natural language processing. *Science* **2015**, *349*, 261–266. [CrossRef] [PubMed]
25. Sykora, M.D.; Jackson, T.W.; OBrien, A.; Elayan, S. Emotive Ontology: Extracting Fine-Grained Emotions from Terse, Informal Messages. In Proceedings of the IADIS International Conference Intelligent Systems and Agents 2013, Prague, Czech Republic, 22–24 July 2013.
26. Shaughnessy, K.; Reyes, R.; Shankardass, K.; Sykora, M.; Feick, R.; Lawrence, H.; Robertson, C. Using geolocated social media for ecological momentary assessments of emotion: Innovative opportunities in psychology science and practice. *Can. Psychol. Can.* **2017**. [CrossRef]
27. Hofmann, W.; Patel, P.V. Survey signal. *Soc. Sci. Comput. Rev.* **2015**, *33*, 235–253. [CrossRef]
28. National Oceanic and Atmospheric Administration Hurricane Sandy. Available online: https://www.weather.gov/okx/HurricaneSandy (accessed on 28 July 2018).
29. NYC Housing Authority Sandy Recovery and Progress. Available online: https://www1.nyc.gov/site/nycha/about/recovery-history.page (accessed on 28 July 2018).

30. Shelton, T.; Poorthuis, A.; Graham, M.; Zook, M. Mapping the data shadows of Hurricane Sandy: Uncovering the sociospatial dimensions of 'big data'. *Geoforum* **2014**, *52*, 167–179. [CrossRef]
31. Kryvasheyeu, Y.; Chen, H.; Obradovich, N.; Moro, E.; Van Hentenryck, P.; Fowler, J.; Cebrian, M. Rapid assessment of disaster damage using social media activity. *Sci. Adv.* **2016**, *2*, e1500779. [CrossRef] [PubMed]
32. Takayasu, M.; Sato, K.; Sano, Y.; Yamada, K.; Miura, W.; Takayasu, H. Rumor diffusion and convergence during the 3.11 Earthquake: A twitter case study. *PLoS ONE* **2015**, *10*, e0121443. [CrossRef] [PubMed]
33. Statista Number of Monthly Active Twitter Users in the United States from 1st Quarter 2010 to 2nd Quarter 2018 (In Millions). Available online: https://www.statista.com/statistics/274564/monthly-active-twitter-users-in-the-united-states/ (accessed on 12 October 2018).
34. Pew Research Center Social Media Fact Sheet. Available online: http://www.pewinternet.org/fact-sheet/social-media/ (accessed on 16 October 2018).
35. Pew Research Center Demographics of Key Social Networking Platforms. Available online: http://www.pewinternet.org/2015/01/09/demographics-of-key-social-networking-platforms-2/ (accessed on 16 October 2018).
36. Sloan, L.; Morgan, J. Who tweets with their location? Understanding the relationship between demographic characteristics and the use of geoservices and geotagging on twitter. *PLoS ONE* **2015**, *10*, e0142209. [CrossRef] [PubMed]
37. Harvard Center for Geographic Analysis Geo-tweet Archive. Available online: http://www.gis.harvard.edu (accessed on 16 October 2018).
38. Harvard Center for Geographic Analysis Twitter Rehydration Script. Available online: https://github.com/cga-harvard/hhypermap-bop/tree/master/BOP-utilities/Twitter_Rehydration (accessed on 16 October 2018).
39. Sykora, M.D.; Jackson, T.W.; OBrien, A.; Elayan, S. National security and social media monitoring: A presentation of the EMOTIVE and related systems. In Proceedings of the 2013 European Intelligence and Security Informatics Conference, Uppsala, Sweden, 12–14 August 2013; pp. 172–175.
40. Ekman, P. Are there basic emotions? *Psychol. Rev.* **1992**, *99*, 550–553. [CrossRef] [PubMed]
41. Anselin, L.; Syabri, I.; Kho, Y. GeoDa: An introduction to spatial data analysis. *Geogr. Anal.* **2006**, *38*, 5–22. [CrossRef]
42. R Development Core Team. *R: A Language and Environment for Statistical Computing*; R Foundation for Statistical Computing: Vienna, Austria, 2013; ISBN 3-900051-07-0.
43. Anselin, L.; Rey, S.J. *Modern Spatial Econometrics in Practice: A Guide to GeoDa, GeoDaSpace and PySAL*; GeoDa Press LLC: Chicago, IL, USA, 2014.
44. Chow, G.C. Tests of equality between sets of coefficients in two linear regressions. *Econometrica* **1960**, *28*, 591. [CrossRef]
45. GeoDa Center for Geospatial Analysis and Computation GeoDaSpace 2013. Available online: https://geodacenter.asu.edu/software (accessed on 16 October 2018).
46. Gammon, C. Why Hurricane Sandy Hit Staten Island So Hard/New York City Hurricanes. Available online: http://www.livescience.com/24616-hurricane-sandy-staten-island-effects.html (accessed on 12 October 2018).
47. Federal Emergency and Management Agency FEMA MOTF Hurricane Sandy Impact Analysis. Available online: http://fema.maps.arcgis.com/home/item.html?id=307dd522499d4a44a33d7296a5da5ea0 (accessed on 10 October 2015).
48. Bloch, M.; Fessenden, F.; McLean, A.; Tse, A. Derek Watkins Surveying the destruction Caused by Hurricane Sandy. Available online: http://www.nytimes.com/newsgraphics/2012/1120-sandy/survey-of-the-flooding-in-new-york-after-the-hurricane.html (accessed on 28 July 2018).
49. Sykora, M.D.; Robertson, C.; Shankardass, K.; Feick, R. Stresscapes: Validating Linkages Between Place and Stress Expression on Social Media. In Proceedings of the 2nd International Workshop on Mining Urban Data, Lille, France, 11 July 2015.
50. Chen, X.; Sykora, M.D.; Jackson, T.W.; Elayan, S. Tweeting Your Mental Health: Exploration of Different Classifiers and Features with Emotional Signals in Identifying Mental Health Conditions. In Proceedings of the 51st Hawaii International Conference on System Sciences, Waikoloa Village, HI, USA, 3–6 January 2018.

15

From Science to Policy and Practice: A Critical Assessment of Knowledge Management Before, During and After Environmental Public Health Disasters

Mélissa Généreux [1,2,*], Marc Lafontaine [3] and Angela Eykelbosh [4]

1 Eastern Townships Integrated University Centre in Health and Social Services—Sherbrooke Hospital University Centre, Sherbrooke, QC J1G 1B1, Canada
2 Department of Community Health Sciences, Faculty of Medicine and Health Sciences, Université de Sherbrooke, Sherbrooke, QC J1H 5N4, Canada
3 Chemical Emergency Preparedness and Response Unit, Environmental Health Science and Research Bureau, Healthy Environments and Consumer Safety Branch, Health Canada, Ottawa, ON K1A 0K9, Canada; marc.lafontaine@canada.ca
4 National Collaborating Centre for Environmental Health, Vancouver, BC V5Z 4C2, Canada; angela.eykelbosh@bccdc.ca
* Correspondence: Melissa.genereux@usherbrooke.ca

Abstract: Canada regularly faces environmental public health (EPH) disasters. Given the importance of evidence-based, risk-informed decision-making, we aimed to critically assess the integration of EPH expertise and research into each phase of disaster management. In-depth interviews were conducted with 23 leaders in disaster management from Canada, the United States, the United Kingdom, and Australia, and were complemented by other qualitative methods. Three topics were examined: governance, knowledge creation/translation, and related barriers/needs. Data were analyzed through a four-step content analysis. Six critical success factors emerged from the analysis: blending the best of traditional and modern approaches; fostering community engagement; cultivating relationships; investing in preparedness and recovery; putting knowledge into practice; and ensuring sufficient human and financial resources. Several promising knowledge-to-action strategies were also identified, including mentorship programs, communities of practice, advisory groups, systematized learning, and comprehensive repositories of tools and resources. There is no single roadmap to incorporate EPH expertise and research into disaster management. Our findings suggest that preparation for and management of EPH disaster risks requires effective long-term collaboration between science, policy, and EPH practitioners at all levels in order to facilitate coordinated and timely deployment of multi-sectoral/jurisdictional resources when and where they are most needed.

Keywords: knowledge transfer; knowledge management; environmental public health; disaster risk management

---

1. Introduction

Canada, like many countries, increasingly faces emergencies and disasters that have public health impacts [1], including large-scale chemical incidents (e.g., the 2013 Lac-Mégantic train derailment) and natural disasters (e.g., the 2016 Fort McMurray wildfires). Such environmental public health (EPH) disasters may cause extensive environmental, human, and material losses, and may sometimes affect entire communities and/or necessitate evacuation and relocation. In addition to acute health risks, a large body of literature indicates that the population burden of psychopathology in the aftermath of EPH disasters is substantial and potentially of long duration [2–5]. EPH disasters may differ from other public health emergencies (e.g., Ebola outbreak, pandemic influenza), as most require both a short-term response (within hours), as well as a longer-term response (including monitoring, remediation and/or restoration efforts) that may stretch over years. And generate a need for multidisciplinary scientific expertise (chemistry, epidemiology, human health risk assessment, mental health, etc.). The increasing frequency and severity of EPH events is thought to be driven by the interactions of complex phenomena such as population and economic growth, land-use, resource scarcity, urbanization, and climate change, all of which are expected to continue into the foreseeable future.

The governance required to prepare for, respond to, and recover from a wide range of EPH disasters—natural or human-induced—is arguably the most complex and critical function of disaster management. Such EPH governance should serve to facilitate and strengthen capacity for risk assessment, surveillance, risk management, public communication, monitoring and evaluation, and mitigation and recovery activities. The components of EPH governance should, therefore, include not just policies, programs, and coordination structures, but should also address gathering and interpretation of relevant and up-to-date information with which to guide action [6].

1.1. Background

As the successor to the Hyogo Framework for Action 2005–2015: Building the Resilience of Nations and Communities to Disasters (HFA), the Sendai Framework for Disaster Risk Reduction 2015–2030 (Sendai Framework), adopted by 187 Member States at the Third United National World Conference on Disaster Risk Reduction, has shifted its emphasis from disaster management to disaster risk management [7]. With 35 explicit references to health, this people-centered framework encourages both risk reduction and resilience strengthening through an all-hazard, all-of-state and all-of-society approach [8]. Science should routinely be used to support disaster risk reduction [9] and, therefore, holds a key place in the Sendai Framework. Knowledge flowing from and to different stakeholders ensures that policy and practice are evidence-based and risk-informed (Figure 1; [10]).

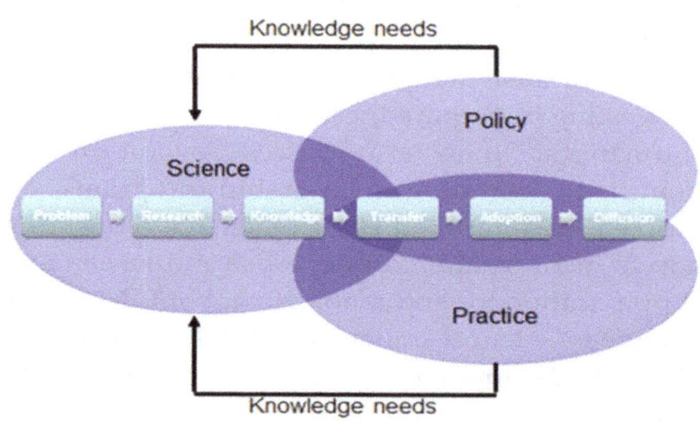

Figure 1. The science-policy-practice continuum (adapted from [10]).

1.2. Knowledge-to-Action (KTA) Process

Evidence-informed decision-making, in emergency management and in all other areas of public health, requires effective knowledge translation to turn research knowledge into action. The Canadian Institutes of Health Research (CIHR) have proposed a cyclical knowledge-to-action (KTA) process [11,12]. This process has been divided into various phases, from the identification of the problem to monitoring and sustaining the use of the available pertinent knowledge. The funnel, located at the heart of this cycle, represents knowledge creation. As it moves through the funnel, knowledge is refined and becomes more easily applicable to end-users. However, once created, knowledge needs to be translated into action. This cycle provides a framework for strategies in knowledge creation and translation.

Various types of knowledge may be utilized within KTA strategies in disaster settings. These include knowledge generated through science, as well as local (community-based) or indigenous knowledge [13]. Too often disaster management practitioners tend to focus on the former, ignoring the latter which is, nevertheless, of great value for disaster management, given local knowledge may provide contextual information not found in science-based information sources. For its part, scientific knowledge refers to primary literature (e.g., first-generation knowledge), knowledge synthesized from literature review (e.g., second-generation knowledge), and also to more user-friendly tools and resources, including decision aids, training modules, practice guidelines, lessons learned, and protocols (e.g., third-generation knowledge) [14]. Knowledge can also be classified as either tacit (i.e., understood or implied knowledge that exists without being stated) or explicit (i.e., formal or codified knowledge that is stated in detail) [15]. Such concepts build notably on the "knowledge creation spiral" theory within organizations, introduced by Nonaka and Takeuchi in 1995, which emphasizes on the importance of involving both the top and front-line employees in knowledge creation process [16]. By integrating top-down and bottom-up approaches, this system enables the creation, accumulation, and translation of tacit and explicit knowledge.

Effective KTA processes must also account for how knowledge is shared and transformed through sharing. Four processes transforming knowledge from one form to another have been identified, namely:

- Socialization;
- Externalization;
- Internalization; and
- Combination.

Socialization consists of sharing of individual tacit knowledge through collaborative methods, like meetings (tacit to tacit). Externalization refers to codifying the tacit knowledge into tools and resources (tacit to explicit). Internalization corresponds to learning by doing, through simulations or exercises (explicit to tacit). Finally, combination can be defined as the extraction and the combination of explicit knowledge, in order to organize it into various forms, such as repositories (explicit to explicit) [17].

1.3. Toward a National Framework

Canada has gained significant expertise and knowledge from recent EPH disasters, including the 2013 Lac-Mégantic train derailment, the 2016 Fort McMurray wildfires, and the 2016 Seaforth Channel diesel spill [18–21]. However, despite this growing expertise, two fundamental challenges remain. First, how can we improve knowledge generation (through research) before, during, and after disasters? Although disasters mobilize public health practitioners in a matter of hours, organizing scientific research efforts, and/or acquiring access to the knowledge generated may take weeks or months. Second, how can we improve dissemination and use of new and existing knowledge? These are especially complex challenges in Canada, in which knowledge-generating entities must cooperate across three levels of government, two official languages, and vast geographic distances. Rather than reinventing the wheel time and time again, how can we ensure that public health actors at all levels know what has been done elsewhere, how can we understand the uncertainties, and how can we integrate it in the face of a disaster?

Given the short time-frames and potentially high human costs that characterize EPH disasters, a national framework is urgently needed to facilitate and integrate knowledge creation and associated research into emergency response and recovery in Canada. Such a framework would allow public health professionals to systematize what has already been done, build on existing assets—such as expertise, evidence, guidelines, lessons learned, resources, training and protocols—and clarify what remains to be achieved through future collaborations.

Our aim was to determine how to better integrate EPH knowledge and assets in disaster settings in Canada [22], using the Sendai Framework as a template [23]. To that end, we conducted a critical assessment of knowledge management (i.e., providing the right information, in the right place, at the right time) before, during, and after EPH disasters in Canada. The following specific objectives were pursued to achieve this goal:

1. Describe various existing models of governance for disaster management, with a focus on the science-policy-practice interface;
2. Identify main resources available and challenges for knowledge management; and
3. Formulate recommendations toward the establishment of a national framework.

2. Materials and Methods

2.1. Design

This project draws heavily on the US National Institutes of Health (NIH) Disaster Research Response (DR2) Program. The DR2 Program is a national framework for research on the medical and public health aspects of disasters and public health emergencies [24,25] which offers data collection tools and resources, training and exercise materials, and research protocols, and facilitates networking between researchers and practitioners responding to environmental emergencies. This project was led in close collaboration with a national steering committee created in 2016, to oversee the development of a Canadian DR2 (CanDR2); the committee is co-chaired by Health Canada and the National Collaborating Centre for Environmental Health (NCCEH) and is composed of representatives from many Canadian and international agencies.

2.2. Sample Selection

Key informants (KIs) involved in preparedness for, response to, and recovery from EPH disasters, both at the local and national (i.e., provincial or federal) levels in Canada and other countries were invited to participate in this initiative.

The KIs identified were experienced emergency planners from health or non-health sectors, medical officers of health, knowledge transfer experts, or academics, who possessed expertise in the management of natural (e.g., floods, winter storms, heat waves, hurricanes, wildfires) or technological (e.g., chemical spills, train derailments) disasters.

At least one representative from each of the provinces of British Columbia, Alberta, Ontario, Québec, and the Atlantic Canada region was sought. These provinces or regions were selected based on their geographic location (dispersed across Canada), their experiences in facing EPH disasters, and the varying size and capacity of their public health workforce. In addition, KIs from the federal level in Canada were invited to participate in this initiative, as well as KIs from governmental or non-governmental organizations in other key English-speaking countries, including the United States, the United Kingdom, and Australia. While we emphasized the importance of diversity across KIs (at all levels, from governmental and non-governmental organizations, from health and non-health sectors), this diversity did not prevent our study from reaching data saturation (i.e., we obtained a sample large enough such that no new data were generated from additional participants).

An initial list of KIs was generated by the CanDR2 Steering Committee and invited to participate through an introductory email briefly describing the project. Nearly all invitees accepted, with a final sample of 23 KIs.

2.3. Data Collection Instrument and Methods

An interview guide containing mostly open-ended questions deemed to be relevant to our objectives was developed and endorsed by the members of the CanDR2 Steering Committee. Four overarching dimensions of the EPH response to disasters were explored, namely (1) governance, (2) knowledge creation, (3) knowledge translation, and (4) barriers and needs related to these processes [26]. The interview guide drew heavily on the World Health Organization (WHO)'s toolkit for assessing health system capacity for crisis management, more specifically on the governance and leadership function. This standardized toolkit is organized according to the six functions of the WHO health system framework. For the first function, that is effective leadership and governance, fourteen essential attributes are described, including programs on preparedness, and research and evidence base [6].

The interview process comprised two parts. In the first part of the interview, seven questions were used to broadly characterize the governance model/strategic framework in each of the jurisdictions under study, in order to obtain an overview of disaster management structures and coordination mechanisms. The second part of the interview specifically addressed knowledge creation (three questions) and knowledge translation processes (five questions). Existing barriers and factors conducive to strengthening of science-policy-practice interface and integration of knowledge into action were assessed throughout the interviews. A specific question on obstacles and strengths was also added at the end of the guide. Each interview lasted approximately 60 min. Interviews were conducted by the project leader in English ($n = 16$) or in French ($n = 7$), either on the telephone ($n = 19$) or face-to-face ($n = 4$), from April to July 2017.

2.4. Other Data Sources

In-depth interviews were complemented by other qualitative methods. The project leader was involved as the public health director or a medical adviser during three large-scale EPH disasters in Canada, namely the 2013 Lac-Mégantic train derailment, the 2016 Fort McMurray wildfires, and the 2017 Quebec flood. Furthermore, she attended 15 scientific fora (conferences, workshops, symposia, etc.) related to EPH disaster management from July 2016 to July 2017. Throughout these meetings and informal discussions with key international experts, additional explanations and good practices were documented. Field notes were taken after each scientific forum. Finally, a wide range of documents and websites suggested by KIs were consulted to deepen the understanding of laws, structure, policies, plans, procedures and programs identified during interviews.

2.5. Analysis

In order to carry out the analysis of the KIs' discourse and other data gathered, we conducted a four-step content analysis: (1) double-reading of transcripts, (2) data coding, (3) data processing, and (4) interpretation of data.

In Step 1, an initial (appropriation) reading of interviews and field notes was used to identify the main ideas characterizing each interview or event. The second (reading served to confirm and clarify these ideas. In Step 2, raw qualitative data were classified into an analysis grid, with a coding structure based on four dimensions established a priori: governance, knowledge creation, knowledge translation, and barriers and needs [26]. In the data processing Step 3, the analysis grid was used to draw out themes and subthemes from the coded transcripts. Data that were conceptually related to one another were first identified within each dimension. This set of data became sub-themes corresponding to ideas or concepts in relation with our subject. Examination of these sub-themes across all four pre-determined dimensions then led to their grouping into cross-cutting themes. The final Step 4 was interpretation of the coded and processed data in the context of our initial objectives [27].

2.6. Integrated Knowledge Translation

In accordance with the principle of integrated knowledge translation, as promoted by CIHR [28], members of the CanDR2 Steering Committee were involved in each step of the project. Early in the process, they contributed in identifying the problem and clarifying the aim of the project, they were invited to comment on the protocol and the interview guide, and they identified a list of potential KIs. Once data were gathered and analyzed, preliminary and final findings were presented and discussed with members of the CanDR2 Steering Committee on two occasions. Presentation of findings and recommendations to various stakeholders (e.g., organizations involved in disaster management in Canada) is also planned in the upcoming months.

3. Results

3.1. Description of the Data

Overall, 16 interviews were conducted among KIs from Canada (n = 16) and other jurisdictions (n = 7) (see Table 1). Fifteen KIs came from the public health or health sector, whereas the remaining KIs came from the municipal sector (n = 4), academia (n = 2), or non-governmental organizations (NGO; n = 2). The sample had balanced representation at the national and local levels, and of both genders. Two KIs represented the indigenous communities' perspective. Interestingly, many KIs had been involved in the management of EPH disasters, including the 2005 explosion and fire at the Buncefield oil storage depot (United Kingdom), the 2009 Black Saturday Bushfires in Victoria (Australia), the 2011 Alberta Slave Lake floods (Canada), the 2012 Neptune Technologies explosion (Canada), the 2013 Lac-Mégantic train derailment (Canada), the 2016 Fort McMurray wildfires (Canada), the 2016 Seaforth Channel diesel spill (Canada), Hurricane Matthew in 2016 (United States), the 2017 New Brunswick ice storm (Canada), the 2017 Quebec flood (Canada), the Flint water crisis (United States), as well as annual flooding in Ontario (Canada).

Table 1. Profiles of KIs interviewed in this study.

ID	Jurisdiction	Sector	Level	Gender
1	British Columbia	Health	National	F
2	British Columbia	Public Health	National	F
3	British Columbia	Public Health	Local	F
4	Alberta	Health	National	F
5	Alberta	Public Health	Local	M
6	Ontario	Health	National	M
7	Ontario	Public Health	Local	M
8	Québec	Municipal	Local	M
9	Québec	Municipal	Local	M
10	Québec	Municipal	Local	M
11	Québec	Academic	National	F
12	Atlantic	Public Health	Local	F
13	Canada	Public Health	National	F
14	Canada	Public Health	National	F
15	Canada	NGO	National	F
16	Canada	Public Health	National	M
17	United States	Public Health	National	F
18	United States	Academic	Local	M
19	United Kingdom	Public Health	National	F
20	United Kingdom	Public Health	National	F
21	United Kingdom	Municipal	Local	F
22	Australia	Public Health	Local	F
23	Australia	NGO	National	M

3.2. Emerging Themes: Critical Success Factors

Six cross-cutting themes, which are here identified as critical factors in successful disaster knowledge management, materialized from the data interpretation, with a range of sub-themes emerging in each category. These sub-themes, which represent the current situation and challenges, are further discussed below.

3.2.1. Blending the Best of Traditional and Modern Approaches

The data revealed that, in Canada and other developed countries, disaster management is well structured at all levels and that, overall, public health authorities are involved in these institutional arrangements. Most structures rely on the incident command system (ICS) for coordinating disaster responses, consider all phases of the disaster management continuum (mitigation, preparedness, response, and recovery) and are supported by laws, policies, plans, and procedures. Routine surveillance and epidemiological investigations are fairly well integrated during the response phase, as are conferences, meetings, training activities, and exercises during the preparedness phase. In short, the above traditional approaches are adequately implemented.

More modern all-hazard approaches [29,30] as promoted in many key documents, including the Sendai Framework [7], are currently integrated into disaster management preparedness and response in some jurisdictions. However, for most KIs in Canada and elsewhere, the Sendai Framework is not known or not a priority. Some KIs nevertheless expressed their desire for a major paradigm shift: "Requirements are based on old emergency management approaches and principles, we need governance from a different perspective" (KI#6). Others emphasized the importance of better understanding the potential risks: "It is important to be involved in risk assessment before a disaster strikes, to better manage risks altogether, as proposed in the Sendai Framework" (KI#9). An observation made at the Fifth Regional Platform for Disaster Risk Reduction in the Americas [31], which was also noted by one KI, is the poor representation of local-level participants of some major countries at this meeting: "Those involved don't share with lower levels, it's the opposite than [sic] what's proposed in the framework" (KI#18). This suggests that even if we are on the right track in implementing modern approaches, additional efforts are required to fully achieve this goal.

3.2.2. Fostering Community Engagement

The importance of identifying and leveraging existing assets or resources at the community level, including local health agencies, and working with existing capacities were strongly valued among KIs. Furthermore, it was indicated that local knowledge should be given consideration in the same manner as scientific knowledge: "We need to hear more from the community, it's really important" (KI#15). However, it was broadly acknowledged that communities typically remain poorly engaged in disaster management and that strategies to foster community engagement while maintaining the efficiency of disaster response and research are yet to be developed [32]. The interviewees indicated that ideally such strategies would provide a mixture of top-down and bottom-up approaches, and mobilize local knowledge and expertise before, during, and after a disaster.

Although leveraging local capacity was recognized as important, KIs also noted that building capacity in small municipalities, rural and Indigenous communities remains a challenge, and that support is required from higher-level governmental and academic institutions. For example, one KI (who has previously responded to a fuel spill) noted that more detailed technical guidance is needed to support local risk assessment: "What kind of environmental and biospecimen sample should be taken? What's needed? How often? What parameters? What detection limits? What should be the benchmarks (or appropriate end-points)?" (KI#3). Developing this type of technical guidance is often beyond the capacity of those responding to the crisis at hand, as such work requires time, research, and multidisciplinary expertise.

3.2.3. Cultivating Relationships

Many of the successes identified by KIs relied on individual leadership (or "champions") and strong interpersonal connections. Beyond structures, plans, and procedures, formal or informal relationships and networks have been identified by the majority of KIs as the most promising avenue to strengthen knowledge management capacities in disaster settings. Indeed, many KIs emphasized the need for breaking down silos between sectors (e.g., first responders vs. public health), practitioners and academics, French-speaking and English-speaking provinces, local and national levels, and even within public health organizations [33]. For example, KI#16 noted that "First Nations communities can ask for support, but this depends a lot on relationships previously built with governmental agencies". As noted by KI#9, "Strong links must be established right from the start between public health and first responders to establish a risk assessment and management strategy." Because public health authorities are well connected with universities in many jurisdictions, it may be possible to build bridges with academics to bring additional expertise to affected communities.

Some KIs mentioned that an overlap exists between academic and public health expertise in the context of EPH disasters, in that both may offer expertise in epidemiology, toxicology, surveillance, risk, and exposure assessment, etc. These two essential partners, therefore, need to clarify their respective roles, in order to unite their efforts and act in a synergistic manner. Building such functional partnerships may unlock latent resiliency, especially if accomplished before a disaster strikes. As expressed by one KI, "We need to connect the dots. We need to better know each other before an event; it is too late to learn during the crisis" (KI#10). Indeed, the power of these "connected dots" was apparent during the response to the 2017 Quebec floods. Within 24 h, an international network of renowned organizations including the US Centers for Disease Control and Prevention (CDC), Public Heath England (PHE), and WHO were bringing concrete support to Quebec public health authorities. This pre-established network permitted rapid access to validated materials, including the Community Assessment for Public Health Emergency Response (CASPER) toolkit in the US [34] and a protocol and questionnaires from the National Study of Flooding and Health in the UK [35].

3.2.4. Investing in Preparedness and Recovery

Although the four phases of disaster management are usually considered in disaster management structures, our data suggested local efforts are (by necessity) oriented toward the short-term. Our interviews suggested that Canadian EPH practitioners, particularly those at the local level, are struggling with one crisis activation after another; some organizations contacted during this study report remaining in near continual response mode in recent years. Consequently, little energy can be allocated to preparedness and recovery. Recovery is perhaps the most difficult task because of the accumulating burden on EPH professionals, including emotional load, fatigue, cumulative workload, and organizational factors, including less effective coordination structure and gradually weakening political commitment. According to one respondent, "we could probably do more between disasters, it is all about prioritization" (KI#5). As a result of this "disaster hangover", long-term monitoring of physical and mental health issues is not routinely carried out, despite the fact that those issues probably have the most significant impact on populations [36].

Another critical area that is typically overlooked in the post-disaster landscape is the identification and sharing of problems and lessons learned. Once the disaster is over, teams are asked to return to their regular tasks as quickly as possible, such that "Practitioners don't have enough time to think, to learn, to gain knowledge" (KI#11). As reported by many KIs, subsequent crises arise and similar problems are again encountered. For example, during the 2017 ice storm in New Brunswick (NB), one KI observed that public health was not as prepared as it could be, noting that "We always have to reinvent the wheel" (KI#12). This strongly expressed desire to improve learning from past events was the most consistent finding across KIs interviewed.

3.2.5. Putting Knowledge into Practice

The interviewees reported the science-policy-practice interface before, during, and after EPH disasters is not as robust as it could be, at either the local or national level in Canada, or in the other countries considered. Several interviewees from local organizations, within and outside the health sector, mentioned working infrequently with researchers due to the demands of day-to-day operations. The lack of systematic mechanisms to incorporate research and expertise into disaster management was also noted. The first challenge identified was "making sure that we are asking the right questions to inform and to learn from a given event" (KI#2). While accessing local data (e.g., environmental monitoring, epidemiological investigations, victim registries, response information, and after action reports) is essential to generate knowledge, as suggested by some KIs, such sharing can be sensitive for partners involved in disaster response, including first responders, local authorities, and non-governmental organizations. Various cultural backgrounds, lack of clarity in respective roles and responsibilities, privacy issues, security clearance, fear of being judged, not having the mandate, and competition might explain this phenomenon. The search of those responsible and/or the causes after disasters is negatively perceived in many countries, which may become a growing obstacle to learning from previous experiences.

Once knowledge is generated, this newly developed evidence has to be transferred from experts and researchers to inform policies and practices. In the aftermath of the Fort McMurray wildfires, "an evaluation of the psychosocial response and recovery was conducted through focus groups and interviews to identify further needs and current gaps" (KI#4). These findings emphasize the importance of having trained, dedicated staff who are tasked with taking on these "additional" data collection and knowledge translation activities.

Another issue commonly reported is the need to adapt scientific knowledge to local context, to make it clear and concise. Ideally, more user-friendly tools and resources would be produced (i.e., third-generation knowledge): "There is a lot of knowledge, amazing amount of information, really good evidence. The challenge is having the time to make it digestible" (KI#15). The same issue has been raised regarding the Sendai Framework, which is much better known among academics than practitioners. Although "it is important, it is not clear how it will materialize" (KI#13). Finally, many local organizations are trying to develop a resource repository, but few have a comprehensive one yet. For example, although the current Canadian Disaster Database (https://www.publicsafety.gc.ca/cnt/rsrcs/cndn-dsstr-dtbs/index-en.aspx) facilitates learning by identifying events geographically and by types, Canada does not currently have a central repository to share resources (tools, reports, etc.) and connect seekers to the experts involved.

3.2.6. Ensuring Sufficient Human and Financial Resources

Unsurprisingly, a recurring theme related to human and financial capacities. With few exceptions, disaster risk management and capacity-building activities are not prioritized, leading to insufficient funding and resources. According to many KIs, having trained, dedicated staff, either in local authorities or in specialized branches at the national level, could certainly help. Local emergency planners or coordinators have been found to play central roles in Canada and elsewhere. Although more focused on acute care than public health, Health Emergency Management BC (HEMBC) has been providing expertise, education, tools, and support since 2004 in BC, being "in charge of strategic planning, priority setting, networking, and performance measures" (KI#1). Another issue raised pertains to disaster research funding, which can be very complex. The first weeks following a disaster offer a window of opportunity that should be exploited, as political commitment and willingness to support research and long-term monitoring activities rapidly decrease thereafter. To secure funds, some KIs proposed that "disaster research should be seen as a national priority, with disaster-specific funding opportunities" (KI#11). Canada does not currently have an expedited research funding or ethical review process in place to address the immediate aftermath of disasters. For example,

CIHR offered $2 million in health research funding after the Fort McMurray wildfires, but this grant competition did not start until October 2016 (i.e., a few months after the fires).

3.3. Promising Knowledge-to-Action Strategies

Throughout the multiple data sources examined, we discovered a wide range of effective solutions already adopted by many countries worldwide to promote the integration of current knowledge into emergency preparedness, response, and recovery. The objective of this project was not to undertake an exhaustive inventory of these solutions, but rather to draw attention to strategies that might be adaptable to the Canadian context. For each country surveyed, the most promising strategies have been categorized according to the four types of KTA processes identified by Rhem [17] (i.e., socialization, externalization, internalization, combination; see Table 2). Few, if any, innovative strategies were found with respect to the internalization process, which refers to learning by doing (e.g., drills or exercises). By contrast, a plethora of socialization strategies have been identified. These strategies, all more creative than the internalization strategies, have two common denominators. First, they draw on human capital. Second, whether they are deployed before, during, or after an EPH disaster, they all promote more effective interplay of science, policy, and practice.

Table 2. Examples of promising KTA strategies.

Socialization	Externalization	Combination
	Canada	
Opportunities for professional growth from mentorships at Canadian Red Cross	Report on lessons learned by the community after the 2016 Seaforth channel spill	User-friendly Sharepoint® with resources and tools shared on an ongoing basis in Alberta
Lessons learned from Slave Lake and Lac-Mégantic integrated into the mental health recovery plan in Fort McMurray	Book on the Lac-Mégantic tragedy sharing lessons learned by health and community networks	Environmental public health response and recovery toolkit in Alberta
Multisectoral debriefing after Neptune Technologie explosion that led to a better response in Lac-Mégantic	Mapping of responsibilities/accountabilities following recommendations at Canadian Red Cross	Emergency preparedness and response working group in NB to facilitate access to documents and resources
During 2017 Quebec floods, meeting with a city previously affected by a major flood to learn from past experiences		
During 2017 Quebec floods, visit of an expert on the ground to share his knowledge		
Provincial symposium organized by HEMBC		
	United States	
Local emergency planning committees (federal mandate)	Rapid Needs Assessment facilitated by CASPER toolkit	Lessons learned database at FEMA
Phone call organized by CDC between 4 states affected after Hurricane Matthew	Central office for all after-action reports at CDC (problems and corrections)	Disaster Lit®: 12,000 records (grey literature) related to public health disasters at NLM

Table 2. *Cont.*

Socialization	Externalization	Combination
Midwest Consortium for Hazardous Waste Worker Training		NIH DR2 Program: Repository of surveys, questionnaires, protocols, guidance, forms
Environmental Justice Summit organized in Flint (Michigan)		
Disaster epidemiology community of practice		
Disaster information specialists at NLM		
	United Kingdom	
Newcastle conference on psychosocial impacts of emergencies	Overview and Scrutiny Committee in Newcastle following after-action reports	Mapping of the Sendai Framework implementation: resources, projects, all sectors
Local resilience forums		
PHE Centre for Radiation, Chemical and Environmental Hazards		
UK Alliance for Disaster Research		
	Australia	
Expert advisory panel/group activated by Chief Public Health Officer	Lessons from the community after 2009 Victoria bushfires	
Mentoring network at the Australian Red Cross		
	The Netherlands	
Expert Group Health Research and Care after Disasters and Environmental Crises		
	Global	
WHO Thematic Platform for Health Emergency and Disaster Risk Management Research Group	International Federation of Red Cross Psychosocial Center website: a lot of very useful resources	Global Public Health Intelligence Network (GPHIN): a web-based early-warning tool
UNISDR Scientific and Technical Advisory Group		Evidence Aid: reliable, up-to-date evidence on interventions in the context of emergencies
WHO collaborating center on chemical incidents		Weekly updates from the PHE Global Hazards Weekly Bulletin

Mentorship programs among employees and/or community members appear well established in the Canadian and Australian Red Cross organizations. For example, a mayor of a city previously devastated by a bushfire could in turn support another mayor currently facing a similar situation by sharing tools and lessons learned. Moreover, in the Netherlands and New South Wales (Australia), expert advisory groups can be activated to assist health authorities dealing with complex issues raised by environmental public health emergencies; depending on the situation, various types of expertise (e.g., environmental health, mental health, epidemiology, toxicology) can be mobilized within these jurisdictions to rapidly provide an overview of current scientific knowledge that might inform decision-making [37].

Various networks or communities of practice, both at national and international levels, have been put in place to better incorporate scientific and/or local knowledge into practice. An example of this is the WHO Thematic Platform for Health Emergency and Disaster Risk Management Research Group, a growing international network of policy-makers, practitioners, and researchers [38]. This initiative, recently underscored at the Global Platform in Cancun in May 2017 [39], is a good example of how the various stakeholders in disaster planning and management can all work together more effectively. An additional benefit of this global network whose members span all time zones is that the group can collectively support the response to a disaster occurring anywhere in the world at any time.

Externalization and combination processes were less frequently reported than socialization. However, two communities have released or are about to release reports on lessons learned after 2009 Victoria (Australia) bushfires [40] and the 2016 Seaforth Channel (Canada) diesel spill for public review and as learning resources.

Various approaches combining KTA processes have been developed. The USA has some of the most promising strategies, including "Lessons Learned Information Sharing", a database set up by the Federal Emergency Management Agency (FEMA), and a comprehensive repository easily available on the National Library Medicine (NLM) website called Disaster Lit®. Through the latter, the NIH has put together 12,000 records of hand-picked documents related to public health disasters from the grey literature, including factsheets, guidelines, assessment tools, training material, reports, web pages, and web sites [41]. Another example is Evidence Aid, an initiative that aims to improve access to evidence on disaster-related health interventions, actions, and policies [42].

The city of Newcastle (UK) has demonstrated an exceptional degree of commitment to emergency/disaster preparedness and response. The city has hired three emergency planners who are fully dedicated to disaster management. Their work is undertaken in a multiagency space (including public health), with joint risk assessment and planning and a community risk register that drives the action plan. After every incident or exercise, a structured debrief is organized, as is often the case in many other jurisdictions; however, in Newcastle such information is also presented as a report to the city council and the "Overview and Scrutiny Committee" (led by the opposition), which together look at all of the council actions. According to KI#21, giving politicians ownership of the report makes the whole process open, transparent, and accountable. Local engagement and leadership has also led to the incorporation of other KTA strategies, including the recent organization of a conference entitled "Psychosocial Impacts of Emergencies" [43]. This event aimed to bring together people from multiple levels and different agencies to foster collaboration, promote community engagement, and raise awareness of the current gaps in disaster risk management.

4. Discussion

Authors translating knowledge to action by closing gaps between knowledge and practice is an iterative, dynamic, and complex process [12]. This project aimed to identify factors influencing this process, and explore solutions to promote the bridge between science, policy, and practice for disaster management. Our results corroborate and expand upon the published literature. Several studies have previously identified similar factors that may limit knowledge translation in disaster preparedness and response, including gaps in basic knowledge, such as the lack of long-term observational and interventional research [44–46], challenges in systematically collating and delivering lessons learned from events, and difficulties in creating and sustaining effective community engagement [47–50]. And as with other studies [15], we also found several factors facilitating the uptake of knowledge, including the importance that knowledge is tailored to local contexts and made actionable. Overall, our interview results support the promotion of interactions between researchers, experts, and users from all sectors to produce, disseminate, and make use of knowledge for the purpose of improving disaster preparedness and management [51–53].

More specifically, five recommendations emerged from the interviews with KIs and field observations:

(1) Community of practice: A pan-Canadian community of practice involving emergency managers, public health practitioners, academics, local champions, Red Cross professionals, and any other stakeholders interested in EPH disasters, should be hosted within a trusted organization to support disaster preparedness. Within this community of practice, local initiatives could be shared and general consensus or understanding could be achieved regarding best practices in disaster response (e.g., risk assessment) and recovery (e.g., long-term monitoring). This would also be the ideal setting for the development of standardized tools for disaster health research as a basis for further action.

(2) Roster of experts: Linked to the above community of practice, a roster of Canadian experts (e.g., researchers, toxicologists, epidemiologists, environmental health, occupational health, and mental health experts) should be created to support disaster response and recovery. We anticipate that this network could be called upon as needed to form scientific advisory groups to assist local authorities dealing with EPH disasters in both the short- and long-term. Such an initiative could also increase collaboration and sharing of expertise between researchers and EPH personnel in the field. Drawing on existing models (such as DR2), it would also lead to the identification of relevant research questions and the development of a research agenda that fits operational objectives [24,37,54].

(3) Knowledge generation: A systematic mechanism to promote retention of learning from past events is required. All types of knowledge gained responding to previous disasters should be valued, whether this is first-, second-, or third-generation scientific knowledge, or local knowledge such as success stories, pilot initiatives, and lessons learned from the field [13]. As part of recovery operations, emergency managers and EPH practitioners should take the time to learn from their experiences and contribute to establishing a solid foundation upon which to can build national capacities. Debriefs should involve multiple sectors and seek the input from members of the community [55]. Standardized templates for after-action reports and a tracking system for correctable issues should be made available. Their use should be legislated after any exercise or real event in order to identify lessons, and most importantly to learn from them locally. The storage of completed templates in a central location (publicly available) would facilitate access to local knowledge and foster vertical and horizontal knowledge translation.

(4) Knowledge transfer: There is an urgent need in Canada (and elsewhere) to gather and synthesize disaster-related knowledge, and to transfer it to other communities, ideally using same central space (i.e., a virtual repository) identified in item (3) above. This knowledge might take the form of research findings, research protocols, practice guidelines, data collection tools and resources, training and exercises materials, lessons learned, etc. Such a virtual repository could be developed de novo, but Canadian documents could also be identified and shared through the extensive repository of tools and resources available from the US (i.e., Disaster Lit®, an NLM resource guide). Moreover, Canadian representatives should be appointed to the NLM Disaster Information Specialist Program, which supports the provision of disaster-related health information resources to the disaster workforce through a network of information professionals and librarians.

(5) Guidance on Sendai Framework: Guidance for a better integration of the Sendai Framework into health emergency management in the Canadian context should be developed. Such guidance would be particularly helpful for a growing number of stakeholders wishing a paradigm shift from disaster management to disaster risk management.

It is hoped our findings and recommendations will contribute to the identification and implementation of concrete solutions that foster the creation and the use of knowledge before, during, and after EPH disasters. Based on the challenges and successes identified during our interviews, we believe that there is no single roadmap to incorporate EPH expertise and research into disaster management. However, one thing is certain: these solutions should be developed not only during but also (or primarily) before and after disasters. The search for solutions should be based on the assumption that various types of knowledge translation processes are necessary [16].

Their complementary nature should be exploited in such a way as to develop a pan-Canadian framework that is adaptable to the needs of each province and territory, and other levels of government or sectors.

Strengths and Limitations

This project is, to the best of our knowledge, the first to critically assess capacity for knowledge management in EPH disaster settings in Canada. Our diverse sample of KIs represented a wide range of Canadian perspectives: rural and urban, indigenous and non-indigenous, anglophone and francophone, and from the east coast to west coast. This sample was further complemented by respondents from other countries to capture perceptions, ideas, and experiences on a broader basis. The measuring instrument (i.e., the interview guide) was based upon a standardized toolkit developed by the WHO to assess capacities for crisis management [6]. Furthermore, examination of qualitative data followed a rigorous protocol that helped to increase the internal validity of the data collected for coding purposes. Finally, a steering committee composed of knowledge users from various backgrounds accompanied the entire process, from the identification of the problem to the validation of potential solutions.

There are inherent limitations to a qualitative approach based primarily on KI interviews. First, the sample size was limited to 23 KIs. Our interviews also gathered opinions and ideas that may have been influenced by many factors including past experiences, recall bias, social desirability, and hidden agendas. In order to minimize the effect of those factors, we used additional sources of information to complement the interview data. Our design has therefore facilitated triangulation of findings and improved both reliability and validity.

5. Conclusions

Generally speaking, critical success factors for public health action include good governance, development of strong and sound partnerships, dedicated capacity and resources, and use of evidence to inform actions. Good governance is perhaps the single most important factor influencing the effectiveness of emergency preparedness, response and recovery. Beyond structures and plans, it is necessary to cultivate relationships and share responsibility for ensuring the safety, health, and well-being of affected communities, while respecting the local culture, capacity, and autonomy. Preparation for and management of EPH disaster risks requires effective long-term collaboration between science, policy, and EPH practitioners at all levels in order to facilitate coordinated and timely deployment of multi-sectoral/jurisdictional resources when and where they are most needed.

Author Contributions: Conceptualization: M.G., M.L., A.E.; methodology: M.G., M.L., A.E.; software: N/A.; validation: N/A.; formal analysis: N/A.; investigation: N/A.; resources: N/A.; data curation: N/A.; writing—original draft preparation: M.G., M.L., A.E.; writing—review and editing: M.G., M.L., A.E.; supervision, N/A.; project administration: co-authors.; funding acquisition: N/A.

References

1. Canadian Disaster Network on Disaster Risk Reduction. *Eighth Annual National Roundtable on Disaster Risk Reduction*; Public Safety Canada: Halifax, NS, Canada, 2017.
2. Galea, S.; Nandi, A.; Vlahov, D. The epidemiology of post-traumatic stress disorder after disasters. *Epidemiol. Rev.* **2005**, *27*, 78–91. [CrossRef] [PubMed]
3. Goldmann, E.; Galea, S. Mental health consequences of disasters. *Annu. Rev. Public Health* **2014**, *35*, 169–183. [CrossRef] [PubMed]
4. Neria, Y.; Nandi, A.; Galea, S. Post-traumatic stress disorder following disasters: A systematic review. *Psychol. Med.* **2008** *38*, 467–480. [CrossRef] [PubMed]

5. Warsini, S.; West, C.; Dip, E.G.; Mills, J.; Usher, K. The psychosocial impact of natural disaster among adult survivors. An integrative review. *Issues Mental Health Nurs.* **2014**, *35*, 420–436. [CrossRef] [PubMed]
6. World Health Organization. *Strengthening Health-system Emergency Preparedness: Toolkit for Assessing Health-system Capacity for Crisis Management*; WHO: Copenhagen, Denmark, 2012.
7. United Nations Office for Disaster Risk Reduction. *Sendai Framework for Disaster Risk Reduction 2015–2030. United Nations Office for Disaster Risk Reduction*; United Nations: Geneva, Switzerland, 2015.
8. Aitsi-Selmi, A.; Murray, V. The Sendai framework: Disaster risk reduction through a health lens. *Bull. World Health Organ.* **2015**, *93*, 362. [CrossRef] [PubMed]
9. Southgate, R.J.; Roth, C.; Schneider, J.; Shi, P.; Onishi, T.; Wenger, D.; Amman, W.; Ogallo, L.; Beddington, J.; Murray, V. Using Science for Disaster Risk Reduction. UNISDR. 2013. Available online: www.preventionweb.net/go/scitech (accessed on 15 January 2019).
10. Spiekermann, R.; Kienberger, S.; Norton, J.; Briones, F.; Weichselgartner, J. The Disaster-Knowledge Matrix—Reframing and evaluating the knowledge challenges in disaster risk reduction. *Int. J. Disaster Risk Reduct.* **2015**, *13*, 96–108. [CrossRef]
11. Graham, I.D.; Logan, J.; Harrison, M.B.; Straus, S.E.; Tetroe, J.; Caswell, W.; Robinson, N. Lost in knowledge translation: Time for a map? *J. Contin. Educ. Health Prof.* **2006**, *26*, 13–24. [CrossRef]
12. Straus, S.E.; Tetroe, J.; Graham, I. Defining knowledge translation. *Can. Med. Assoc. J.* **2009**, *181*, 165–168. [CrossRef]
13. Mercer, J.; Kelman, I.; Taranis, L.; Suchet-Pearson, S. Framework for integrating indigenous and scientific knowledge for disaster risk reduction. *Disaster* **2010**, *34*, 214–239. [CrossRef]
14. Brouwers, M.; Stacey, D.; O'Connor, A. Knowledge creation: Synthesis, tools and products. *Can. Med. Assoc. J.* **2009**, *182*, 68–72. [CrossRef]
15. Seneviratne, K.; Baldry, D.; Pathirage, C. Disaster knowledge factors in managing disasters successfully. *Int. J. Strateg Prop. M.* **2010**, *14*, 376–390. [CrossRef]
16. Nonaka, I.; Takeuchi, H. *The Knowledge Creating Company*; Oxford University Press: Oxford, UK, 1995.
17. Rhem, A.J. "Sound the Alarm!": Knowledge management in emergency and disaster preparedness. In *Knowledge Management in Practice*; Taylor and Francis Group: Abingdon, UK, 2017.
18. Eykelbosh, E.; Kosatky, T. Oil spills: Treating patients, counselling communities. *B. C. Med. J.* **2017**, *59*, 61–64.
19. Généreux, M.; Petit, G.; Maltais, D.; Roy, M.; Simard, R.; Boivin, S.; Shultz, J.M.; Pinsonneault, L. The public health response during and after the Lac-Mégantic train derailment tragedy: A. case study. *Disaster Health* **2015**, *2*, 1–8. [CrossRef] [PubMed]
20. Géreux, M.; Petit, G.; Lac-Mégantic Community Outreach Team; O'Sullivan, T. Public health approach to supporting resilience in Lac-Mégantic: The EnRiCH Framework. In *Health 2020 Priority Area Four: Creating Supportive Environments and Resilient Communities. A Compendium of Inspirational Examples*; Erio, Z., Ed.; World Health Organization: Geneva, Switzerland, 2018; pp. 156–162.
21. Généreux, M.; Petit, G.; Roy, M.; Maltais, D.; O'Sullivan, T. The "Lac-Mégantic tragedy" seen through the lens of The EnRiCH Community Resilience Framework for High-Risk Population. *Can. J. Public Health* **2018**, *109*, 261–267. [CrossRef] [PubMed]
22. *CIHR Best Brain Exchange Report: Integrating Environmental Health Research into Chemical Emergency/Disaster Management. CIHR*; The Science, Knowledge Translation & Ethics Branch; Public Safety Canada: Ottawa, ON, Canada, 2016.
23. Wahlström, M. New Sendai framework strengthens focus on reducing disaster risk. *Int. J. Disaster Risk Sci.* **2015**, *6*, 200–201. [CrossRef]
24. Miller, A.; Yeskey, K.; Garantziotis, S.; Arnesen, S.; Bennett, A.; O'Fallon, L.; Thompson, C.; Reinlib, L.; Masten, S.; Remington, J.; et al. Integrating health research into disaster response: The new NIH disaster research response program. *Int. J. Environ. Res. Public Health* **2016**, *13*, 676. [CrossRef]
25. National Institute of Health. NIH Disaster Research Response (DR2). 2017. Available online: https://dr2.nlm.nih.gov/ (accessed on 15 January 2019).
26. Andreani, J.C.; Conchon, F. Fiabilité et validité des enquêtes qualitatives: Un état de l'art en marketing. *Revue Française du Marketing* **2005**, *201*, 5–21. (In French)
27. Feldman, M.S. *Strategies for Interpreting Qualitative Data*; Sage Publications: Thousand Oaks, CA, USA, 1994.
28. Canadian Institutes of Health Research. *Guide to Knowledge Translation Planning at CIHR: Integrated and End-of-Grant Approaches*; Canadian Institutes of Health Research: Ottawa, ON, Canada, 2012.

29. Federal Emergency Management Agency. *National Preparedness Goal*, 2nd ed.; US Department of Homeland Security: Washington, DC, USA, 2015.
30. Public Safety Canada. *An Emergency Management Framework for Canada*, 2nd ed.; Emergency Management Policy Directorate; Public Safety Canada: Ottawa, ON, Canada, 2011.
31. Government of Canada. 5th Regional Platform for Disaster Risk Reduction in the Americas. 2017. Available online: http://eird.org/rp17/ (accessed on 15 January 2019).
32. Lichtveld, M.; Kennedy, S.; Krouse, R.Z.; Grimsley, F.; El-Dahr, J.; Bordelon, K.; Sterling, Y.; White, L.; Barlow, N.; DeGruy, S.; et al. From design to dissemination: Implementing community-based participatory research in post-disaster communities. *Am. J. Public Health* **2016**, *106*, 1235–1242. [CrossRef]
33. Généreux, M.; Pinsonneault, L.; Roy, M. Fostering partnerships between public health functions within health and social services organizations: A perspective from the province of Quebec (Canada). *J. Prev. Med. Care* **2016**, *1*, 23–27. [CrossRef]
34. Centers for Disease Control and Prevention. *Community Assessment for Public Health Emergency Response (CASPER) Toolkit*, 2nd ed.; CDC: Atlanta, GA, USA, 2012.
35. Waite, T.D.; Chaintarli, K.; Beck, C.R.; Bone, A.; Amlôt, R.; Kovats, S.; Reacher, M.; Armstrong, B.; Leonardi, G.; Rubin, J.; Oliver, I. The English national cohort study of flooding and health: Cross-sectional analysis of mental health outcomes at year one. *BMC Public Health* **2017**, *17*, 129. [CrossRef]
36. Géreux, M.; Maltais, D. Three years after the tragedy: How the Le Granit community is coping. In *Bulletin d'information de la direction de santé publique de l'Estrie*; Vision Santé publique: Sherbrooke, QC, Canada, 2017.
37. Alting, D.; Duckers, M.L.; Yzermans, J. The expert group health research and care after disasters and environmental crises: An analysis of research questions formulated by Dutch health authorities for the expert group between 2006 and 2016. *Prehosp. Disaster Med.* **2017**, *32*, S197. [CrossRef]
38. Lo, S.T.T.; Chan, E.Y.Y.; Chan, G.K.W.; Murray, V.; Abrahams, J.; Ardalan, A.; Kayano, R.; Wai Yau, J.C. Health emergency and disaster risk management (Health-EDRM): Developing the research field within the Sendai Framework paradigm. *Int. J. Disaster Risk Sci.* **2017**, *8*, 145–149. [CrossRef]
39. WHO. *WHO statement to the 2017 global platform for disaster risk reduction*; WHO: Geneva, Switzerland, 2017.
40. McAllan, C.; McAllan, V.; McEntee, K.; Gale, B.; Taylor, D.; Wood, J.; Thompson, T.; Elder, J.; Mutsaers, K.; Leeson, W.; et al. Lessons Learned by Community Recovery Committees of the 2009 Victorian Bushfires Advice We offer to Communities Impacted by Disaster. Available online: https://www.redcross.org.au/getmedia/7f796fb7-958f-4174-98da-00b6e0182856/Lessons-Learned-by-Community-Recovery-Committees-of-the-2009-Victorian-Bushfires-v1-0.pdf.aspx (accessed on 15 January 2019).
41. Norton, E. A toolkit for disaster preparedness & response information. *World Association for Disaster and Emergency Medicine Webinar*. 2017. Available online: https://wadem.org/wp-content/uploads/2017/02/toolkit-nlm-2-23-17-norton.pdf (accessed on 11 February 2019).
42. Gerdin, M.; Clarke, M.; Allen, C.; Kayabu, B.; Summerskill, W.; Devane, D.; MacLachlan, M.; Spiegel, P.; Ghosh, A.; Zachariah, R.; et al. Optimal evidence in difficult settings: Improving health interventions and decision making in disasters. *Plos Med.* **2014**, *11*, e1001632. [CrossRef] [PubMed]
43. Newcastle City Council. Psychosocial Impacts of Emergencies. 2017. Available online: http://www.fuse.ac.uk/media/sites/researchwebsites/fuse/eventdocs/Psychological%20impacts%20of%20emergencies.pdf (accessed on 15 January 2019).
44. Birnbaum, M.L.; Daily, E.K.; O'Rourke, A.P. Research and evaluations of the health aspects of disasters, Part VII: The Relief/Recovery Framework. *Prehosp. Disaster Med.* **2016**, *31*, 195–210. [CrossRef] [PubMed]
45. Chan, E.Y.Y.; Murray, V. What are the health research needs for the Sendai Framework? *Lancet* **2017**, *390*, E35–E36. [CrossRef]
46. Tsutsumi, A.; Takashi, I.; Ito, A.; Thronicroft, G.; Patel, V.; Minas, H. Mental health mainstreamed in new UN disaster framework. *Lancet Psychiatr.* **2015**, *2*, 679–680. [CrossRef]
47. Gamboa-Maldonado, T.; Marshak, H.H.; Sinclair, R.; Montgomery, S.; Dyjack, D.T. Building capacity for community disaster preparedness: A call for collaboration between public environmental health and emergency preparedness and response programs. *J. Environ. Health.* **2012**, *75*, 24–29.
48. Jong, S.V.Z. *Let's Talk Oil Spill Risk. Lessons Learned from Coastal Communities in British Columbia, Canada*; Routledge: Kentuck, AL, USA, 2016.

49. Leadbeater, A. Community leadership in disaster recovery: A case study. *Aust. J. Emerg. Manag.* **2013**, *28*, 41–47.
50. Svendsen, E.R.; Whittle, N.; Wright, L.; McKeown, R.E.; Sprayberry, K.; Heim, M.; Caldwell, J.J.; Gibson, J.; Vena, J. GRACE: Public health recovery methods following an environmental disaster. *Int. Arch. Occup. Environ. Health* **2010**, *65*, 77–85. [CrossRef]
51. Dar, O.; Buckley, E.J.; Rokadiya, S.; Huda, Q.; Abrahams, J. Integrating health into disaster risk reduction strategies: Key considerations for success. *Am. J. Public Health* **2014**, *104*, 1811–1816. [CrossRef]
52. Lurie, N.; Manolio, T.; Patterson, A.P.; Collins, F.; Frieden, T. Research as a part of public health emergency response. *N. Engl. J. Med.* **2013**, *368*, 1251–1255. [CrossRef] [PubMed]
53. Yeskey, K.; Miller, A. Science unpreparedness. *Disaster Med. Public Health Prep.* **2015**, *9*, 444–445. [CrossRef] [PubMed]
54. Decker, J.A.; Kiefer, M.; Reissman, D.B. A decision process for determining whether to conduct responder health research following disasters. *Am. J. Disaster Med.* **2013**, *8*, 25–33. [CrossRef] [PubMed]
55. Gibson, T.; Wisner, B. "Let's talk about you ... ": Opening space for local experience, action and learning in disaster risk reduction. *Disaster Prev. Manag. Int. J.* **2016**, *25*, 664–684. [CrossRef]

16

Alternative Leadership in Flexible Surge Capacity—The Perceived Impact of Tabletop Simulation Exercises on Thai Emergency Physicians Capability to Manage a Major Incident

Phatthranit Phattharapornjaroen [1,2], Viktor Glantz [1], Eric Carlström [3,4], Lina Dahlén Holmqvist [5] and Amir Khorram-Manesh [1,6,*]

1 Institute of Clinical Sciences, Department of Surgery, Sahlgrenska Academy, Gothenburg University, 40530 Gothenburg, Sweden; phatthranit.pha@mahidol.edu (P.P.); gusglavi@student.gu.se (V.G.)
2 Department of Emergency Medicine, Center of Excellence, Ramathibodi Hospital, Mahidol University, Bangkok 10400, Thailand
3 Institute of Healthcare Sciences, Sahlgrenska Academy, Gothenburg University, 40100 Gothenburg, Sweden; eric.carlstrom@gu.se
4 USN School of Business, University of South-Eastern Norway, P.O. Box 235, 3603 Kongsberg, Norway
5 Institute of Medicine, Department of Molecular and Clinical Medicine, Sahlgrenska University Hospital, 40530 Gothenburg, Sweden; lina.holmqvist@vgregion.se
6 Department of Research and Development, the Swedish Armed Forces Center for Defense Medicine, Västra Frölunda, 42676 Gothenburg, Sweden
* Correspondence: amir.khorram-manesh@surgery.gu.se

Abstract: Flexible surge capacity aims to activate and utilize other resources than normally are surged in a community during the primary and secondary surge capacity. The presence of alternative leadership, skilled and knowledgeable in hospital and prehospital emergency management, is invaluable. Thai emergency physicians work at both levels, emphasizing their important role in emergency management of any source in a disaster-prone country. We aimed to investigate Thai emergency physicians' ability in terms of knowledge and preparedness to manage potential emergencies using tabletop simulation exercises. Using an established method for training collaboration, two training courses were arranged for over 50 Thai emergency physicians, who were divided into three teams of prehospital, hospital, and incident command groups. Three scenarios of a terror attack along with a bomb explosion, riot, and shooting, and high building fire were presented, and the participants' performance was evaluated regarding their preparedness, response and gained knowledge. Two senior observers followed the leadership characteristic in particular. Thai physicians' perceived ability in command and control, communication, collaboration, coordination, and situation assessment improved in all groups systematically. New perspectives and innovative measures were presented by participants, which improved the overall management on the final day. Tabletop simulation exercise increased the perceived ability, knowledge, and attitude of Thai emergency physicians in managing major incidents and disasters. It also enabled them to lead emergency management in a situation when alternative leadership is a necessity as part of the concept of a flexible surge capacity response system.

Keywords: disasters; emergencies; flexible surge capacity; leadership; Thailand; 3LC

1. Introduction

Major Incidents and Disasters (MID) affect societies and their inhabitants and result in medical and nonmedical consequences due to the imbalance between the needs and available resources [1].

MID management is a multiprofessional process of organizing and managing the available resources and responsibilities for dealing with all humanitarian aspects of MID, specifically in mitigation, preparedness, response, and recovery phases to lessen the impact of emergencies [2]. Some strategies for MID management include establishing command and control, reliable and efficient ways of communication, information, organization, warning systems, stockpiling of resources, and the development of response plans for the mobilization and management of resources such as personnel, equipment, volunteers, and emergency facilities. The efficiency of the organizational structure in the response is paramount for the outcome of the event [2,3].

The initial approach to proper management of MID is to increase the management system's capacity, i.e., Surge Capacity (SC). Three broad areas of healthcare demand SC in response to a MID [4]. Firstly, Public Health Surge Capacity (the ability of the public health system to increase capacity for patient care, epidemiological investigation, laboratory services, mass fatality management, etc.). Secondly, Healthcare Facility-Based Surge Capacity (augments the response within the healthcare facility structure, e.g., triage-tent on hospital grounds). Finally, Community-based Surge Capacity (the public effort to support and augment the healthcare system). The four essential elements of SC, i.e., Staff, Stuff, Structure, and System (4S), should rapidly and effectively be surged in the affected areas. Staff refers to available/alternative personnel, Stuff refers to available/alternative equipment, Structures refer to Alternate Care Facilities (ACF), and systems are procedures and guidelines that govern the emergency management process [5,6].

The expansion of a MID necessitates a new surge capacity (secondary SC), which underlines the need for extra efforts to obtain additional resources still available within the management system [7–9]. Nevertheless, a further expansion of the incident demands new approaches, policies, and adjustable preparedness within the community to scale up and down resources in a fast, smooth, and productive way, i.e., "flexible surge capacity" (FSC) [10]. The concept of FSC is concordant with the new paradigm of proactivity in disaster management and emphasizes on risk reduction rather than focusing on pure relief operations to reduce vulnerability and increase resilience within communities [11]. Therefore, risk assessment and focus on all four elements of SC is necessary for achieving an FSC. Although the disaster management cycle should incorporate, recognize, and value the participation of affected communities [12], it is necessary that adequate infrastructure is in place to ensure access to emergency services [13]. In this perspective, the readiness of hospitals is essential and among necessary measures, staff pools and new staff categories are needed to replace the regular staffing structure, and to reduce the risk of lacking qualified staff, e.g., leadership.

Although many functions and measures are necessary for proper and successful MID management, the command and control (C2) function remains the most critical function [14,15]. C2 emphasizes the leaderships' characteristics to command, control, communicate, collaborate, and coordinate [2,6,14,15]. Such ability offers an excellent opportunity for the leaders to attain a mutual goal, assess the situation from different perspectives, overview all necessary measures, successfully sort out all injuries, treat them adequately and distribute them equally to designated medical facilities. Most hospitals have an emergency management committee, which consists of predesignated positions and staff. Such a group of professionals needs to be trained to act decisively and quickly during crises. Previous studies have, however, shown that these committees suffer from the rarity of MID, and thus, neither have the experience nor are trained enough to act as needed [15,16]. There is a lack of experience and knowledge about the management process and collaboration with other partners, particularly in hospital and prehospital arenas. One specialty with the ability and knowledge to connect hospitals and prehospital organizations is Emergency Medicine [17].

Thailand is a disaster-prone country with a westernized healthcare system. Emergency Medicine residency training in Thailand started in 2004, during which the first Tsunami hit its southern part and caused mass casualties and structural devastation. One of the outcomes of this deadly event was understanding the needs for organizational and structural changes, and proper knowledge in command and control within the disaster management system. Since then, many educational initiatives such as MIMMS (Major Incident Medical Management and Support), and MRMI (Medical Response to Major Incidents) have been established and yearly conducted to raise the theoretical and practical knowledge of all staff [18–21]. Thai Emergency Physicians (EP), work within and outside the hospitals and are the point of contact and the first line of medical assessment [19,20]. This role requires the right level of structural and organizational knowledge of MID management and merits a more responsible and critical role in response to major emergencies. One way to obtain such knowledge is through tabletop simulations training [21].

The Three-Level Collaboration (3LC) training model is used to train small groups of commanders up to hundreds of participants in the management of MID. The development of the 3LC model was based on hypothesizing that the collaborative elements in a mutual task help reduce the organizational barriers [21]. The method has been compared with traditional exercises in several studies [22–24]. In one of these, the 3LC method improved collaboration as well as learning. At the 3LC exercise, 94.3% of the personnel perceived the exercise to be focused on collaboration. The traditional exercises reported a corresponding figure of 75.6%. The majority of the participants answered that they learned something new during the exercises (78.5%, traditional 64.9%). They also felt that the exercises had an impact on real-life activities during daily work (80.4%, traditional 61.7%) [24]. Organizational capabilities and limitations are enlisted to promote interplay with no hierarchical authority, and to promote the ability to switch between different collaboration strategies as demanded by the specific situation. Collaboration training offers a chance to not only exhibit stability (the quality that one develops through drill and practice), but also to practice transitions, overlaps, fearlessness, improvisation, creative thinking, and the ability to handle unexpected situations. Such education is beyond the repeated learning that comes from the drill in control and command structures and other mechanical structures.

2. Aim

This study aimed to evaluate the progress of knowledge and learning outcomes of a group of Thai EPs before and after 3LC simulation exercise in seven documented and essential areas (CSCATTT): Command and control, Safety, Communication, Triage, Treatment, and Transport, which according to MIMMS concept are essential elements to lead and manage a MID [18].

3. Method

3.1. Population

All EPs voluntarily registered to an Incident Command System course at a major hospital in Bangkok, Thailand. Participants who were present during the entire course session were included. Consequently, those who could not present or left the course for a few hours were excluded. Otherwise, there were no exclusion criteria, and all staff working with MID, including nurses could take part in the course.

3.2. Course Design

Two two-day courses with the same structure consisting of a short introduction and a scenario simulation exercise on the first day, followed by two more scenarios on day two. A round of discussion and comments for the whole course took place at the end of the course. Participants were divided into three groups of (1) a prehospital team (Operational), (2) emergency departments command group (Tactical), and (3) hospital command group (Strategical).

There was a rotation between different groups, which enabled all participants to try different positions to reach consensus in the whole group of participants to achieve similarities rather than differences. No instruction was given about participants' posts in each group, and they had to figure out what they need and how to use all competences, based on the given lectures and earlier knowledge in MIMMS. Three different scenarios (1) fire in a tall building, (2) a terrorist attack and a bomb explosion, and (3) riots, including shooting, were presented to the groups during rotation (Appendix A). After each scenario, the participants in each group had to present their results. Each group received comments from supervisors and other participants. At the end of the presentations, and according to the 3LC model, the participants in each group had to gather again and discuss what they could do better if they had a new opportunity. Each group presented the results of this round, and other participants and supervisors could comment on their findings. Finally, each group gathered to discuss the necessary knowledge and functions and guidelines for each position to be taken home as the quality, which is needed for operational, tactical, and strategic levels. Besides, two supervisors followed each group and evaluated their performance based on MIMMS-CSCATT concept (see below) [18].

3.3. Pre- and Post-Course Test

The pre- and post-course tests were conducted to evaluate the gained knowledge in each participant [25]. The tests were designed using the learning objectives established for the course, i.e., crucial factors for successful management of MID incorporated in CSCATTT (Command and control, Security, Communication, Assessment, Triage, Treatment, Transport), a well-known model used in MIMMS courses internationally [18]. Both tests consist of the same items. The test aimed for each participant's self-assessment in knowledge about the subjects of CSCATTT, displayed as a Likert scale, in which No knowledge was represented by 0%, while 100% was full knowledge. Participants were asked to mark the grade of their understanding in each topic on a five-level Likert Scale. A nonparametric test, Wilcoxon signed rank test, was chosen to compare the means.

3.4. Observational Evaluation

All groups were observed based on a Participant Observation model with a focus on the leadership in all groups [26–28]. Among various signs of good leadership, the following points were mainly observed to evaluate the leadership: Communication and Decision-making ability, Accountability, Delegation, and Empowerment of others. Two observers collected and noted their observations, which were discussed after each scenario to reach a consensus. The observer registered if a commander was identified and appointed during the incident and if the appointed commander possessed the control. The observer did also register if the commander ensured successful medical management, i.e., built a team of multiple staff overcoming a potentially chaotic situation and if the team reached a subtactical, tactical, or operational level [18]. The data were recorded as Event Sampling, which allows focusing on one specific subject. All other types of behavior were ignored [26–28].

3.5. Observational Evaluation

As part of 3LC simulation training, group discussions took place after each scenario. Besides confirming and discussing the results and improvement measures, these discussions also aimed to discuss the observational findings in each occasion. The process aimed to pair data collected by observation to the discussion and interviews to unearth individual motivations or behaviors that were not immediately obvious in a group setting [24–28].

4. Results

There were 56 participants registered, however, only 52 could complete the course. The four physicians excluded (two females and two males) had to go back to work due to emergencies, and were not presented at all levels of simulation training. A sum of 52 EPs took part in the entire course on two occasions. Nurses were also invited to these courses, but none were registered due to hesitance of the spoken language of the course (English). There were 36 females and 16 males. The age of the participants ranged between 26–35 years, with a range of experience between 1–10 years as EP. The majority of participants were from the hospitals in Bangkok. However, 16 physicians were from hospitals in other parts of Thailand. The pre- and post-training tests were conducted before and after the session.

a. Command and control (C2): There was an increasing knowledge of C2 after the course. Around 20% of the EPs ($n = 10$) had little or very little knowledge about C2, and 46% ($n = 24$) had medium knowledge. At the end of the course, there was a shift to the positive end, where the majority of our participants had a good to a very good understanding of C2 function ($n = 49$, 94%) (Figure 2). The change was statistically significant ($p = 0.00$, $z = -5.436$).

b. Safety: There was an increasing knowledge of safety issues after the course. Around 15% of the EPs ($n = 8$) had no or very little knowledge about safety issues, and 44% ($n = 23$) had medium knowledge. At the end of the course, there was a shift to the positive end, where the majority of our participants had a good to a very good understanding of safety issues ($n = 50$, 96%) (Figure 3). The change was statistically significant ($p = 0.00$, $z = -6.056$).

c. Communication: There was an increasing knowledge of communication ways and difficulties after the course. Around 21% ($n = 11$) of the EPs had none or very little knowledge about communications issues, and 44% ($n = 23$) had medium knowledge. At the end of the course, there was a shift to the positive end, where the majority of our participants had a good to a very good understanding of safety issues ($n = 48$, 92%) (Figure 4). The change was statistically significant ($p = 0.00$, $z = -5.872$).

d. Assessment: There was an increasing knowledge about the importance of the assessment during a major incident after the course. Around 17% ($n = 9$) of the EPs had no or very little knowledge about assessment and its association with the incident management, and 48% ($n = 25$) had medium knowledge. At the end of the course, there was a shift to the positive end, where the majority of our participants had a good to a very good understanding of assessment issues ($n = 48$, 92%) (Figure 5). The change was statistically significant ($p = 0.00$, $z = -5.464$).

e. Triage: There was an increasing knowledge about the importance of triage and associated dilemmas during a major incident after the course. Around 17% ($n = 9$) of the EPs had no or very little knowledge about triage and its role during incident management, and 30% ($n = 16$) had medium knowledge. Although 29 EPs reported a good or very good knowledge, there was still a shift to the positive end at the end of the course, where the majority of our participants had a good to a very good understanding of triage issues ($n = 46$, 88%) (Figure 6). The change was statistically significant ($p = 0.00$, $z = -4.585$).

f. Treatment: There was an increasing knowledge about the treatment alternatives and options at the right time and right place during a major incident after the course. Around 17% ($n = 9$) of the EPs had none or very little knowledge about the treatment given during incident management, and 28% ($n = 15$) had medium knowledge. Although 28 EPs reported good or very good knowledge, there was still a shift to the positive end at the end of the course, where the majority of the participants had good to a very good understanding of triage issues ($n = 37$, 71%) (Figure 7). The change was statistically significant ($p = 0.00$, $z = -5.287$).

g. Transport: There was an increasing knowledge about the importance of triage and associated dilemmas during a major incident after the course. Around 21% ($n = 11$) of the EPs had none or very little knowledge about triage and its role during incident management, and 32% ($n = 17$) had medium knowledge. At the end of the course, there was a shift to the positive end, where the majority of our participants had a good to a very good understanding of assessment issues ($n = 38$, 73%) (Figure 8). The change was statistically significant ($p = 0.00$, $z = -5.634$).

h. Observations: Two critical observations were reported (Figure 1). Both observers collected their documented results in which they had specifically commented on the ability of decision-making, communication, accountability, empowerment of other group member and delegation of tasks. Consensus was made and the groups were exposed to the observers' understanding to unearth individual motivations or behaviors that were not immediately obvious in a group setting [24,25].

a. During the exercises, each team selected its leader with three leadership styles, without any previous knowledge and spontaneously;

   i. Consensus leadership (G3): The leader tried to reach consensus with other members before any decision. Slower decision-making process.

   ii. Passive leadership (G2): The leader laid back and observed other members and only interrupted if needed. Decisions were made, but sometimes not of the leader.

   iii. Active Leadership (G1): The leader had the last word in every decision and continuously directed the group. Less delegation and empowerment.

b. Each group developed its communication method consisting of a mobile telephone, paper-based messages, and signs.

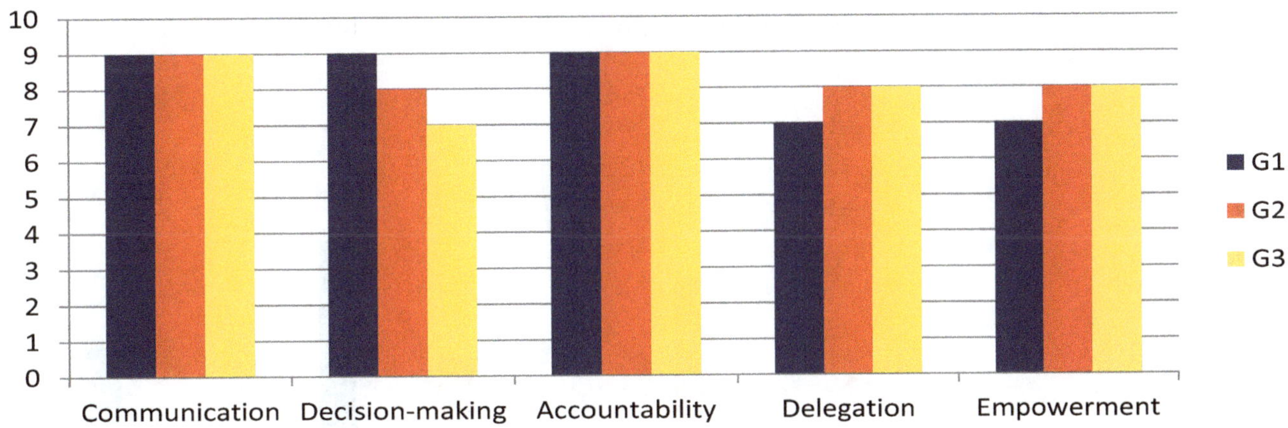

Figure 1. Shows the results of the leadership characteristics during the exercise.

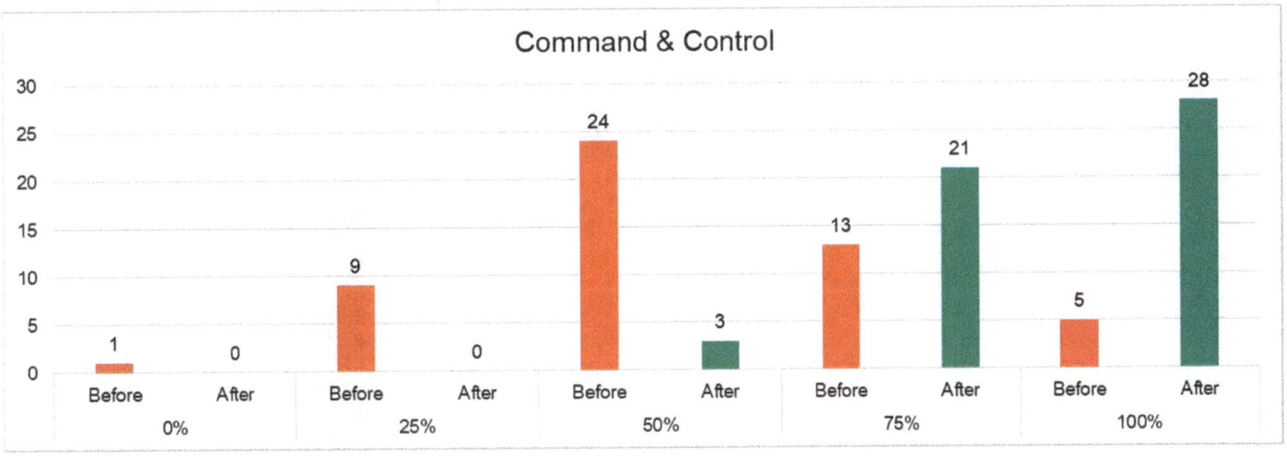

Figure 2. Shows the results of the pre-, and post-test in Command and Control.

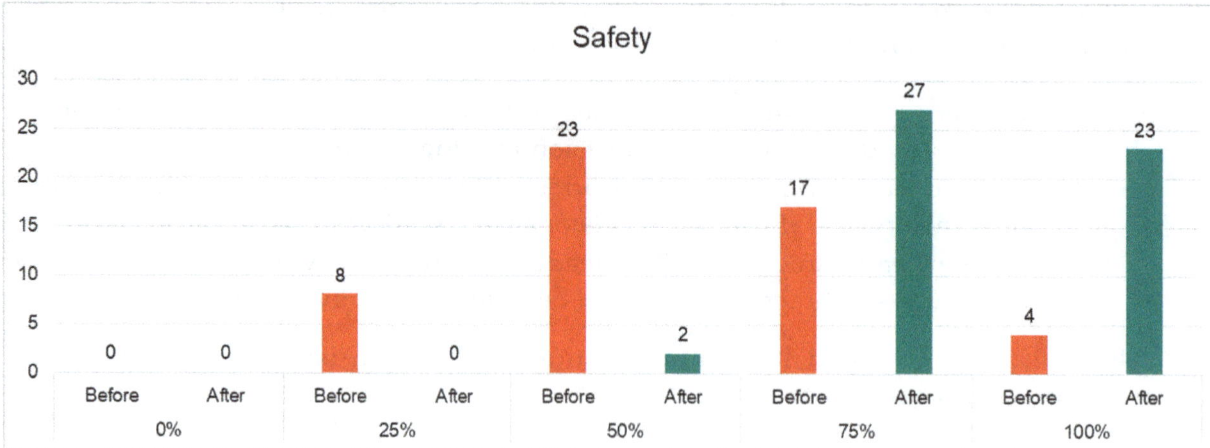

Figure 3. Shows the results of the pre-, and post-test in Safety issues.

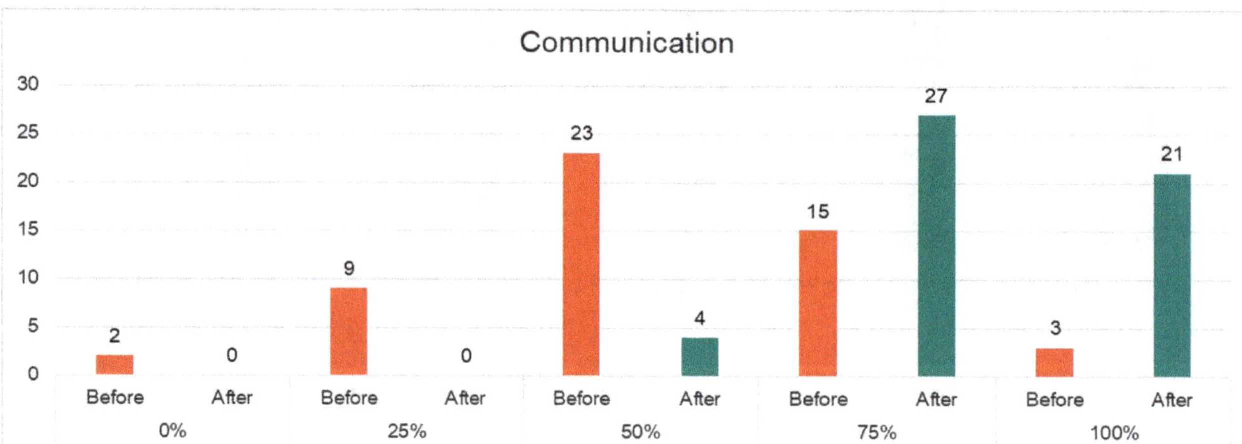

Figure 4. Shows the results of the pre-, and post-test in Communication.

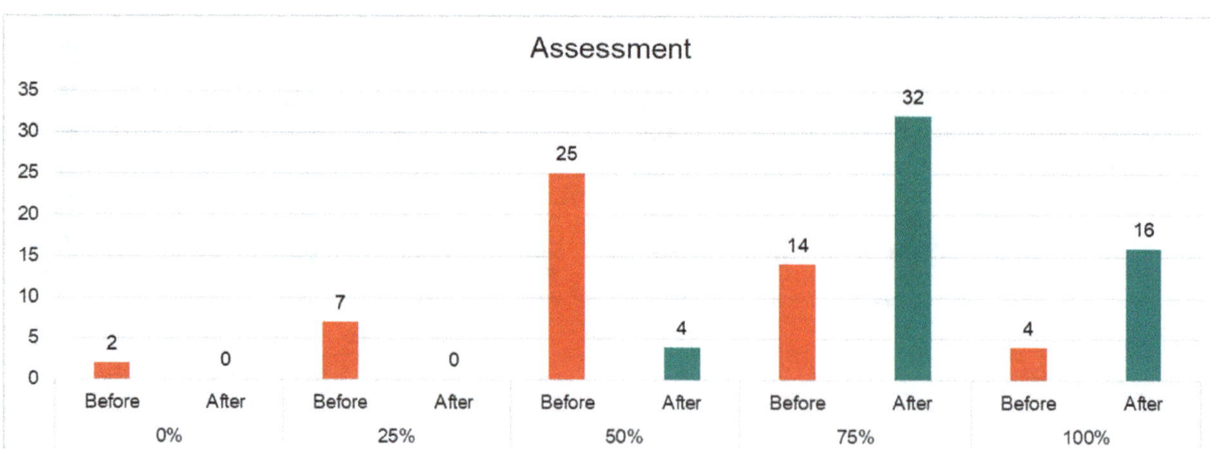

Figure 5. Shows the results of the pre-, and post-test in situation Assessment.

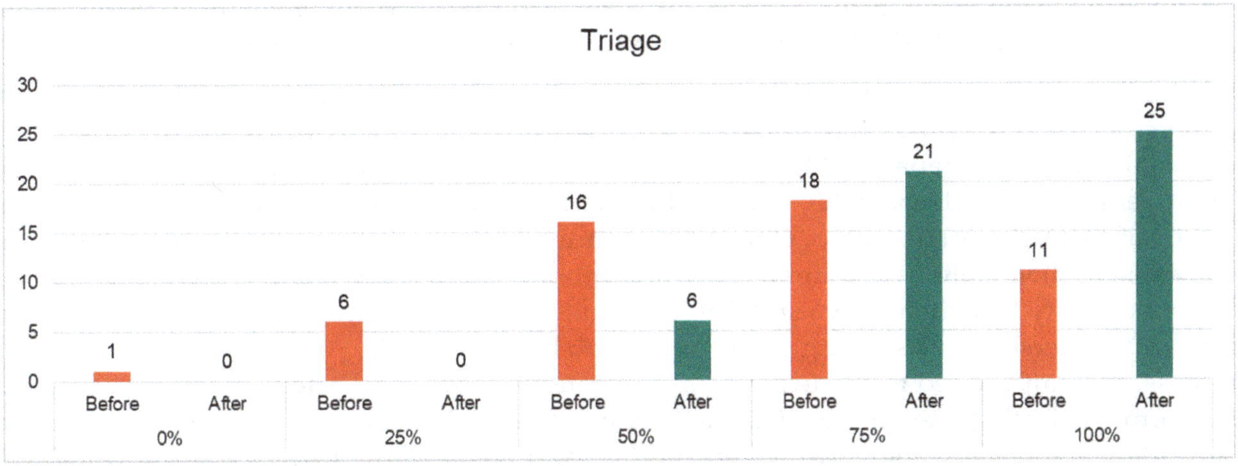

Figure 6. Shows the results of the pre-, and post-test in Triage.

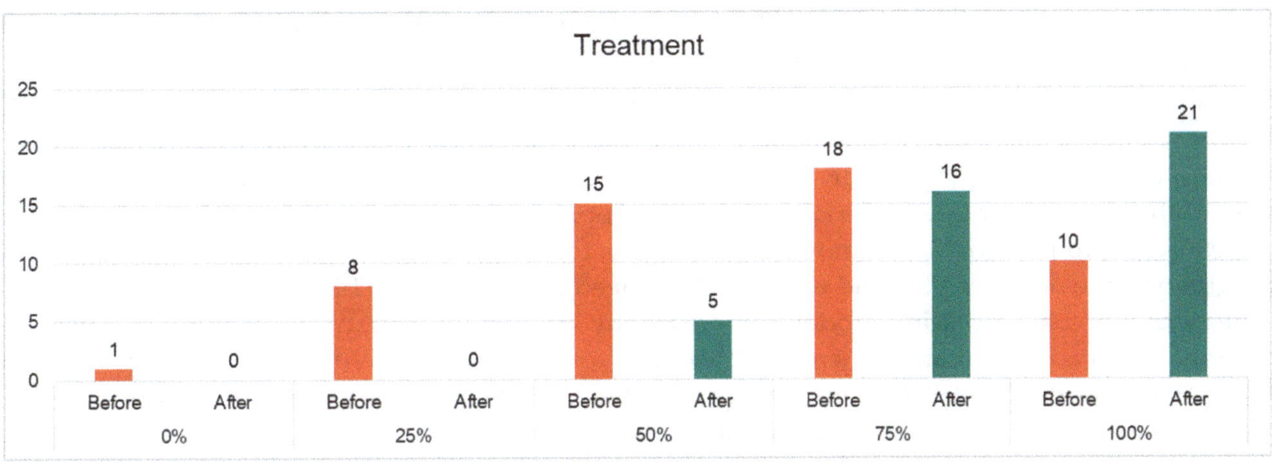

Figure 7. Shows the results of the pre-, and post-test Treatment issues.

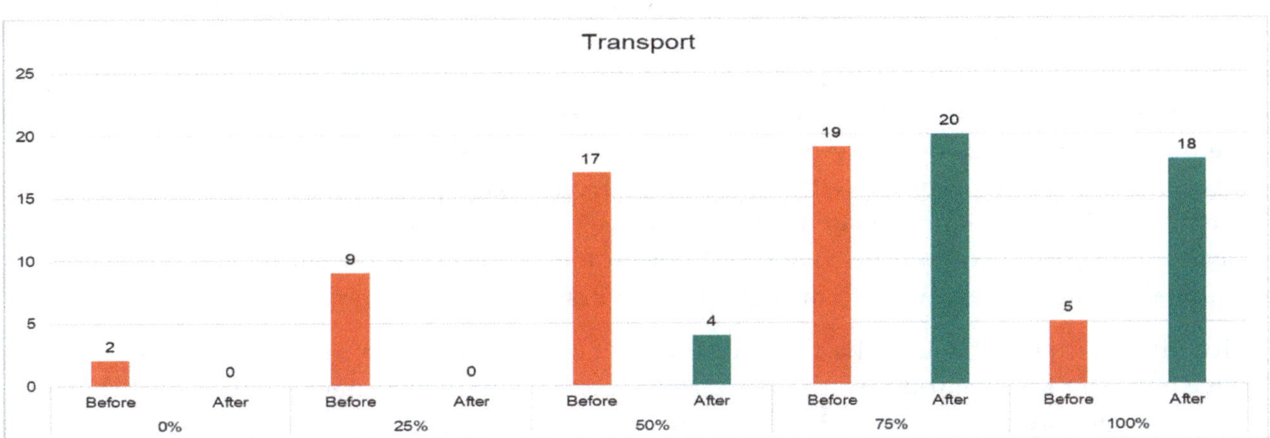

Figure 8. Shows the results of the pre-, and post-test Transport issues.

5. Discussion

The essential raise of knowledge among Thai EPs was registered in Command and control, Safety, Communication, and situation Assessment. At the same time, the understanding of the subject areas, Triage, Treatment, and Transport did not develop to the same extent. All changes were statistically significant. Since these physicians are working at both hospital and prehospital levels, it is not surprising that the grade of their knowledge in strict medical areas, e.g., Triage, Treatment, and Transport, is higher than other subjects within CSCATTT, which specifically deal with leadership characteristics.

Earlier studies have discussed the medical and nonmedical aspects of MID management, showing critical shortcomings in the latter [15]. Disaster and major incidents are rare, but they need to be mitigated and managed if they occur. In successful management, collaboration is one crucial factor that demands skilled leadership and reliable communication. In this group of EPs with no earlier experience of MID, the collaborative elements in a mutual task helped to reduce the organizational barriers, enlisted their abilities and limitations, and promoted interplay with no hierarchical authority, as well as the ability to switch between different collaboration strategies as demanded by the specific situation and leadership styles. The groups grew up to be more stable, practiced transitions, overlaps, fearlessness, and improvised to create new ways of handling the unexpected situation by discovering different communication alternatives. During training, their ability to try out the situation developed their confidence, increased their trust to each other, and reduced the internal fear of doing wrong. They could test a model, evaluate its effect in the next stage, create a new approach, test it, and develop their approach continuously [21,23,24,29]. All these elements are necessary for successful teamwork at the time of emergency. The ultimate requirement is to act in a flexible surge capacity (FSC) when hospitals and communities must activate their resources, respectively [10].

Choosing EPs as one of the major players in MID management is a natural selection [17,19,20]. In countries such as Thailand, they work at both hospital and prehospital levels and thus have a logical connection to both entities [19,20]. In a changing world, when resources may not be enough to match the needs, there must be more material and personal options than what is offered by standard disaster plans. FSC aims to provide new innovative solutions to these shortcomings [10]. Other reports have high lightened the need for FSC and discussed the need for ACF [30]. This paper tried to examine the possibility of using a simulation model to increase the knowledge and understanding of a new set of professionals to lead MID management. Training EPs for the next MID will strengthen the whole chain of disaster management and partly accommodate the WHO´s policy of proactivity and increase the strength and ability of communities to handle the first waves of MID impacts since EPs are one group, who will face upcoming incidents [17,19]. Other measures within the community, such as civilians' empowerment as immediate responders, and the necessity of creating new guidelines and systems have been reported elsewhere [31–33]. Altogether, they facilitate the concept of FSC (Flexible Surge Capacity). Using the elements of CSCATTT as a model enables a direct assessment of critical features that need to be in place during MID management [18]. These elements are part of educational initiatives given to all healthcare staff, and are not only perceived abilities and knowledge but also what they practice in every-day missions, and emphasize the importance of medical and nonmedical aspects of MID management. In a future with limited resources and expanding needs, civilian help can be decisive in creating Resilience in each society [31–33]. The same method and elements can be used to educate other groups of people to act at different levels of management or maybe increase their awareness about any given event to mitigate the adverse outcomes of any incidents [15,30–34].

Moynihan [29] emphasizes the value of trying it out, i.e., to test a model to cope with an event, evaluate the effect of the model in the next stage, create a new approach, test it, and develop the method continuously. Through the 3LC-exercise, the EPs practiced their ability to make a concerted and coherent assessment of which collaboration form is applicable at a given time. The collaboration is not a static activity but subject to construction, deconstruction, and reconstruction, depending on what is appropriate for a specific time, place, or event. The 3LC exercise illustrates the primary goal of practicing the different forms of collaboration and switching between them by including asymmetries in the scenarios [21–24]. For instance, the police can arrive first at the scene and begin caring for victims with serious injuries, or understaffed emergency rescue services have to get help from the police and paramedics at a fire incident. The exercise also reveals the need for a joint assessment and the importance of knowing both prehospital and hospital fields. The latter offers a valuable opportunity to increase the collaborative segment of MID management. At the same time, decisions can be made based on knowledge about the different organizations' limitations and capabilities [15,16].

6. Limitations

This study did not compare the 3LC and traditional types of exercises. In earlier studies, 3LC had a significant impact on perceived collaboration, learning as well as performance. Based on these findings, before and after design control was chosen (pre- and post-test) [22–25]. Measuring the perceived effects of exercises, using a self-assessment tool, may be considered as a limitation. The possibility of over- or underreporting cannot be ignored. However, there are some advantages with the tool too, such as it encourages the participants to reflect over their own learning progress and performance, to be more responsible for their own learning, to develop their judgment skills while they have no pressure of peer evaluation, make participants more autonomous learners and finally make them aware of their weaknesses and strength. To verify the causality and generalizability of the results, a study that is not just based on a written test would give additional insightful and important information.

As an alternative, a comparative design, including a control group, should be considered in future studies. However, pre- and post-test scores provide information on whether or not participants have learned from the training. Besides, a well-designed pre- and post-test can help trainers understand which concepts or competencies were well taught during the training and which ones need additional time, or need to be covered using alternative methods [25,33]. Pre- and post-tests may not be the best tools to use for every type of training but still offer a good overview of the tested group's advancement. Wishing to understand what knowledge can be credited to the training itself, using a pre- and post-test methodology is essential. As shown statistically in this study, the knowledge of EPs in all areas of CSCATT increased significantly. Another limitation was that the data collection occurred immediately after the exercises and not supplemented with data collected weeks or months after the exercises [27,28].

An alternative method of evaluating learning, such as the observation of skills demonstrated in a role-play, might be more appropriate in some situations. In this study, we combined the Participant observation method as a complement to the pre- and post-course tests [26–29]. It is a variant of the natural observations model. Still, the researcher joins in and becomes part of the group they are studying to get a more in-depth insight into their activities. In this overt observation model, the researchers revealed their identity and purpose to the group and asked permission to observe. There are some limitations to this model. It can be challenging to get time/privacy for recording, which means observers have to wait until they are alone and rely on their memory, which is a problem as they may forget details and are unlikely to remember direct quotations. Furthermore, if the researcher becomes too involved, they may lose objectivity and become bias, and thus reduce the validity of the data.

The participants in this study were all physicians, while other staff such as nurses, paramedics, administrators, etc. are also important parts of a hospitals' MID management. This study was the first step in a series of studies that are planned to evaluate the concept of FSC, and physicians were simply chosen due to their actual position within the Thai healthcare and their knowledge in English. It is clear that other knowledgeable staff could also possess the leadership position [34].

Finally, although statistically significant results were obtained in this study, the number of included EPs can be challenged. However, for everyone working within healthcare, it is clear that a larger number of physicians cannot be gathered at the same time for any kind of exercise or training. This is a challenging fact that affects all types of education and training within all healthcare systems [21,35]. Similar argument is true concerning the provision of a control group. It is hard to get enough healthcare workers in a training session, and still harder to have one third of them as a control group.

Simulation exercises emerged as a solution to this issue since reality-based exercises demand not only a large number of participants but also cost a lot and often evaluate just one part of the disaster management chain [21,35].

7. Conclusions

In conclusion, the findings in this report indicate that the ability in all elements of CSCATTT, particularly expertise in command and control, communication, collaboration and coordination, and situation assessment, improved in all groups of EPs systematically and after each scenario. The 3LC method also enabled all participants to create new perspectives and innovative measures, which improved the overall management of scenarios on the final day. The 3LC increases the ability, knowledge, and attitude of Thai emergency physicians in managing MID. It also enables them to lead emergency management in an unexpected situation, as alternative leaders in a flexible surge capacity-response system [10,30].

Author Contributions: Conceptualization, A.K.-M.; data curation, P.P.; formal analysis, P.P., V.G., E.C. and A.K.-M.; investigation, P.P. and A.K.-M.; methodology, E.C. and A.K.-M.; project administration, P.P.; resources, P.P., A.K.-M.; supervision, A.K.-M.; validation, L.D.H.; writing—original draft, P.P.; writing—review & editing, V.G., E.C., L.D.H. and A.K.-M. All authors have read and agreed to the published version of the manuscript.

Acknowledgments: The authors would like to thank Yohan Robinson for his support to this project.

Appendix A

Appendix A.1. Scenarios, 3LC Exercises, Bangkok, Thailand

Scenario 1: A bomb

On 15 September 2017, the dispatch center contacted and informed you about a Bomb found 5 km from your hospital. There was another hospital 200 m next to the scene. More than 100 people were injured. Mange situation based on CSCATTT.

Around 30 min after the first contact, a second bomb is found at the middle of the scene. How would you manage the scene now?

Scenario 2: A Fire in a Tall Building

On 15 December 2017, the dispatch center contacted and informed you that there was a fire on the fifth floor of an 11 floors apartment 5 km away from your hospital. More than 50 people were injured. How do you manage the situation based on CSCATTT?

Around 30 min after the fire incident and when there is a crowd and gathering of people, a truck drives into the treatment zones inside the area, and hit many people.

Scenario 3: Riot and Active Shooter

On 15 May 2015, you were on a night shift at the hospital and saw Riots on the news; the place of the incident was 5 km from your hospital. Some people starts shooting and ambulances started and kept bringing injured people to your hospital. How would you manage your emergency department based on CSCATTT?

One of the injured victim had a bomb strapped on his chest. How would you manage the situation? Would you evacuate your emergency department?

References

1. WHO. Hospital Emergency Response Checklist. An All-Hazards Tool for Hospital Administrators and Emergency Managers. 2011. Available online: http://www.euro.who.int/__data/assets/pdf_file/0008/268766/Hospital-emergency-response-checklist-Eng.pdf (accessed on 25 June 2020).
2. Vitalii, S.; Khorram-Manesh, A.; Nyberg, L. Disaster cycle and management. In *Handbook of Disaster and Emergency Management*; Khorram-Manesh, A., Ed.; Kompendiet: Göteborg, Sweden, 2017; Chapter 2; pp. 23–29.
3. United Nations International Strategy for Disaster Reduction (UNISDR). *Terminology on Disaster Risk Reduction*; United Nations: Geneva, Switzerland, 2009. Available online: https://www.unisdr.org/files/7817_UNISDRTerminologyEnglish.pdf (accessed on 25 June 2020).
4. Hick, J.; Christian, M.; Sprung, C. Surge Capacity and Infrastructure considerations for mass critical care. *Intensive Care Med.* **2010**, *36*, 11–20. [CrossRef]
5. Barbich, D.; Koenig, K. Understanding Surge Capacity: Essential Elements. *Acad. Emerg. Med.* **2006**, *6*, 1098–1102. [CrossRef] [PubMed]
6. Kaji, A.; Koenig, K.L.; Bey, T. Surge capacity for healthcare systems: A conceptual framework. *Acad. Emerg. Med.* **2006**, *13*, 1157–1159. [CrossRef] [PubMed]
7. Bonnet, C.; Peery, B.; Cantrill, S.; Pons, P.; Haukoos, J.; McVaney, K.; Colwell, C. Surge capacity: A proposed conceptual framework. *Am. J. Emerg. Med.* **2007**, *25*, 297–306. [CrossRef] [PubMed]
8. Runkle, J.D.; Brock-Martin, A.; Karmus, W.; Svendsen, E.R. Secondary Surge Capacity: A framework for understanding long-term access to primary care for medically vulnerable populations in disaster recovery. *Am. J. Public Health* **2012**, *102*, 24–32. [CrossRef] [PubMed]
9. Adams, L.M. Exploring the concept of surge capacity. *Issues Nurs.* **2009**, *14*, 2. [CrossRef]
10. Khorram-Manesh, A. Flexible Surge Capacity—Public Health, Public Education, and Disaster Management. *Health Promot. Perspect* **2020**, *10*, 175–179. [CrossRef]
11. The Lancet Editorial. Disaster prevention should be equal. *Lancet Glob. Health* **2017**, *5*, 1047. [CrossRef]
12. Krolik, M. Exploring a rights-based approach to disaster management. *Aust. J. Emerg. Manag.* **2013**, *28*, 44–48. Available online: https://knowledge.aidr.org.au/resources/ajem-oct-2013-exploring-a-rights-based-approach-to-disaster-management/ (accessed on 14 July 2020).
13. Rice, K.; Felizzi, M.V.; Hagelgans, D. Human Rights-Based Approach to Disaster Management: Valparaiso, Chile. *J. Hum. Rights Soc. Work* **2017**, *2*, 117–127. [CrossRef]
14. Prytz, E.G.; Rybing, J.; Carlström, E.; Khorram-Manesh, A.; Jonson, C.O. Exploring prehospital C2-work during a mass gathering event. *Int. J. Emerg. Serv.* **2015**, *4*, 227–241. [CrossRef]
15. Khorram-Manesh, A.; Lönroth, H.; Rotter, P.; Wilhelmsson, M.; Aremyr, J.; Berner, A.; Nero Andersson, A.; Carlström, E. Non-medical aspects of civilian-military collaboration in management of major incidents. *Eur. J. Trauma Emerg. Surg.* **2017**, *43*, 595–603. [CrossRef]
16. Khorram-Manesh, A.; Hedelin, A.; Örtenwall, P. Regional coordination in medical emergencies and major incidents; plan, execute and teach. *Scand. J. Trauma Resusc. Emerg. Med.* **2009**, *17*, 32. [CrossRef]
17. Kahn, C.A.; Koenig, K.L.; Schultz, C.H. Emergency physician disaster deployment: Issues to consider and model policy. *Prehosp. Disaster Med.* **2017**, *32*, 462–464. [CrossRef]
18. Sammut, J.; Cato, D.; Homer, T. Major Incident Medical Management and Support (MIMMS): A practical multiple casualty, disaster-site training course for all Australian healthcare personnel. *Emerg. Med.* **2001**, *13*, 174–180. [CrossRef]
19. Sittichanbuncha, Y.; Prachanukool, T.; Sarathep, P.; Sawanyawisuth, K. An emergency medical service in Thailand—Providers perspectives. *J. Med. Assoc. Thai* **2014**, *97*, 1016–1021.
20. Khorram-Manesh, A.; Angthong, C.; Pangma, A.; Sulannakarn, S.; Burivong, R.; Jarayabhand, R.; Örtenwall, P. Hospital Evacuation; Learning from the Past? Flooding of Bangkok 2011. *BJMMR* **2014**, *4*, 395–415. [CrossRef]
21. Khorram-Manesh, A.; Berlin, J.; Carlström, E. Two validated ways of the ability of decision-making in emergencies, Results from a literature review. *Bull. Emerg. Trauma* **2016**, *4*, 186–196.
22. Sorensen, J.; Magnussen, L.I.; Torgersen, G.E.; Christiansen, A.M.; Carlstrom, E. Percieved Usefulness of Maritime Cross-Border Collaboration Exercises. *Arts Soc. Sci. J.* **2018**, *9*, 1–5. [CrossRef]

23. Magnussen, L.I.; Carlström, E.; Sörensen, J.L.; Torgersen, G.E.; Hagenes, E.F.; Kristiansen, E. Learning and Usefulness stemming from collaboration in a maritime crisis management exercise in Northern Norway. *Disaster Prev. Manag.* **2018**, *27*, 129–140. [CrossRef]
24. Berlin, J.; Carlström, E. The three level collaboration exercise—Impact of learning and usefulness. *J. Conting. Crisis Manag. (JCCM)* **2015**, *23*, 257–265. [CrossRef]
25. Aykal, G.; Kespali, M.; Aydin, Ö.; Esen, H.; Yegin, A.; Gungör, F.; Yilmaz, N. Pre-Test and Post-Test Applications to Shape the Education of Phlebotomists in a Quality Management Program: An Experience in a Training Hospital. *J. Med. Biochem.* **2016**, *35*, 347–353. [PubMed]
26. Takala, E.P.; Pehkonen, I.; Forsman, M.; Hansson, G.Å.; Mathiassen, S.E.; Neumann, W.P.; Sjögaard, G.; Veiersted, K.B.; Westgaard, R.H.; Winkel, J. Systematic evaluation of observational methods assessing biomechanical exposures at work. *Scand. J. Work Environ. Health* **2010**, *36*, 3–24. [CrossRef] [PubMed]
27. Luna-Reyes, L.F.; Lines Andersen, D. Collecting and analyzing qualitative data for system dynamics: Methods and models. *Syst. Dyn. Rev.* **2004**. [CrossRef]
28. Lofland, J.; Lofland, L.H. *Analyzing Social Setting: A Guide to Qualitative Observation and Analysis*, 2nd ed.; Wadsworth: Belmont, CA, USA, 1984.
29. Moynihan, D.P. Learning under uncertainty: Networks in crisis management. *Public Admin. Rev.* **2008**, *68*, 350–365. [CrossRef]
30. Glantz, V.; Phattharapornjaroen, P.; Carlström, E.; Khorram-Manesh, A. Regional Flexible Surge Capacity—A flexible response system. *Sustainability* **2020**, *12*, 5984. [CrossRef]
31. World Health Organization (WHO). Sustainable Development Goals (SDGs). Available online: https://www.who.int/sdg/en/ (accessed on 25 June 2020).
32. Khorram-Manesh, A.; Plegas, P.; Peyravi, M.; Carlström, E. Immediate Response to Major Incidents: Defining an immediate responder! *Eur. J. Trauma Emerg. Surg.* **2019**. [CrossRef]
33. Khorram-Manesh, A.; Berlin, J.; Ljung Roseke, L.; Aremyr, J.; Sörensson, J.; Carlström, E. Emergency Management and Preparedness Training for Youth (EMPTY): The Results of the First Swedish pilot Study. *Disaster Med. Public Health Prep.* **2018**, *12*, 685–688. [CrossRef]
34. Khorram-Manesh, A. *Learning to Respect Diversity, Gender Equality, and Collaboration: A childhood Agenda or the Content of a Leadership Development Program*; Magnussen, L.I., Ed.; Disaster, Diversity, and Emergency Preparation; IOS Press: Amsterdam, The Netherlands, 2019; pp. 11–18. [CrossRef]
35. Jahangirian, M.; Naseer, A.; Stergioulas, L.; Young, T.; Eldabi, T.; Brailsford, S.; Patel, B.; Harper, P. Simulation in health-care: Lessons from other sectors. *Oper. Res. Int. J.* **2012**, *12*, 45–55. [CrossRef]

17

Narrative Review on Health-EDRM Primary Prevention Measures for Vector-Borne Diseases

Emily Ying Yang Chan [1,2,3,4,5,*], Tiffany Sze Tung Sham [3,4], Tayyab Salim Shahzada [3,4], Caroline Dubois [4], Zhe Huang [1,3], Sida Liu [1,4], Kevin K.C. Hung [1,3,5], Shelly L.A. Tse [3], Kin On Kwok [3], Pui-Hong Chung [3], Ryoma Kayano [6] and Rajib Shaw [7]

1 Collaborating Centre for Oxford University and CUHK for Disaster and Medical Humanitarian Response (CCOUC), The Chinese University of Hong Kong, Hong Kong SAR, China; huangzhe@cuhk.edu.hk (Z.H.); sida.liu@gxfoundation.hk (S.L.); kevin.hung@cuhk.edu.hk (K.K.C.H.)
2 Nuffield Department of Medicine, University of Oxford, Oxford OX37BN, UK
3 JC School of Public Health and Primary Care, Faculty of Medicine, The Chinese University of Hong Kong, Hong Kong SAR, China; tiffany.sham@link.cuhk.edu.hk (T.S.T.S.); tayyabshahzada@link.cuhk.edu.hk (T.S.S.); shelly@cuhk.edu.hk (S.L.A.T.); kkokwok@cuhk.edu.hk (K.O.K.); chungpuihong@cuhk.edu.hk (P.-H.C.)
4 GX Foundation, Hong Kong SAR, China; caroline.dubois@gxfoundation.hk
5 Accident & Emergency Medicine Academic Unit, The Chinese University of Hong Kong, Prince of Wales Hospital, Hong Kong SAR, China
6 World Health Organization Centre for Health Development, Kobe 651-0073, Japan; kayanor@who.int
7 Graduate School of Media and Governance, Keio University, Fujisawa 252-0882, Japan; shaw@sfc.keio.ac.jp
* Correspondence: emily.chan@cuhk.edu.hk

Abstract: Climate change is expanding the global at-risk population for vector-borne diseases (VBDs). The World Health Organization (WHO) health emergency and disaster risk management (health-EDRM) framework emphasises the importance of primary prevention of biological hazards and its value in protecting against VBDs. The framework encourages stakeholder coordination and information sharing, though there is still a need to reinforce prevention and recovery within disaster management. This keyword-search based narrative literature review searched databases PubMed, Google Scholar, Embase and Medline between January 2000 and May 2020, and identified 134 publications. In total, 10 health-EDRM primary prevention measures are summarised at three levels (personal, environmental and household). Enabling factor, limiting factors, co-benefits and strength of evidence were identified. Current studies on primary prevention measures for VBDs focus on health risk-reduction, with minimal evaluation of actual disease reduction. Although prevention against mosquito-borne diseases, notably malaria, has been well-studied, research on other vectors and VBDs remains limited. Other gaps included the limited evidence pertaining to prevention in resource-poor settings and the efficacy of alternatives, discrepancies amongst agencies' recommendations, and limited studies on the impact of technological advancements and habitat change on VBD prevalence. Health-EDRM primary prevention measures for VBDs require high-priority research to facilitate multifaceted, multi-sectoral, coordinated responses that will enable effective risk mitigation.

Keywords: health-EDRM; primary prevention; vector-borne disease; biological hazards; climate change; narrative review

1. Introduction

Vector-borne diseases (VBDs) are viral, parasitic and bacterial illnesses transmitted to humans through vectors such as mosquitoes, sand flies and ticks. Common VBDs affecting human health include malaria, yellow fever, dengue, Zika, chikungunya, Lyme disease, tick-borne encephalitis, leishmaniasis and African trypanosomiasis [1]. The complacency towards and reduced emphasis on vector control [2] and the redirection of health resources, together with population growth, urbanisation and globalization, have contributed to the increased frequency of VBD outbreaks in tropical areas of the world in the past decade [2]. With the impact of climate change on ecological and human living environment, the burden of VBDs has expanded from tropical and subtropical areas to temperate regions, placing 80% of the world's population at risk [3]. This shift in the human vulnerability profile has been attributed to rising temperatures, which favour the migration and geographical expansion of disease vectors [4]. Furthermore, altered precipitation patterns favour larval breeding and have accelerated VBD spread [5]. Contact patterns between humans and pathogens, vectors or hosts may also be altered by climate change in an unpredictable manner [4]. Increased occurrences of natural hazards, such as floods and cyclones, pose a further risk of VBD outbreaks [4]. Geographical areas that were previously unaffected are now facing growing risks [6,7], but are often underequipped in disaster prevention, preparedness and response capacities.

The World Health Organization (WHO) estimates that VBDs currently account for over 17% of the global burden of infectious diseases [1]. As indicated in the Global Burden of Disease Study [8], VBDs have substantial disability weights [9] and can be detrimental to the socioeconomic development of communities. Malaria is a disease which accounts for more than 50% of total deaths caused by VBD [10], and high-risk countries have on average a gross domestic product per capita growth that is over five times lower than countries not affected by the disease [11]. The economic burden of VBDs stems from increased household expenditure on disease prevention and management, lost income from minimised productivity due to sickness or care for the ill [3], damages to crops and livestock by disease vectors [2], and other impacting factors. The United Nations Sustainable Development Goals (SDG) emphasise good health and well-being (SDG 3) [12]. Collaborative initiatives and investments prioritising prevention and treatment research by international bodies in recent decades, such as efforts by the Global Fund [13], have contributed to the alleviation of the global disease burden induced by VBDs [10].

The WHO health-emergency and disaster risk management (health-EDRM) framework was developed in 2018 as an integrated approach for the utilisation and management of resources in addressing current and emerging risks to public health, with the aim of promoting joint action and coherence in implementing other global strategies such as the International Health Regulations (2005), the Sendai Framework for Disaster Risk Reduction 2015–2030, the Paris Agreement on Climate Change, and the Sustainable Development Goals 2015–2030 [14]. Overall, the framework guides the structured analysis and management of health risks brought on by emergencies and disasters, focusing on risk mitigation through hazard and vulnerability reduction, preparedness, response, and recovery measures [14,15]. Health-EDRM emphasises the significance of community involvement to mitigating and counteracting the potential negative impacts of hazardous events such as VBD outbreaks, which are considered biological hazards [14].

The concept of prioritising health in disaster risk management policies was already recognised in the Sendai Framework for Disaster Risk Reduction 2015–2030 [16]. Health actors at all levels have engaged with each other and the WHO in the implementation and monitoring of disaster risk reduction. WHO offices at the regional level, and country governments, have incorporated disaster risk management policies in the health sector, which is an important step in contextualising actions for implementation [17]. The Sendai Framework has been crucial in highlighting health as a core dimension of disaster risk management, and has paved the way for the establishment of the WHO Health-EDRM Research Network, strengthening research and knowledge-sharing globally, allowing for the enhancement of evidence-based policies and practices [17]. There is a crucial need for multi-sectoral, coordinated approaches between the countries' governments, health systems and other stakeholders, especially in the area of recording and reporting against the framework [17]. Additionally, systems need to reinforce the recognition of prevention and recovery within disaster management [17].

The health-EDRM framework outlines a hierarchisation of health risk prevention into primary, secondary and tertiary prevention [14,18]. Primary prevention mitigates against the onset of disease through health promotion targeted at behavioural modification and health risk reduction. Secondary prevention involves inhibiting disease progression through strategies such as screening and early detection. Tertiary prevention focuses on treatment and rehabilitation in order to minimise disabilities and complications [18,19]. Taking into consideration financial, clinical and infrastructural costs, primary prevention can effectively alleviate the burden of VBDs in a community, if necessary through measures that address a wide spectrum of VBDs, such as targeting diseases transmittable through multiple vectors [20] or focusing on vectors that are capable of transmitting multiple diseases [1]. Primary prevention measures often offer the most cost-effective outcomes and enhance health protection through increased community resilience against diseases where treatment is unavailable or access to healthcare is complicated. Secondary and tertiary prevention measures require significant human resources and health infrastructural support, and may therefore be costly, with higher programmatic risks, causing further economic stress on impacted communities.

There is a large amount of available evidence and research concerning clinical treatment approaches to some VBDs, such as Malaria. However, other VBDs, such as dengue, chikungunya, tick-borne encephalitis, Japanese encephalitis, yellow fever and leishmaniasis, lack standardised or straightforward treatments, and rely primarily on therapeutic interventions built on symptom management [21]. There are ongoing clinical trials in these areas, such as vaccine development for Zika and chikungunya, research into rapid malaria tests, as well as drug trials for chikungunya [22].

This narrative literature review examines published evidence on health-EDRM primary prevention measures for VBD risk mitigation, maps the contextual effectiveness or limitations of each preventive measure, and aims to identify areas of research that need be strengthened in order to develop effective strategies for VBD prevention. The strength of the available scientific evidence is evaluated for each of the prevention measures. Based on the health-EDRM framework, which emphasises the context-based determination of intervention efficacy, analysis of enabling and limiting factors is also included for each measure [14].

2. Materials and Methods

A keyword search-based narrative literature review was conducted using the databases PubMed, Google Scholar, Embase, Medline and ScienceDirect. The search was conducted in May 2020 and included English language-based international peer-reviewed articles, online reports, electronic books and press releases, as well as grey literature by institutions such as the WHO, the United Nations, the Global Fund, the United Nations Children's Fund, the International Energy Agency, the World Bank, the United States Centres for Disease Control and Prevention, the U.S. Food and Drug Administration, and the Hong Kong Centre for Health Protection, published between January 2000 and May 2020. The snowballing search methodology was also applied. Specific keywords and phrases used can be found in Appendix A. The emergence, primary prevention, associated risk factors and management of VBDs were reviewed in order to generate 10 core primary prevention measures for discussion.

With reference to the Oxford Centre for Evidence-Based Medicine (OCEBM) 2009 Levels of Evidence (Figure 1) criteria, the identified papers were categorised into their respective levels according to strength of evidence based on the study design and methodology [23]. Reviewed literature that could not be categorised using the OCEBM Levels of Evidence was classified as 'Others', which includes, but is not limited to, news articles or releases, books, textbooks, position papers, guidelines, case reports and organisational reports.

Level	Therapy/Prevention, Aetiology/Harm
1a	Systematic Review (SR) (with homogeneity) of Randomised Controlled Trials (RCTs)
1b	Individual RCT (with narrow Confidence Interval)
1c	All or none
2a	SR (with homogeneity) of cohort studies
2b	Individual cohort study (including low quality RCT; e.g., <80% follow-up)
2c	'Outcomes' Research; Ecological studies
3a	SR (with homogeneity) of case-control studies
3b	Individual Case-Control Study
4	Case-series (and poor-quality cohort and case-control studies)
5	Expert opinion without explicit critical appraisal, or based on physiology, bench research or 'first principles'

Figure 1. The Oxford Centre for Evidence-Based Medicine (OCEBM) 2009 Levels of Evidence (adapted from www.cebm.net) [23].

3. Results

The search identified 134 relevant publications, all of which were included in the results analysis.

Using the identified research, 10 core bottom-up primary prevention measures were proposed and discussed based on the health-EDRM framework. Five personal protection practices (wear protective clothing when outdoors, avoid heading outdoors to vector-prone areas and during peak biting conditions, apply insect repellent, sleep under bed nets, receive prophylactic vaccinations and chemoprophylaxis), three environmental management practices (use insect-killing traps, manage stagnant water appropriately, manage waste appropriately), and two customary household practices (minimise household entry points, cover exposed foodstuffs) were included. Tables 1 and 2 (personal), Table 3 (environmental) and Table 4 (customary household) highlight relevant health risk, desired behavioural change, potential co-benefits, enabling and limiting factors, alternatives, and strength of evidence available in published literature with regard to these primary prevention measures. Table 5 categorises all 134 reviewed publications according to the OCEBM Levels of Evidence [23]. Of note, a number of the reviewed articles report an assessment of more than one primary prevention measure. The review results indicate that approximately 60% of the studied literature relate to personal protection, 24% to environmental management, and merely 16% focus on customary household practices. Measures such as outdoor avoidance, sleeping under bed nets and receiving prophylactic vaccinations and chemoprophylaxis are amongst the most commonly reported studies. Details on the precise breakdown of each reviewed reference can be found in Table S1.

Table 1. Personal Protection Practices as Health Emergency and Disaster Risk Management (Health-EDRM) Primary Prevention Approaches against Vector-borne Diseases (VBDs) (Part 1).

Parametres	Wear Protective Clothing When Outdoors	Avoid Heading Outdoors to Vector-Prone Areas and During Peak Biting Conditions	
		Vector-Prone Areas	Peak Biting Conditions
Risk	• Disease vectors have landing preferences for exposed skin over fabric. This is evident in studies on the Human Landing Catch (HLC) technique—HLC participants wear protective clothing to limit the area of exposed skin that attracts vectors [24]. • There is often a greater risk of VBD transmission outdoors compared to indoors, as seen for malaria [25], chikungunya [26], and tick-borne disease transmission [27].	• Specific locations such as secondary forests and rubber plantations are at a high risk of VBD transmission, such as dengue and Japanese encephalitis [28].	• The time of the day and weather influence VBD exposure risk. Mosquitoes infected with *Plasmodium*, the parasite that causes malaria, are most active from dusk to dawn [29–31]. • There are positive correlations between temperature and the number of dengue [32] and tick-borne encephalitis [33] transmission incidences, as well as between temperature, humidity, rainfall and the number of malaria transmission incidences [34].
Behavioural Change	• Wear protective clothing, long-sleeve tops, and long trousers to minimise skin exposure and create a physical barrier against bites from vectors such as mosquitoes [31] and ticks [35]. • Wear light-coloured clothing [21]. • Wear loose-fitting and tightly-woven clothes to avoid vector bites through the clothing when it is pulled tight to the skin [36]. • Tuck trousers into socks and boots to further reduce skin exposure. Seal clothing junctions with adhesive tape as an additional precaution under extreme infestation pressure [36].	• Avoid vector-prone or VBD-endemic areas if possible [21,31,36,37].	• Avoid or minimise outdoor activities during hot and humid seasons, unless necessary [37]. • Avoid or minimise outdoor activities during specific periods of a day, such as from dusk to dawn in malaria-endemic areas if possible [21,31,36].
Co-benefit(s)	• Protects skin from sun exposure and lowers risk of sunburn [38,39]. • Protects skin from scratches and infections [39].	• Reduces hazardous risks such as tiger [40] and bear [41] attacks in rubber plantations and secondary forests respectively.	• Protects individuals from heat exhaustion and further progression to heat stroke under exposure to high temperatures [42,43]. • Protects individuals from health risks such as increased cardiovascular disease mortality under exposure to high humidity [44]. • Protects individuals from fall-related injuries, which are more prevalent during the rainy season [45].
Enabling Factor(s)	• Availability and affordability of protective clothing [46]. • Suitability of the weather—cool and dry weather is favourable where additional clothing is unlikely to cause discomfort.	• Ability and flexibility to stay indoors for long periods without great discomfort; adequate household space is favourable. • Ability to make informed decisions on specific local habitats and conditions to avoid; the risk variability of different environments and the non-exhaustive list of prone areas and peak biting conditions above should be noted.	

Table 1. *Cont.*

<table>
<tr><th rowspan="2">Parametres</th><th rowspan="2">Wear Protective Clothing When Outdoors</th><th colspan="2">Avoid Heading Outdoors to Vector-Prone Areas and During Peak Biting Conditions</th></tr>
<tr><th>Vector-Prone Areas</th><th>Peak Biting Conditions</th></tr>
<tr><td rowspan="2">Limiting Factor(s) and/or Alternative(s)</td><td rowspan="2">• Lack of protective clothing [46].
• Presence of fabric holes in clothing: The holes serve as entry points for disease vectors to come into contact with skin. Holes may develop under the attack by fabric pests such as clothes moth larvae [47].
• Unfavourable circumstances: In scorching areas and for labour-intensive occupations, heavy protective clothing may cause discomfort or impair human body heat exchange with the environment and cause heat stress [46,48].</td><td colspan="2">• Unfavourable circumstances: Staying indoors for long periods in poor, crowded living environments such as slums [49] may cause great discomfort.</td></tr>
<tr><td>• Occupational limitations: Those such as farmers and rubber plantation workers do not have the flexibility to avoid prone areas.</td><td>• Occupational limitations: Those with night shifts such as security guards and police officers do not have the flexibility to avoid heading outdoors at night.
• Unfavourable circumstances: For populations in areas which are typically sultry (hot and humid), such as the tropics [50], risk mitigation is more challenging.</td></tr>
<tr><td>Strength of Evidence</td><td>• The effectiveness of wearing protective clothing as a physical barrier against vector bites is well-supported by evidence.
• While light-coloured clothing may enhance tick detection [37], it may also attract more ticks [51] and increase tick-borne disease risk. Findings on vector landing preferences on this matter are dated and inconsistent.</td><td>• The positive correlation between larvae breeding and the extent of vegetation cover [52] is well-supported by evidence.
• The assertion that rubber latex collection cups in plantations are potential breeding sites for common vectors, especially during the rainy season [53], is well-researched.</td><td>• The negative correlation between humidity and mosquito desiccation risk, as well as the positive correlations between temperature and larvae breeding, adult vector development and virus replication, are well-supported by evidence [54,55].
• The relationship between temperature, humidity, rainfall, and vector transmission incidences is well-supported by evidence.
• Research on the relationship between time of the day and peak biting conditions is limited to malaria-transmitting mosquitoes. Minimal evidence is available on other VBDs and disease vector types such as ticks and sand flies.</td></tr>
</table>

Table 2. Personal Protection Practices as Health-EDRM Primary Prevention Approaches against VBDs (Part 2).

Parametre	Apply Insect Repellent	Sleep Under Bed Nets	Receive Prophylactic Vaccinations and Chemoprophylaxis
Risk	• Vector landing rate is an indication of human biting rate of disease vectors [56], which is positively correlated with the risk of vector bites and subsequently VBD transmission.	• Specific mosquito species tend to have higher biting rates at night [30]. • An overwhelming majority of malaria vector bites occur when people are in bed [57].	• The immune status of a population largely influences its sensitivity to diseases [58]. • Immunologically-unprotected populations are particularly susceptible to infectious diseases [58].
Behavioural Change	• Apply insect repellent on exposed surfaces (skin or clothing, but not on both simultaneously) in vector-prone areas, especially when outdoors [21,31,36,37]. • Use repellent containing DEET, a common active ingredient that repels rather than kills mosquitoes [59,60] and ticks [61], thus minimising their chance of landing. • Apply permethrin, another common active ingredient, to clothing. The chemical retains its effectiveness for up to six washings [62]. • Use roll-on repellents as opposed to sprays [63]; the former minimises repellent dispersion to nearby foodstuffs and more effectively concentrates the repellent.	• Sleep under bed nets in vector-prone areas [21,37]. • Use bed nets, which offer an immediate physical barrier, to prevent disease vector entrance. Some bed nets are treated with insecticides, creating an additional chemical barrier to repel vectors. • Ensure that bed net fabric is not in contact with the user [64] and no entry points are available for vectors [36]. • Check the bed nets for holes, which may severely reduce their efficacy [64–66]. • Select quality bed nets, which is essential to successfully prevent VBD transmission. Compared to conventionally-treated bed nets made by regularly dipping into insecticides [67], long-lasting insecticide-treated bed nets manufactured in factories have high efficacy and durability. Thus, the latter is recommended for long-term usage in vector-prone areas [67,68].	• Receive the appropriate and up-to-date vaccine for those living in or travelling to vector-prone areas [21,37]. Vaccination is a form of active immunisation achieved through exposing an unimmunised individual to a pathogenic agent. The immune system is stimulated, and long-term immunity is achieved through triggering cell- or antibody-mediated immunity [69]. • Receive the appropriate chemoprophylaxis recommended for those living in or travelling to vector-prone areas. Chemoprophylaxis is 'the administration of a drug to prevent the development of a disease' [70].
Co-benefit(s)	• No other health co-benefits to note beyond its intended use.	• Protects individuals from household pests such as rodents and cockroaches during sleep [64,71]. • Prevents dust from landing on bed sheets and coverings [64]. • Provides a sense of security through a closed sleeping environment, in particular for individuals living in open shelters.	• Provides individuals with the opportunity to interact with health workers, access health services, and receive health education when visiting healthcare units for prophylaxis, in particular for remote, rural populations living in endemic areas.
Enabling Factor(s)	• Availability and affordability of insect repellents. • Proper education on the correct use of insect repellents.	• Availability and affordability [72] of bed nets and related equipment for bed net hanging: Specific materials such as ropes and sticks [73] may be required to set up the bed nets. • Availability of space to hang the bed net. • Proper education on the correct use of bed nets [72].	• Availability and affordability of vaccinations and chemoprophylaxis. • Awareness and acceptance towards vaccinations and chemoprophylaxis. • Accessibility of adequate and appropriate healthcare services.

Table 2. *Cont.*

Parametre	Apply Insect Repellent	Sleep Under Bed Nets	Receive Prophylactic Vaccinations and Chemoprophylaxis
Limiting Factor(s) and/or Alternative(s)	• Lack of access to insect repellents: In resource-deprived areas, other potentially effective natural alternatives include eucalyptus-based repellents [74,75], neem [74] and citronella [74]. • Potential health hazards: The active ingredients of insect repellents may cause allergy [76].	• Lack of access to quality insecticide-treated bed nets: In resource-deprived areas, basic untreated bed nets, although not to the same extent, still offer significant protection from vectors as a physical barrier [77]. They may be constructed at home using mesh-like materials. • Physical deterioration [64–66]: Damaged bed nets have significantly reduced efficacies. Proper maintenance of bed nets is important. • Thermal discomfort [78,79]: Bed nets may attenuate airflow and cause discomfort to users, especially in hot and humid areas—this can be overcome with better designs. • Inconvenience: The hanging [72,80] and washing [80] of bed nets may be considered troublesome. • Complacency: People may underestimate the local severity and danger of VBDs [80], thus hold a complacent attitude towards the need for bed nets.	• Vaccination hesitancy: ○ People may lack confidence in and be fearful towards vaccines (e.g., needle phobia), especially with the misunderstanding that vaccines pose a risk of infection [81]. ○ Vaccination may go against traditions and beliefs in specific social contexts or religions [81], such as in ultra-orthodox Jewish communities [82]. ○ People may underestimate the local severity and danger of VBDs, thus hold a complacent attitude towards the need for prophylaxis [81]. ○ People may have a preference for community-perceived alternatives to vaccines, such as alcohol, religious prayers and traditional remedies [81]. • Lack of access [83] to prophylactic strategies: Inadequate vaccine supply, poor road terrain and inconvenient transport to immunisation centres, limited service delivery points, and insufficient health workers may hamper vaccination rates in developing countries [84]. Mobile immunisation campaigns may be preferred to reach poorly accessible areas [81]. • Proper health educational interventions [81] and extensive vaccination programmes are crucial to enhance prophylaxis.

Table 2. *Cont.*

Parametre	Apply Insect Repellent	Sleep Under Bed Nets	Receive Prophylactic Vaccinations and Chemoprophylaxis
Strength of Evidence	• Compared to other active ingredients in commercially-available insect repellents, DEET is well-supported to have a longer duration of efficacy [85]. • Research on the safety of DEET has yielded conflicting findings. While some studies demonstrate potential harms such as the pro-angiogenic properties of DEET [86], others suggest that DEET imposes minimal to no evident health risks under proper usage [87], even when applied on vulnerable groups such as children and pregnant women [88]. • Recommendations on the appropriate DEET concentration are inconsistent across international organisations and governments. Limited studies suggest that a higher DEET concentration indicates a longer duration of effectiveness, yet does not necessarily indicate higher insect-repelling ability [60,88]. More extensive research is necessary to establish a uniform DEET concentration recommendation across institutions. • The strength of evidence available to support the efficacy of local natural alternatives is variable and may be conflicting, as in the case of citronella [74,85]. • Local natural alternatives may also be subject to less stringent safety testing, as in the case of neem, which may cause dermatitis if used undiluted [74].	• The strength of evidence available to support the efficacy of bed nets is strong. • Bed nets demonstrate high potential for vector bite prevention in [89] vector-prone areas, such as for dengue and Japanese encephalitis [71,79]. The introduction of insecticide-treated bed nets has contributed to the substantial reduction in malaria transmission across sub-Saharan Africa [90]. • Regarding bed net coverage, studies demonstrate that insecticide-treated bed net use in nearby compounds had a protective effect for child mortality and other health hazards in compounds lacking the bed nets, which suggests that high coverage of bed net use not only provides protection to individuals, but also has an area-wide effect on the mosquito population [91]. There is also evidence of the importance of widespread bed net coverage in the whole population for equitable community-wide benefits of protecting vulnerable target groups, such as young children and pregnant women, rather than merely exclusive bed net coverage amongst the vulnerable [92]. • Bed net efficacy may be compromised under improper usage, such as incomplete net tucking and bed net sharing [64]. There is also evidence [64,93] of instances of mosquitoes biting through insecticide-treated bed nets, especially when users are in physical contact with the net fabric. There may further be a reduction in irritancy and toxicity of the insecticide-treated nets to mosquitoes after they feed on insecticide-treated bed net users [93], although further research is necessary to fully support this possibility.	• The strength of evidence available to support the efficacy of VBD prophylaxis is variable. • Some VBDs such as yellow fever [94,95], tick-borne encephalitis [96,97] and Japanese encephalitis [98,99] have highly efficacious vaccines that are well-supported by evidence. • Some VBDs have limited prophylactic strategies available: ○ RTS,S, the only vaccine against malaria shown to be protective in young children, has been demonstrated to prevent 4 out of 10 cases of malaria in clinical trials [83]. Although RTS,S only offers partial protection and is a supplementary primary prevention strategy [83], pilot vaccination programmes have been or will be launched in three countries in sub-Saharan Africa [83,100]. ○ Malaria chemoprophylaxis, especially under long-term usage, may be associated with health risks, rare fatalities, adverse drug reactions and inadequacies [101,102], thus excluding chemoprophylaxis as a safe option for long-term travellers and populations in malaria-endemic locations and limiting its recommended use to short-term travellers [103]. Individualised strategies, such as sequential regimens with different medications for chemoprophylaxis, will have to be recommended instead [103]. Besides, vivax malaria relapses cannot be prevented with current first-line chemoprophylactic regimens [103]. ○ Dengvaxia, the only U.S. Food and Drug Administration (FDA)-approved vaccine against dengue fever [104], demonstrated poor efficacy [105], and may increase the risk of severe dengue symptoms in seronegative patients infected for the first time after vaccination, since it acts like a first dengue infection [105].

Table 3. Environmental Management Practices as Health-EDRM Primary Prevention Approaches against VBDs.

Parametre	Use Insect-Killing Traps	Manage Stagnant Water Appropriately	Manage Waste Appropriately
Risk	• VBDs are transmitted to humans via living organisms such as mosquitoes, sand flies, and ticks [21].	• Water bodies and still water are the most common mosquito larval habitats [52]; their prevalence increases the risk of disease transmission, as noted for VBDs such as Zika [106], chikungunya [107], and malaria [108]. • Specific disaster occurrences may also increase VBD health risks. Under climate change, extreme weather events such as flooding and heavy rainfall may increase habitats for common vectors [20].	• Accumulation and decomposition of solid waste attracts common houseflies, especially in areas with no centralised waste management systems and with open dumpsites [109]. • Improper waste disposal augments the risk of VBD outbreaks.

Table 3. *Cont.*

Parametre	Use Insect-Killing Traps	Manage Stagnant Water Appropriately	Manage Waste Appropriately
Behavioural Change	• Use insect-killing traps in areas with high-vector density [36]. Traps work by attracting and killing vectors. • Select the appropriate trap for the context. Traps eliminate vectors by different mechanisms, such as emitting blue UV-light irradiation to increase reactive oxygen species production and damage DNA structures [110], and electrocuting insects on a high voltage grid. • Dispose of dead insect bodies with care and proper hygiene such as thorough handwashing with soap and water after waste handling as they may carry VBDs and be hazardous.	• Practice long-term habitual draining and elimination of stagnant water in containers inside and outside of households [21,31]. • Take note of disaster-associated VBD health hazards in disaster-prone areas. • Ensure that drinking water is stored in proper, sealed environments which are free of breeding potential.	• Practice long-term habitual proper disposal of waste [21]. • Practice specific waste management strategies such as the separation of organic and inorganic waste and the disposal of solid waste in open dumpsites away from water bodies, which are potential larval breeding grounds [111]. • Microbial pathogens are prevalent in accumulated solid waste, and unprotected handling may result in infected wounds and sepsis [109,112]. Protect hands with gloves and/or use assistive tools such as clamps or tongs when handling waste. Wash hands thoroughly with clean water and soap after waste handling to minimise infection risk.
Co-benefit(s)	• UV-light traps serve as an alternative light source due to their luminescent property.	• Reduces the hazardous risk of slipping due to stagnant water on flooring [113]. • Reduces the risk of mould development which has respiratory repercussions [114].	• Encourages the separation of household waste which eases landfill burdens and reduces health hazards such as respiratory diseases and congenital abnormalities associated with proximity to landfills [115]. • Reduces the arbitrary disposal of hazardous household waste [115]. • Reduces surface water and groundwater pollution, air contamination, and greenhouse gas emissions (e.g., methane) from open waste dumping sites [116].
Enabling Factor(s)	• Availability and affordability of insect-killing traps. • Proper education on the correct use of insect-killing traps.	• Availability of direct household water supply. • Availability and affordability of tightly-sealed water containers.	• A well-coordinated waste management system [117]. • Availability and affordability of waste bags and bins.
Limiting Factor(s) and/or Alternative(s)	• Lack of electricity: Insect-killing traps often rely on electricity to function. Taking the case of sub-Saharan Africa, nearly 600 million people have no access to electricity [118]. Passive non-electricity-requiring traps using fipronil-laced honey or toxic honey baits [119] to kill mosquitoes can potentially serve as alternatives. • Lack of access to insect-killing traps: In resource-deprived areas, cheaper alternatives such as sticky paper traps with adhesive killing mechanisms can be used. However, their insect-trapping efficacy may be limited to closed environments such as greenhouses only [120].	• Lack of water supply: It would be a challenge to avoid stagnant water accumulation in communities that lack direct household water supply—for these communities, it is common to store collected water from community standpipes and rivers [121]. Under such circumstances, tightly-sealed water containers are recommended for water storage. • Lack of tightly-sealed water containers: For communities with only open plastic bottles or buckets available for water storage, larvicides can be added to the stagnant water. It is important to monitor the safety of the practice and educate people on the proper usage of larvicides [122].	• Lack of a well-coordinated waste management system: Insufficient waste collection points and inadequate waste bins around the community, especially in developing countries [116] and resource-deprived areas, serve as barriers to proper waste disposal [123].

Table 3. *Cont.*

Parametre	Use Insect-Killing Traps	Manage Stagnant Water Appropriately	Manage Waste Appropriately
Strength of Evidence	• A comparatively large amount of evidence on the working mechanisms and efficacy of insect-killing traps is available. A variety of attractants are used in insect-killing traps, such as blue UV-light [124], carbon dioxide [125], octenol [126] and heat [127], all of which are scientifically proven to draw insects. • Studies have shown that different commercial insect-killing traps have varying efficacies in trapping and killing vectors such as the *Aedes* species, which can transmit chikungunya and Zika viruses [128]. Some traps can potentially target sand flies in addition to mosquitoes [129]. • On the safety of different killing mechanisms, limited studies have demonstrated that the UV light in traps is non-hazardous to humans [130], whereas the electrocution of insects may potentially release bacteria and viruses [131]. • Studies on whether or not pathogens remain in the infected dead insects' bodies, and evidence-based guidelines on the proper disposal of dead insect bodies, are limited.	• A comparatively large amount of evidence on the effectiveness of proper stagnant water management on VBD risk reduction is available. The aquatic characteristics of larval habitats are well-evidenced, and extensive research has been conducted regarding areas that are prone to stagnant water accumulation. Numerous studies demonstrate that household water containers, holes and furrows in discarded tyres [132], mud pots [116], and blocked drainage systems [109] are common larval breeding grounds. • Case studies that evaluate the VBD outbreak risk associated with disaster occurrences that favour water accumulation are abundant. Taking the case of Djibouti, the country was suffering from pre-existing malaria and chikungunya outbreaks; studies reflect that heavy rain and floods in late 2019 further exacerbated the situation and exposed those affected to VBD risks [133].	• A comparatively large amount of evidence on VBD prevalence in areas with improper solid waste accumulation is available. Items such as tyres, porcelain, plastic materials, and open coconut shells are commonly suggested to 'provide breeding sites, burrows and food for vectors' [134,135]. Such studies often link back to the favourability of larval breeding under stagnant water accumulation in waste materials [116,132]. There is also extensive research on how open dumping sites exacerbate VBD risks [116,134]. • Evidence of the effectiveness of putting proper waste management into practice in communities and its relation to VBD risk reduction is minimal.

Table 4. Customary Household Practices as Health-EDRM Primary Prevention Approaches against VBDs.

Parametre	Minimise Household Entry Points		Cover Exposed Foodstuffs
	Wall Cracks	Door and Window Openings	
Risk	• Household entry points such as wall cracks as well as open doors and windows provide opportunities for vector entrance, contributing to the risk of indoor infestation. • A significant number of vectors may accumulate in the cracks if they remain unrepaired [140].	• Entry points through open doors and windows have large surface areas and are more prone to the entrance of disease vectors [141].	• Common vectors such as flies are attracted to odours and chemicals released by exposed foodstuffs, such as the volatile fermentation products [136] of ripe fruits associated with the breeding of yeast in the fruit [137]. • Disease vectors may contaminate exposed foodstuffs in open containers via direct contact or droppings, which contribute to health hazards such as a high incidence of diarrhoea in children under six [138]. • If uncooked food with pathogens such as *Salmonella* and *E. Coli* are left uncovered, houseflies may serve as vectors and expose humans to the risk of food-borne pathogenic infections [139].

Table 4. *Cont.*

Parametre	Minimise Household Entry Points		Cover Exposed Foodstuffs
	Wall Cracks	Door and Window Openings	
Behavioural Change	• Household improvements to minimise entry points are effective in reducing infestation from vectors such as *Aedes aegypti*, which transmit the Zika and chikungunya viruses [142]. The risk of malaria transmission from the *Anopheles* mosquito is similarly reduced [143].		• Practice the covering of exposed foodstuffs with food covers or nets to prevent food contamination by flies [111], especially in contexts without refrigerators.
	• Repair cracks to seal potential vector entry points [21].	• Install door and window screens and close windows in the early evening to reduce indoor disease vector density [21,36,144,145].	
Co-benefit(s)	• Protects individuals from household pests such as rodents [146,147] and cockroaches [148].		• Protects exposed foodstuffs from household pests such as rodents [149].
	• Reduces water leakage [150], such as during heavy rainfall.	• Enhances household safety, such as decreasing the risk of theft or burglary [151].	
Enabling Factor(s)	• Availability and affordability of crack-repairing materials. • Knowledge about crack-repairing, or accessibility to professional services.	• Availability and affordability of door and window screens. • Knowledge about door and window screen installation, or accessibility to professional services.	• Availability and affordability of food covers.
Limiting Factor(s) and/or Alternative(s)	• Contextual limitations: Household modifications do not apply to the homeless and the impoverished living in open, unstable shelters. • Universal applicability: Household modification recommendations may not apply to all settings due to housing differences [152]. • Professional requirement: Crack-repairing and door and window screen installation using modern methods often require professional tools and skills as well as long-term maintenance strategies.		• Lack of access to quality food covers: In resource-deprived areas, clean pieces of cloth, lids, or any materials that can serve as physical barriers should be used as alternatives for covering exposed foodstuffs.
	• Lack of access to modern crack-repairing materials: In resource-deprived areas, mud and lime mixtures may serve as alternatives, although they may be more costly in the long-term [153]. • Less well-off populations that cannot afford modern building materials [154] may use other locally-available alternatives.	• Lack of access to door and window screen installation services: The installation of door and window screens involves significant renovation work that is often costly and unaffordable for impoverished populations [155].	

Table 4. *Cont.*

Parametre	Minimise Household Entry Points		Cover Exposed Foodstuffs
	Wall Cracks	Door and Window Openings	
Strength of Evidence	• While there is available evidence on the effects of crack-repairing on VBD risk reduction, studies on the detailed evaluation of different crack-repairing methods remain limited. • Materials such as cement, modern crack-fillers, and a mixture of mud and lime are scientifically proven to be efficacious in reducing indoor vector density. • There are few studies on other more cost-effective alternatives for populations in resource-deprived areas. Mud is a locally-available alternative, but there are limited studies on whether crack-repairing with mud alone is potentially correlated with an increased risk of vector entrance [156].	• A comparatively large amount of evidence on the efficacy of proper door and window screen installation, as well as the closing of windows, in reducing indoor vector density is available. • Given that variations exist in screening designs, further research on their specific efficacies is necessary [141].	• A comparatively large amount of evidence of the potential health risks associated with disease vectors if foodstuffs are exposed and not covered or stored well is available. • Research on the efficacy of the use of food covers, and that of potential alternatives in resource-deprived areas, is limited.

Table 5. Overview of Health-EDRM Primary Prevention Approaches against VBDs in the Reviewed Articles, Categorised by the Oxford Centre for Evidence-Based Medicine (OCEBM) Levels of Evidence. (Please see Table S1 for details.).

Category	Intervention	Number of Reviewed Articles under Each Category in the OCEBM Levels of Evidence											
		1a	1b	1c	2a	2b	2c	3a	3b	4	5	Others *	Total
Personal Protection Practices	Wear Protective Clothing When Outdoors	0	2	0	0	0	0	0	1	4	4	3	14
	Avoid Heading Outdoors to Vector-Prone Areas and During Peak Biting Conditions	0	0	0	0	0	0	0	0	3	16	4	23
	Apply Insect Repellent	0	1	0	0	0	0	0	0	2	9	5	17
	Sleep Under Bed Nets	2	2	0	0	2	0	1	0	5	7	3	22
	Receive Prophylactic Vaccinations and Chemoprophylaxis	1	0	0	1	0	0	1	0	3	8	6	20
Environmental Management Practices	Use Insect-Killing Traps	0	1	0	0	0	0	0	0	0	8	5	14
	Manage Stagnant Water Appropriately	0	0	0	0	2	0	0	0	1	11	1	15
	Manage Waste Appropriately	0	0	0	1	1	0	0	0	1	4	2	9
Customary Household Practices	Minimise Household Entry Points	1	3	0	1	1	0	0	1	6	3	2	18
	Cover Exposed Foodstuffs	0	0	0	0	1	0	0	1	2	2	1	7
Total		4	9	0	3	7	0	2	3	27	72	32	159 **

* 'Others' includes but is not limited to news articles or releases, books, textbooks, position papers, guidelines, case reports and organisational reports.** Of the 134 publications reviewed, some included findings on more than one primary prevention measure, and are counted more than once in Table 5.

4. Discussion

VBDs are classified as biological hazards under the WHO health-EDRM framework [14] and their associated health risks should be managed according to the disaster management cycle (prevention, mitigation, preparedness, response and recovery), which encompasses both top-down and bottom-up interventions [157,158]. Top-down interventions require well-driven bottom-up initiatives to achieve effective primary prevention and to modify community health risk reduction-related measures [159]. Both the WHO health-EDRM framework [14] and the WHO global vector control response 2017–2030 framework [3] emphasise community engagement and mobilisation in enhancing protection against VBDs. The scientific effectiveness and feasibility of the community-level implementation of the 10 proposed primary prevention measures in this review can each be influenced by distinctive external factors, particularly with regards to access to financial or material resources.

Health promotion enables people to have more control over the improvement of their health outcomes, and is done through enhancing health literacy, encouraging behavioural change, and developing supportive policies [160]. There are numerous models which explore behavioural change as a result of education-based health promotion, one of which is the 'knowledge, attitudes, practices model', which prompts behavioural changes through knowledge enhancement [160]. In the case of vaccinations and chemoprophylaxis, it is critical for health interventions to enhance individual knowledge and awareness on why and how to receive prophylaxis as a primary prevention mechanism against VBDs, particularly in addressing misconceptions which underestimate the danger of VBDs [81]. Behaviour can be changed through addressing attitudes, such as misunderstandings [81], perception of social norms, cultural traditions and religious beliefs, for example in the case of ultra-orthodox Jewish communities who do not practice vaccination [81,82]. Finally, the behavioural change theory should consider how to promote practice. The viability and efficacy of the practice itself is favoured or limited by a variety of factors; policies will have to address barriers to accessing, and augmenting motivation in, the community [159].

The enabling and limiting factors that impact the effective uptake of primary prevention measures are closely interlinked. This review identified a number of determinants of success, including adequate resources, risk awareness, and well-coordinated supportive systems. A number of primary prevention measures rely on the availability and affordability of material resources, such as insect repellents, protective clothing, UV lamps, household building materials and bed nets (which additionally require space and equipment to set up [73]). Resource-deprived communities, which are at a higher risk of facing vulnerability, may lack the necessary material or financial resources. Materials must be accompanied by knowledge of their appropriate use. Inadequate information can lead to the improper maintenance of vector-prevention commodities, subsequently compromising their efficacy. For example, damaged bed nets with holes and improper bed net usage have been shown to lead to outcomes worse than no usage at all [64–66]. Some measures may also be affected by other health conditions, such as allergic reactions to insect repellent active ingredients [76], while others may be limited by cultural concerns, as demonstrated in the case of vaccination hesitancy in certain religious communities [81,82]. The feasibility of certain measures, such as the avoidance of outdoors, is dependent on an individual's personal, professional and socioeconomic situation. Avoidance of going outdoors into vector-prone areas and during peak biting conditions can be impractical, such as in farming populations that need to spend long periods outdoors, and in tropical areas where the climate is 'peak-biting'—hot and humid—all year long [50]. Similarly, there may be cases where access to a fully enclosed shelter or household improvements are not feasible, such as for those who are homeless or living in temporary shelters. Beyond resource access, proper education and personal circumstances, some primary prevention measures rely heavily on infrastructural and systemic support. Ensuring community access to vaccinations and chemoprophylaxis requires functioning health systems able to provide the necessary services, including an adequate supply of vaccines or medicine, trained health workers for administration and education, and an established clinic (fixed or mobile) from where the vaccine or drug can be distributed. Health system infrastructure is a critical enabling factor lacking in many rural or resource-poor contexts [84]. The environmental management of vectors also requires a robust and coordinated top-down waste management system [109,117], with multi-sectoral collaboration [161] between the health, environmental and civil engineering sectors, as well as other local and national-level authorities. Authorities should ensure the sufficiency of waste collection points such as waste bins [123], which can affect proper waste disposal, and the supply of electricity [118], which can affect the use of insect-killing traps, particularly in developing contexts [116]. Therefore, the success or failure of a community's uptake of primary prevention measures is shaped by the availability of material resources and information, supportive health and civil infrastructure, policy formulation, geographical climate, individual or professional flexibilities, and social contexts. Nonetheless, it should always be noted that each measure offers its contribution towards VBD prevention, and the measures serve as an alternative to one another. When one measure cannot be carried out, the practice of other measures is not necessarily impeded.

In comparing the strength of evidence of the reviewed literature (Table 5, please see Table S1 for details), the largest proportion (45%) fell into Level 5 classification, which covers a wide range of study designs and methodologies, such as entomological studies, observational exploratory studies, experimental studies, modelling studies, qualitative studies, and expert opinions. 20% of the reviewed literature was categorised into 'Others', which includes but is not limited to news releases, reports by international organisations like the WHO, and textbooks. Level 4 publications, such as cross-sectional mixed method studies, behavioural surveys, household surveys, questionnaires, interventional studies and case series studies contributed a relatively large portion (17%), with many addressing the knowledge, perceptions, acceptance and opinions of populations with regards to VBD-prevention measures. Regarding individual primary prevention measures, evidence is most lacking at all levels with regard to the practices of covering exposed foodstuffs (4%) and proper waste management (6%). The literature relevant to sleeping under bed nets and minimising household entry points was significantly stronger in study design. There is published evidence on the risk reduction relating to wearing protective clothing and the management of stagnant water; however, while a multitude of studies emphasised the impact of primary prevention measures on VBD health risk reduction, a limited number of studies focused on the impact of the measure itself on disease prevention efficacy or outcome. For instance, many studies demonstrate the potential VBD-related health risks of exposed foodstuffs [136–139] and household entry points [140,141]; however, there are limited studies that demonstrate the effectiveness of covering food or household crack-repairing on disease incidence reduction within a community [156]. Similarly, for solid waste management, while evidence on the health risks [134,135] associated with improper solid waste accumulation is available, there is a lack of in-depth comparative studies between different waste management system models and their strengths and weaknesses.

The methodology used for this review is limited in that it does not include non-English-based literature, non-electronically-accessible literature, grey literature outside of those areas deliberately searched, any publications before 2000, or any publication not identified due to incompatibility with the keywords used for the literature search. Notably, publications documenting experiences from low-resource VBD-endemic settings that are not readily accessible via mainstream databases or online platforms may not have been included in this review.

Certain areas were found to be lacking in the updated evidence. On the efficacy of light-coloured clothing, while the WHO provides recommendations for protective wear against VBDs [21], the search generated no clear evidence, that had been updated within the past two decades, to support the rationale behind vector landing preferences on darker surfaces, and vice versa. Recommendations concerning the appropriate concentration of DEET in insect repellent are often inconsistent across international organisations and governments. More extensive research is needed to better establish the correlation between DEET concentration, repellent strength and duration of efficacy. In addition, while there are various observational studies on the correlation between modern technological advancements, such as air conditioning, and decreased disease vector bites [162–165], there is limited updated scientific evidence available on the precise impacts of such advancements on changes to vector habitat. Addressing these research gaps will facilitate better-grounded and more evidence-based institutional guidelines.

The best available evidence is always evolving, requiring the continuous updating of guidelines and recommendations. The ongoing research on VBD prophylactic strategies is very active, as well as that on the development of insecticide resistance regarding insecticide-treated bed nets [166,167] and insect repellents [168]. In light of the many different designs, parameters, sample sizes and investigation methods used, it is often difficult to evaluate and compare related studies, thus resulting in a lack of standardisation in guidelines. For instance, a variety of attraction and killing mechanisms, as well as door and window screen designs [141], are used in different studies to evaluate insect-killing trap and household modification efficacies. Efforts to achieve increased consistency in the methodology of published research are crucial to making comparative analyses between studies on different VBD-prevention commodities possible [169–172].

Three areas are particularly lacking in the published evidence. Firstly, there has been minimal research done on available alternatives to the proposed practices. Taking the case of insect repellents, numerous studies are available to prove the efficacy [59–61,85] and explore the potential safety concerns [86–88] of DEET. However, the strength of research supporting the repellence of natural alternatives like plant oils is variable [74]. For instance, limited and conflicting findings on citronella efficacy were identified [74,85], and potential health hazards, like dermatitis under high-concentration neem-oil use, are indicated, with less stringent safety testing conducted compared to DEET [74]. Secondly, limited research is available on other disease vectors such as sand flies and ticks. A bulk of the literature identified in this analysis focuses on mosquitoes—the discussions on common vector breeding grounds [52,106–108] and the efficacy of insect-killing traps seldom involve other disease vectors [128]. There is a need for research into effective methods to better understand the breeding habitat ecology of sand flies in immature stages, which will facilitate the development of targeted control strategies such as source reduction, which are not yet possible as sand fly larvae can be difficult to detect, in contrast to other vectors such as mosquitoes [173–175]. Similarly, in the case of insect-killing traps, only limited studies demonstrate their potential in targeting sand flies in addition to mosquitoes [129], and evidence on tick elimination by the traps is lacking entirely. Thirdly, research on the spectrum of VBDs is disproportionately distributed; studies are oftentimes skewed towards more prevalent VBDs, such as malaria. While consideration is given to other VBDs such as Zika or tick-borne encephalitis, this literature review occasionally extrapolates the primary prevention measures proposed for the more extensively-researched diseases so as to apply them to other VBDs as well—for example, the determination of the time of day with peak biting conditions was based on *Plasmodium*-infected (malaria) mosquitoes being active from dusk to dawn [29–31]. Further research on these three areas is necessary in order to develop comprehensive and informed guidelines or policies that can be implemented in varying contexts to mitigate against the risk and alleviate the disease burden of VBDs.

This review has identified major research gaps in the current published literature relating to health-EDRM primary prevention measures for VBDs (Table 6). Strengthening the available evidence in these areas will create a scientific basis on which governments, policy-makers and community stakeholders can develop effective, targeted and achievable strategies for protecting at-risk populations against VBDs. Aspects of the WHO health-EDRM framework can be applied to address these research gaps. Increasing capacities for information and knowledge management can support collection, analysis and dissemination across multiple sectors, allowing for the comparative evaluation of available evidence, as well as the development of consistent guidelines and recommendations [14]. This is particularly important for any research undertaken in resource-poor contexts, which will provide necessary evidence towards developing effective and targeted VBD prevention measures in such contexts. The framework highlights the need for more multifaceted and multisectoral approaches, the lessons of which will lead to the further development of evidence-based strategies [14].

Table 6. Major Research Gaps in Current Published Literature Relating to Health-EDRM Primary Prevention Measures for VBDs.

	Research Gaps
1	Current studies on health-EDRM primary prevention measures for VBDs mostly focus on health risk reduction practices, yet efficacy evaluation on actual disease reduction is lacking.
2	Available literature is mostly classified as cross-sectional studies. Evidence on efficacy of the prevention measure based on randomised controlled studies or extensive cohort studies is limited.
3	Comparative evaluations for variations of certain primary prevention measures, such as efficacy of different insect-killing mechanisms or household modification materials, are limited.
4	Research outcomes are skewed towards certain vectors (e.g., mosquitoes). Research evidence on other vectors such as sand flies or ticks is limited.
5	Research outcomes are skewed towards certain VBDs (e.g., malaria). Research evidence on other VBDs such as Zika, chikungunya, or tick-borne encephalitis is limited.
6	Research and evidence on available alternatives to the proposed practices (e.g., using natural substitutes as opposed to chemical-based insect repellents) is limited.
7	Updated research on evidence relating technological advancements and the rapid change of ecological and human living environments to behavioural practices against VBDs is limited.
8	Consistency in recommendations from research papers, policies, and frontline international agencies (e.g., as in DEET concentration recommendations) is lacking.
9	Literature highlighting the effectiveness of multi-faceted, multi-sectoral and coordinated responses in enabling effective risk mitigation for population-level protection is lacking.

All 10 primary prevention measures require sustainable, continuous implementation and maintenance in order to be truly effective in preventing VBDs. Primary prevention measures focusing on stagnant water, waste management and the covering of exposed foodstuffs offer the long-term co-benefit of mitigating risks arising from other biological hazards under the health-EDRM framework [14], such as water-borne and food-borne diseases [139]. Practising continuous primary prevention is particularly necessary as long as certain VBDs do not have standardised effective treatment options, and if vector-elimination is not feasible. Some preventive measures face more complex challenges in practise without adequate health or governance infrastructure. Others are more easily implemented, but are nonetheless reliant on materials such as insect repellents or bed nets, which can be an obstacle in resource-poor settings where the population is already facing vulnerability to impoverishment or disease. It is crucial for policymakers to ensure that systems are able to identify and assess needs, and provide the necessary support for the sustainable and fair distribution of resources. Empowering bottom-up initiatives requires well-coordinated top-down policies [83] that effectively disseminate resources and information, especially in resource-deprived, rural, or health-illiterate populations. A strong, accessible health system is key to providing materials and education to the at-risk population. Centralised, coordinated and well-regulated infrastructure, such as a uniform waste management system [176], can significantly enhance the efficacy of primary prevention practices.

Climate change and its associated consequences, such as changing weather patterns and increased disaster occurrences [18], have shifted the epidemiological patterns of VBDs, as well as the volume and spread of the at-risk population, thus affecting the development policies and strategies for mitigating the VBD burden on health systems. Rising temperatures and unpredictable precipitation patterns, for example, lengthen peak-biting periods and further complicate the capacity for outdoor avoidance, especially in tropical areas which are sultry throughout the year. The increased incidence of hydro-meteorological hazards such as floods and cyclones brings about more extreme rainfall, as well as increased humidity and water accumulation [18], and impact stagnant water management, thus possibly facilitating further larval habitat development for disease vectors [18]. Insect vectors cannot regulate their internal temperatures and are very sensitive to changes, which has caused them to invade new areas in order to adapt [177]. This puts previously unexposed populations at risk, who may lack protective immunity or the experience, resources or services necessary to mitigate the prevalence of disease [6]. The WHO health-EDRM framework stresses the importance of strengthening health systems, with an increased emphasis on climate change adaptation [14], to reducing health risks associated with hazardous events, including VBD outbreaks. It is important for governing bodies to consider the associated challenges of climate change during policy formulation, with the inclusion of climate change scenarios in disaster risk assessments [18]. Considering the limitation of the predicted impact of climate change on VBD transmission, governing bodies should enhance individual capacities and community resilience in cases of sudden VBD surges [178]. For instance, early warning systems should be in place to communicate the health risks associated with seasonal VBD outbreaks to vulnerable populations in advance [18]. As such, primary prevention measures that emphasise the broader aspects of environmental management, resource distribution and public education must not be overlooked. Public education, to encourage early symptom identification and subsequent health-seeking behaviours, can serve as a steppingstone in propagating secondary and tertiary VBD intervention amongst vulnerable populations.

In light of the growing burden of VBDs and emerging public health threats, a progressive primary prevention model is key to disaster risk reduction, as encompassed in the four priorities set out in the Sendai Framework for Disaster Risk Reduction (risk understanding, governance, preparedness and resilience) [16]. In terms of disaster risk understanding, a thorough examination of the enabling and limiting circumstances is required in at-risk populations, including local disease prevention capacity, specific VBD characteristics, and risk drivers such as climate change [16,18]. Disaster governance should be strengthened through stakeholder involvement and multi-sectorial collaboration, as well as through adopting a well-coordinated top-down approach to empowering bottom-up community initiatives in a sustainable manner. Resilience enhancement should be driven by global investments in innovation and research, for instance the development of better prophylactic strategies and better vector-prevention commodity designs for utilisation against VBDs. Finally, disaster preparedness can be reinforced through raised awareness, secured healthcare accessibility and health-seeking behaviour encouragement, so as to better equip vulnerable populations facing future VBD outbreaks.

5. Conclusions

This narrative study identified 10 health-EDRM primary prevention measures against VBDs. Resource availability, risk awareness and systemic support were identified as the core enabling factors for the success of these measures. Resources, health and civil infrastructure, policy formulation, geographical climate and socioeconomic factors were the core sources of limitations, which necessitate the need to consider alternatives. Evidence supporting the effectiveness of alternative preventive measures is lacking, in particular with regards to prevention in resource-poor settings. Similarly, evidence related to preventive measures focusses heavily on mosquitoes, whereas research on effective prevention against diseases transmitted by other vectors such as sand flies and ticks is lacking. At a global level, the necessity of VBD prevention increases with the growing impact of climate change and globalisation.

Health risks associated with VBDs will remain an ongoing biological hazard to communities, and thus sustainability of practice is crucial. As recommended by the WHO health-EDRM framework, in addition to the health sector, the successful adoption of primary prevention measures against VBDs requires a multi-faceted, multi-sectoral and coordinated response, encompassing sectors such as meteorology for hazard prediction, education for health awareness and promotion, and the environmental and civil engineering sectors for waste collection and water management.

In conclusion, this review has shown that evidence of the effectiveness and management of primary prevention practices is focused on a narrow spectrum of VBDs and vector types. In order to fill research gaps, the scope of VBD research should be broadened, and standardised protocols should be adopted so as to better prepare communities for disaster risk mitigation and to build the capacities of populations that are vulnerable with regards to health-EDRM practices.

Supplementary Materials:
Table S1: Relevant Intervention(s), Study Design, Relevant Key Finding(s) and/or Conclusion of Each Reviewed Article Referenced ($n = 134$).

Author Contributions: Conceptualization, E.Y.Y.C. and C.D.; methodology, T.S.T.S. and T.S.S.; formal analysis, T.S.T.S; T.S.S.; writing—original draft preparation, E.Y.Y.C.; T.S.T.S.; T.S.S.; C.D.; writing—review and editing, Z.H.; S.L.; K.K.C.H.; S.L.A.T.; K.O.K.; P.-H.C.; R.K.; R.S.; supervision, E.Y.Y.C.; funding acquisition, E.Y.Y.C. All authors have read and agreed to the published version of the manuscript.

Appendix A. Keywords Used for Literature Search

'bed nets', 'blue-light irradiation', 'bottom-up approach', 'breeding sites', 'carbon dioxide', 'cement', 'chemoprophylaxis', 'chikungunya', 'climate change', 'clothes moth larvae', 'clothes wear and tear', 'cockroaches', 'crack repair', 'dengue', 'diethyltoluamide (DEET) ', 'disease burden', 'door screening', 'doors and windows burglary', 'electricity access', 'fall injury water', 'floods', 'food decay', 'food fermentation', 'food mould and fungi', 'food-borne pathogens', 'forests', 'health hazards', 'health-EDRM', 'heat stroke', 'heat-seeking ability', 'heavy rain', 'household waste management', 'housing improvements', 'humidity', 'immunisation', 'infectious disease', 'insect repellents', 'insect traps', 'insecticide-treated nets', 'Japanese encephalitis', 'larval habitats', 'larvicides', 'lime', 'living environment', 'long clothing', 'long-lasting insecticide-treated nets', 'malaria', 'mosquito larvae', 'mosquito traps', 'mosquitoes', 'mould development water', 'mud', 'natural repellents', 'octenol', 'pesticide', 'primary prevention', 'protective behaviour', 'protective clothing', 'rodents', 'rubber plantations', 'sand flies', 'solid waste management', 'sticky traps', 'sunburns', 'temperature', 'tick-borne diseases', 'tick-borne encephalitis', 'ticks', 'top-down approach', 'tropical climates', 'ultraviolet irradiation', 'vaccination', 'vaccine complacency', 'vaccine hesitancy', 'VBDs', 'vector attraction', 'vector biting', 'vector contamination', 'vector exposure risk', 'vector human movement', 'vector landing preference', 'vector light clothing', 'vector net', 'vector traps', 'vectors', 'wall cracks', 'waste management', 'waste mismanagement', 'water storage', 'water supply', 'West Nile virus', 'window screening', 'yellow fever', 'Zika'.

References

1. Vector-Borne Diseases. Available online: https://www.who.int/news-room/fact-sheets/detail/vector-borne-diseases (accessed on 31 May 2020).
2. Lemon, S.M.; Sparling, P.F.; Hamburg, M.A.; Relman, D.A.; Choffnes, E.R.; Mack, A. *Vector-Borne Diseases: Understanding the Environmental, Human Health, and Ecological Connections*; The National Academies Press: Washington, DC, USA, 2008; pp. 1–27. ISBN 9780309108973.
3. WHO. *Global Vector Control Response 2017–2030*; World Health Organization: Geneva, Switzerland, 2017; ISBN 9789241564090.
4. Wu, X.; Lu, Y.; Zhou, S.; Chen, L.; Xu, B. Impact of climate change on human infectious diseases: Empirical evidence and human adaptation. *Environ. Int.* **2016**, *86*, 14–23. [CrossRef] [PubMed]
5. Hoshen, M.B.; Morse, A.P. A weather-driven model of malaria transmission. *Malar. J.* **2004**, *3*. [CrossRef]
6. Caminade, C.; McIntyre, K.M.; Jones, A.E. Impact of recent and future climate change on vector-borne diseases. *Ann. N. Y. Acad. Sci.* **2019**, *1436*, 157–173. [CrossRef] [PubMed]
7. Fouque, F.; Reeder, J.C. Impact of past and on-going changes on climate and weather on vector-borne diseases transmission: A look at the evidence. *Infect. Dis. Poverty* **2019**, *8*. [CrossRef] [PubMed]
8. Mathers, C. Global Burden of Disease. In *International Encyclopedia of Public Health*; Academic Press: Cambridge, MA, USA, 2016; ISBN 9780128037089.
9. James, S.L.; Abate, D.; Abate, K.H.; Abay, S.M.; Abbafati, C.; Abbasi, N.; Abbastabar, H.; Abd-Allah, F.; Abdela, J.; Abdelalim, A.; et al. Global, regional, and national incidence, prevalence, and years lived with disability for 354 Diseases and Injuries for 195 countries and territories, 1990-2017: A systematic analysis for the Global Burden of Disease Study 2017. *Lancet* **2018** *392*, 1859–1922. [CrossRef]

10. World Health Organization. *World Malaria Report 2019*; World Health Organization: Geneva, Switzerland, 2019; ISBN 9789241565721.
11. Mccarthy, D.; Wolf, H.; Wu, Y. *Malaria and Growth*; The World Bank: Washington, DC, USA, 2000; pp. 2–26. [CrossRef]
12. United Nations. *The Sustainable Development Goals Report 2019*; United Nations: New York, NY, USA, 2019.
13. The Global Fund: Malaria. Available online: https://www.theglobalfund.org/en/malaria/ (accessed on 31 May 2020).
14. WHO. *Health Emergency and Disaster Risk Management: Overview*; World Health Organization: Geneva, Switzerland, 2019; ISBN 9789241516181.
15. World Health Organisation. *Emergency Risk Management for Health—Overview*; World Health Organization: Geneva, Switzerland, 2013.
16. World Health Organization. *Sendai Framework for Disaster Risk Reduction 2015–2030*; World Health Organization: Geneva, Switzerland, 2015.
17. Wright, N.; Fagan, L.; Lapitan, J.M.; Kayano, R.; Abrahams, J.; Huda, Q.; Murray, V. Health Emergency and Disaster Risk Management: Five Years into Implementation of the Sendai Framework. *Int. J. Disaster Risk Sci.* **2020**, *11*, 206–217. [CrossRef]
18. Chan, E.Y.Y.; Shaw, R. *Public Health and Disasters: Health Emergency and Disaster Risk Management in Asia*; Springer: Berlin/Heidelberg, Germany, 2020.
19. Boslaugh, S. Prevention: Primary, Secondary, and Tertiary. In *Encyclopedia of Epidemiology*; SAGE Publications, Inc.: Thousand Oaks, CA, USA, 2008; pp. 839–840.
20. Alison, M. Global Health Impacts of Vector-Borne Diseases. In *Global Health Impacts of Vector-Borne Diseases*; The National Academies Press: Washington, DC, USA, 2016; pp. 1–59.
21. World Health Organization. *A Global Brief on Vector-Borne Diseases*; World Health Organization: Geneva, Switzerland, 2014; p. 9.
22. World Health Organisation. *International Clinical Trials Registry Platform*; World Health Organization: Geneva, Switzerland, 2006.
23. OCEBM Levels of Evidence Working Group. "The Oxford 2009 Levels of Evidence". Oxford Center for Evidence-Based Medicine. Available online: https://www.cebm.net/index.aspx?o=5653 (accessed on 10 August 2020).
24. Achee, N.L.; Youngblood, L.; Bangs, M.J.; Lavery, J.V.; James, S. Considerations for the use of human participants in vector biology research: A tool for investigators and regulators. *Vector-Borne Zoonotic Dis.* **2015**, *15*, 89–102. [CrossRef]
25. Saavedra, M.P.; Conn, J.E.; Alava, F.; Carrasco-Escobar, G.; Prussing, C.; Bickersmith, S.A.; Sangama, J.L.; Fernandez-Miñope, C.; Guzman, M.; Tong, C.; et al. Higher risk of malaria transmission outdoors than indoors by Nyssorhynchus darlingi in riverine communities in the Peruvian Amazon. *Parasites Vectors* **2019**, *12*. [CrossRef]
26. Nakkhara, P.; Chongsuvivatwong, V.; Thammapalo, S. Risk factors for symptomatic and asymptomatic chikungunya infection. *Trans. R. Soc. Trop. Med. Hyg.* **2013**, *107*, 789–796. [CrossRef]
27. Wallace, J.W.; Nicholson, W.L.; Perniciaro, J.L.; Vaughn, M.F.; Funkhouser, S.; Juliano, J.J.; Lee, S.; Kakumanu, M.L.; Ponnusamy, L.; Apperson, C.S.; et al. Incident Tick-Borne Infections in a Cohort of North Carolina Outdoor Workers. *Vector-Borne Zoonotic Dis.* **2016**, *16*, 302–308. [CrossRef]
28. Tangena, J.A.A.; Thammavong, P.; Lindsay, S.W.; Brey, P.T. Risk of exposure to potential vector mosquitoes for rural workers in Northern Lao PDR. *PLoS Negl. Trop. Dis.* **2017**, *11*. [CrossRef] [PubMed]
29. Ndoen, E.; Wild, C.; Dale, P.; Sipe, N.; Dale, M. Dusk to dawn activity patterns of anopheline mosquitoes in West Timor and Java, Indonesia. *Southeast Asian J. Trop. Med. Public Health* **2011**, *42*, 550–561. [PubMed]
30. Van Bortel, W.; Trung, H.D.; Hoi, L.X.; Van Ham, N.; Van Chut, N.; Luu, N.D.; Roelants, P.; Denis, L.; Speybroeck, N.; D'Alessandro, U.; et al. Malaria transmission and vector behaviour in a forested malaria focus in central Vietnam and the implications for vector control. *Malar. J.* **2010**, *9*. [CrossRef] [PubMed]
31. Loeb, M.; Elliott, S.J.; Gibson, B.; Fearon, M.; Nosal, R.; Drebot, M.; D'Cuhna, C.; Harrington, D.; Smith, S.; George, P.; et al. Protective behavior and West Nile virus risk. *Emerg. Infect. Dis.* **2005**, *11*, 1433–1436. [CrossRef] [PubMed]

32. Bhatt, S.; Gething, P.W.; Brady, O.J.; Messina, J.P.; Farlow, A.W.; Moyes, C.L.; Drake, J.M.; Brownstein, J.S.; Hoen, A.G.; Sankoh, O.; et al. The global distribution and burden of dengue. *Nature* **2013**. [CrossRef]
33. Tokarevich, N.; Tronin, A.; Gnativ, B.; Revich, B.; Blinova, O.; Evengard, B. Impact of air temperature variation on the ixodid ticks habitat and tick-borne encephalitis incidence in the Russian Arctic: The case of the Komi Republic. *Int. J. Circumpolar Health* **2017**, *76*. [CrossRef]
34. Chowdhury, F.R.; Ibrahim, Q.S.U.; Shafiqul Bari, M.; Jahangir Alam, M.M.; Dunachie, S.J.; Rodriguez-Morales, A.J.; Ismail Patwary, M. The association between temperature, rainfall and humidity with common climate-sensitive infectious diseases in Bangladesh. *PLoS ONE* **2018**, *15*, e0199579. [CrossRef]
35. Vázquez, M.; Muehlenbein, C.; Cartter, M.; Hayes, E.B.; Ertel, S.; Shapiro, E.D. Effectiveness of personal protective measures to prevent lyme disease. *Emerg. Infect. Dis.* **2008**, *14*, 210–216. [CrossRef]
36. Barnard, D.R. *Global Collaboration for Development of Pesticides for Public Health (GCDPP) Repellents and Toxicants for Personal Protection*; World Health Organization: Geneva, Switzerland, 2000; Volume 46, pp. 408–418.
37. Donohoe, H.; Pennington-Gray, L.; Omodior, O. Lyme disease: Current issues, implications, and recommendations for tourism management. *Tour. Manag.* **2015**, *46*, 408–418. [CrossRef]
38. Linos, E.; Keiser, E.; Fu, T.; Colditz, G.; Chen, S.; Tang, J.Y. Hat, shade, long sleeves, or sunscreen? Rethinking US sun protection messages based on their relative effectiveness. *Cancer Causes Control* **2011**. [CrossRef]
39. Szykitka, W. *Big Book of Self-Reliant Living: Advice and Information on just about Everything You Need to Know to Live on Planet Earth*; The Lyons Press: Guilford, CT, USA, 2010; p. 65.
40. Harahap, R. Sumatran Tigers Seen on Plantation in Riau. Available online: https://www.thejakartapost.com/news/2019/02/28/sumatran-tigers-seen-on-plantation-in-riau.html (accessed on 31 May 2020).
41. Takahata, C.; Nielsen, S.E.; Takii, A.; Izumiyama, S. Habitat selection of a large carnivore along human-wildlife boundaries in a highly modified landscape. *PLoS ONE* **2014**, *9*, e0086181. [CrossRef] [PubMed]
42. Gu, S.; Wang, A.; Bian, G.; He, T.; Yi, B.; Lu, B.; Li, X.; Xu, G. Relationship between weather factors and heat stroke in Ningbo city. *Chin. J. Endem.* **2016**, *37*, 1131–1136. [CrossRef]
43. Kenny, G.P.; Wilson, T.E.; Flouris, A.D.; Fujii, N. Heat exhaustion. In *Handbook of Clinical Neurology*; Elsevier: Amsterdam, The Netherlands, 2018; pp. 505–529.
44. Zeng, J.; Zhang, X.; Yang, J.; Bao, J.; Xiang, H.; Dear, K.; Liu, Q.; Lin, S.; Lawrence, W.R.; Lin, A.; et al. Humidity may modify the relationship between temperature and cardiovascular mortality in Zhejiang province, China. *Int. J. Environ. Res. Public Health* **2017**, *14*, 1383. [CrossRef] [PubMed]
45. Lin, L.W.; Lin, H.Y.; Hsu, C.Y.; Rau, H.H.; Chen, P.L. Effect of weather and time on trauma events determined using emergency medical service registry data. *Injury* **2015**, *46*, 1814–1820. [CrossRef]
46. Crawshaw, A.F.; Maung, T.M.; Shafique, M.; Sint, N.; Nicholas, S.; Li, M.S.; Roca-Feltrer, A.; Hii, J. Acceptability of insecticide-treated clothing for malaria prevention among migrant rubber tappers in Myanmar: A cluster-randomized non-inferiority crossover trial. *Malar. J.* **2017**, *16*. [CrossRef]
47. Ruiu, L.; Floris, I. Susceptibility of environmentally friendly sheep wool insulation panels to the common clothes moth tineola bisselliella in laboratory assays. *Insects* **2019**, *10*, 379. [CrossRef]
48. Gao, C.; Kuklane, K.; Östergren, P.O.; Kjellstrom, T. Occupational heat stress assessment and protective strategies in the context of climate change. *Int. J. Biometeorol.* **2018**, *62*, 359–371. [CrossRef]
49. Unger, A.; Riley, L.W. Slum health: From understanding to action. *PLoS Med.* **2007**, *4*, 1561–1566. [CrossRef]
50. Sobel, A.H. Tropical Weather. *Nat. Educ. Knowl.* **2012**, *3*, 2.
51. Stjernberg, L.; Berglund, J. Detecting ticks on light versus dark clothing. *Scand. J. Infect. Dis.* **2009**, *37*, 361–364. [CrossRef]
52. Dejenie, T.; Yohannes, M.; Assmelash, T. Characterization of Mosquito Breeding Sites in and in the Vicinity of Tigray Microdams. *Ethiop. J. Health Sci.* **2011**, *21*, 57–66. [CrossRef] [PubMed]
53. Sumodan, P.K. Species diversity of mosquito breeding in rubber plantations of Kerala, India. *J. Am. Mosq. Control Assoc.* **2012**, *28*, 114–115. [CrossRef] [PubMed]
54. Mackensie, J.S.; Lindsay, M.D.; Broom, A.K. Effect of climate and weather on the transmission of Ross River and Murray Valley encephalitis viruses. *Microbiol. Aust.* **2000**, *21*, 40.
55. Reinhold, J.M.; Lazzari, C.R.; Lahondère, C. Effects of the environmental temperature on Aedes aegypti and Aedes albopictus mosquitoes: A review. *Insects* **2018**, *9*, 158. [CrossRef]
56. Eldridge, B.F.; Edman, J.D.; Moncayo, A.C. Medical Entomology: A Textbook on Public Health and Veterinary Problems Caused by Arthropods. *J. Med. Entomol.* **2000**, *116*, 15086–15095. [CrossRef]

57. Sherrard-Smith, E.; Skarp, J.E.; Beale, A.D.; Fornadel, C.; Norris, L.C.; Moore, S.J.; Mihreteab, S.; Charlwood, J.D.; Bhatt, S.; Winskill, P.; et al. Mosquito feeding behavior and how it influences residual malaria transmission across Africa. *Proc. Natl. Acad. Sci. USA* **2019**. [CrossRef]
58. Sutherst, R.W. Global Change and Human Vulnerability to Vector-Borne Diseases. *Clin. Microbiol. Rev.* **2004**, *17*, 136–167. [CrossRef]
59. Leal, W.S. The enigmatic reception of DEET—The gold standard of insect repellents. *Curr. Opin. Insect Sci.* **2014**, *6*, 93–98. [CrossRef]
60. CDC, Centers for Disease Control and Prevention. *Fight the Bite for Protection from Malaria Guidelines for DEET Insect Repellent Use*; CDC: Atlanta, GA, USA, 2005; p. 1.
61. Staub, D.; Debrunner, M.; Amsler, L.; Steffen, R. Effectiveness of a repellent containing DEET and EBAAP for preventing tick bites. *Wilderness Environ. Med.* **2002**, *13*, 12–20. [CrossRef]
62. Onyett, H.; Bortolussi, R.; Bridger, N.A.; Finlay, J.C.; Martin, S.; McDonald, J.C.; Robinson, J.L.; Salvadori, M.I.; Vanderkooi, O.G.; Allen, U.D.; et al. Preventing mosquito and tick bites: A Canadian update. *Paediatr. Child Health* **2014**, *19*, 326–328. [CrossRef]
63. Tips for Using Insect Repellents. Available online: https://www.chp.gov.hk/en/features/38927.html (accessed on 31 May 2020).
64. Msellemu, D.; Shemdoe, A.; Makungu, C.; Mlacha, Y.; Kannady, K.; Dongus, S.; Killeen, G.F.; Dillip, A. The underlying reasons for very high levels of bed net use, and higher malaria infection prevalence among bed net users than non-users in the Tanzanian city of Dar es Salaam: A qualitative study. *Malar. J.* **2017**, *16*. [CrossRef] [PubMed]
65. Ochomo, E.O.; Bayoh, N.M.; Walker, E.D.; Abongo, B.O.; Ombok, M.O.; Ouma, C.; Githeko, A.K.; Vulule, J.; Yan, G.; Gimnig, J.E. The efficacy of long-lasting nets with declining physical integrity may be compromised in areas with high levels of pyrethroid resistance. *Malar. J.* **2013**, *12*. [CrossRef] [PubMed]
66. Shah, M.P.; Steinhardt, L.C.; Mwandama, D.; Mzilahowa, T.; Gimnig, J.E.; Bauleni, A.; Wong, J.; Wiegand, R.; Mathanga, D.P.; Lindblade, K.A. The effectiveness of older insecticide-treated bed nets (ITNs) to prevent malaria infection in an area of moderate pyrethroid resistance: Results from a cohort study in Malawi. *Malar. J.* **2020**, *19*. [CrossRef] [PubMed]
67. Insecticide-Treated Bed Nets. Available online: https://www.cdc.gov/malaria/malaria_worldwide/reduction/itn.html (accessed on 31 May 2020).
68. Jayanti, P.; Acharya, I.A. A Study on Efficacy of LLINS As Compared To In-Use ITNs Amongst Troops in a Malaria Endemic Area. *J. Trop. Dis.* **2015**, *3*. [CrossRef]
69. Clem, A.S. Fundamentals of vaccine immunology. *J. Glob. Infect. Dis.* **2011**, *3*, 73–78. [CrossRef]
70. McBride, W.J.H. Chemoprophylaxis of tropical infectious diseases. *Pharmaceuticals* **2010**, *3*, 1561–1575. [CrossRef] [PubMed]
71. Wilson, A.L.; Dhiman, R.C.; Kitron, U.; Scott, T.W.; van den Berg, H.; Lindsay, S.W. Benefit of Insecticide-Treated Nets, Curtains and Screening on Vector Borne Diseases, Excluding Malaria: A Systematic Review and Meta-analysis. *PLoS Negl. Trop. Dis.* **2014**, *8*. [CrossRef]
72. Xu, J.W.; Liao, Y.M.; Liu, H.; Nie, R.H.; Havumaki, J. Use of bed nets and factors that influence bed net use among jinuo ethnic minority in southern China. *PLoS ONE* **2014**, *9*, e0103780. [CrossRef]
73. Das, M.L.; Singh, S.P.; Vanlerberghe, V.; Rijai, S.; Rai, M.; Karki, P.; Sundar, S.; Boelaert, M. Population preference of net texture prior to bed net trial in Kala-Azar-endemic areas. *PLoS Negl. Trop. Dis.* **2007**, *1*. [CrossRef]
74. Maia, M.F.; Moore, S.J. Plant-based insect repellents: A review of their efficacy, development and testing. *Malar. J.* **2011**, *10*. [CrossRef]
75. Batish, D.R.; Singh, H.P.; Kohli, R.K.; Kaur, S. Eucalyptus essential oil as a natural pesticide. *For. Ecol. Manag.* **2008**, *256*, 2166–2174. [CrossRef]
76. McHenry, M.; Lacuesta, G. Severe allergic reaction to diethyltoluamide (DEET) containing insect repellent. *Allergy, Asthma Clin. Immunol.* **2014**, *10*. [CrossRef]
77. Nelson, K.E.; Williams, C.M. *Infectious Disease Epidemiology: Theory and Practice*; Jones & Bartlett Publishers: Burlington, MA, USA, 2008; pp. 1014–1015.
78. Von Seidlein, L.; Ikonomidis, K.; Bruun, R.; Jawara, M.; Pinder, M.; Knols, B.G.J.; Knudsen, J.B. Airflow attenuation and bed net utilization: Observations from Africa and Asia. *Malar. J.* **2012**, *11*. [CrossRef] [PubMed]

79. Ntonifor, N.H.; Veyufambom, S. Assessing the effective use of mosquito nets in the prevention of malaria in some parts of Mezam division, Northwest Region Cameroon. *Malar. J.* **2016**, *15*. [CrossRef] [PubMed]
80. Pulford, J.; Hetzel, M.W.; Bryant, M.; Siba, P.M.; Mueller, I. Reported reasons for not using a mosquito net when one is available: A review of the published literature. *Malar. J.* **2011**, *10*. [CrossRef]
81. Pugliese-Garcia, M.; Heyerdahl, L.W.; Mwamba, C.; Nkwemu, S.; Chilengi, R.; Demolis, R.; Guillermet, E.; Sharma, A. Factors influencing vaccine acceptance and hesitancy in three informal settlements in Lusaka, Zambia. *Vaccine* **2018**, *36*, 5617–5624. [CrossRef]
82. Muhsen, K.; Abed El-Hai, R.; Amit-Aharon, A.; Nehama, H.; Gondia, M.; Davidovitch, N.; Goren, S.; Cohen, D. Risk factors of underutilization of childhood immunizations in ultraorthodox Jewish communities in Israel despite high access to health care services. *Vaccine* **2012**, *30*, 2109–2115. [CrossRef]
83. The Lancet Infectious Diseases Malaria vaccination: A major milestone. *Lancet Infect. Dis.* **2019**, *19*, 559. [CrossRef]
84. Malande, O.O.; Munube, D.; Afaayo, R.N.; Annet, K.; Bodo, B.; Bakainaga, A.; Ayebare, E.; Njunwamukama, S.; Mworozi, E.A.; Musyoki, A.M. Barriers to effective uptake and provision of immunization in a rural district in Uganda. *PLoS ONE* **2019**, *14*, e0212270. [CrossRef]
85. Rodriguez, S.D.; Drake, L.L.; Price, D.P.; Hammond, J.I.; Hansen, I.A.; Liu, N. The efficacy of some commercially available insect repellents for Aedes aegypti (Diptera: Culicidae) and Aedes albopictus (Diptera: Culicidae). *J. Insect Sci.* **2015**, *15*. [CrossRef]
86. Legeay, S.; Clere, N.; Hilairet, G.; Do, Q.T.; Bernard, P.; Quignard, J.F.; Apaire-Marchais, V.; Lapied, B.; Faure, S. The insect repellent N,N-diethyl-m-Toluamide (DEET) induces angiogenesis via allosteric modulation of the M3 muscarinic receptor in endothelial cells. *Sci. Rep.* **2016**, *6*. [CrossRef] [PubMed]
87. Swale, D.R.; Bloomquist, J.R. Is DEET a dangerous neurotoxicant? *Pest Manag. Sci.* **2019**, *75*. [CrossRef] [PubMed]
88. Koren, G.; Matsui, D.; Bailey, B. DEET-based insect repellents: Safety implications for children and pregnant and lactating women. *Can. Med. Assoc. J.* **2003**, *169*, 209–212.
89. Lenhart, A.; Orelus, N.; Maskill, R.; Alexander, N.; Streit, T.; McCall, P.J. Insecticide-treated bednets to control dengue vectors: Preliminary evidence from a controlled trial in Haiti. *Trop. Med. Int. Heal.* **2008**, *13*, 56–57. [CrossRef] [PubMed]
90. Bhatt, S.; Weiss, D.J.; Cameron, E.; Bisanzio, D.; Mappin, B.; Dalrymple, U.; Battle, K.E.; Moyes, C.L.; Henry, A.; Eckhoff, P.A.; et al. The effect of malaria control on Plasmodium falciparum in Africa between 2000 and 2015. *Nature* **2015**, *526*, 207–211. [CrossRef] [PubMed]
91. Hawley, W.A.; Phillips-Howard, P.A.; Ter Kuile, F.O.; Terlouw, D.J.; Vulule, J.M.; Ombok, M.; Nahlen, B.L.; Gimnig, J.E.; Kariuki, S.K.; Kolczak, M.S.; et al. Community-wide effects of permethrin-treated bed nets on child mortality and malaria morbidity in western Kenya. *Am. J. Trop. Med. Hyg.* **2003**, *68*, 121–127. [CrossRef]
92. Killeen, G.F.; Smith, T.A.; Ferguson, H.M.; Mshinda, H.; Abdulla, S.; Lengeler, C.; Kachur, S.P. Preventing childhood malaria in Africa by protecting adults from mosquitoes with insecticide-treated nets. *PLoS Med.* **2007**, *4*, 1246–1258. [CrossRef]
93. Hauser, G.; Thiévent, K.; Koella, J.C. The ability of Anopheles gambiae mosquitoes to bite through a permethrin-treated net and the consequences for their fitness. *Sci. Rep.* **2019**, *9*. [CrossRef]
94. World Health Organization. Vaccines and vaccination against yellow fever WHO Position Paper—June Note de synthèse: Position de l' OMS sur les vaccins et la vaccination contre la fièvre jaune, juin 2013. *Relevé Épidémiologique Hebdomadaire* **2013**, *88*, 269–284.
95. Gotuzzo, E.; Yactayo, S.; Córdova, E. Review article: Efficacy and duration of immunity after yellow fever vaccination: Systematic review on the need for a booster every 10 years. *Am. J. Trop. Med. Hyg.* **2013**, *89*, 434–444. [CrossRef]
96. WHO Publication. Vaccines against tick-borne encephalitis: WHO position paper—Recommendations. *Vaccine* **2011**, *86*, 241–256. [CrossRef]
97. Bogovic, P. Tick-borne encephalitis: A review of epidemiology, clinical characteristics, and management. *World J. Clin. Cases* **2015**. [CrossRef] [PubMed]
98. World Health Organization. Japanese Encephalitis Vaccines: WHO position paper, February 2015—Recommendations. *Vaccine* **2016**, *90*, 69–88. [CrossRef]

99. Hegde, N.R.; Gore, M.M. Japanese encephalitis vaccines: Immunogenicity, protective efficacy, effectiveness, and impact on the burden of disease. *Hum. Vaccines Immunother.* **2017**, *13*, 1320–1337. [CrossRef] [PubMed]
100. Malaria Vaccine Pilot Launched in Malawi. Available online: https://www.who.int/news-room/detail/23-04-2019-malaria-vaccine-pilot-launched-in-malawi (accessed on 31 May 2020).
101. Jover, J.A.; Leon, L.; Pato, E.; Loza, E.; Rosales, Z.; Matias, M.A.; Mendez-Fernandez, R.; Díaz-Valle, D.; Benitez-del-Castillo, J.M.; Abasolo, L. Long-term use of antimalarial drugs in rheumatic diseases. *Clin. Exp. Rheumatol.* **2012**, *30*, 380–387.
102. Schwartz, E. Prophylaxis of Malaria. *Mediterr. J. Hematol. Infect. Dis.* **2012**, *4*. [CrossRef]
103. Chen, L.H.; Wilson, M.E.; Schlagenhauf, P. Prevention of malaria in long-term travelers. *J. Am. Med. Assoc.* **2006**, *296*, 2234–2244. [CrossRef]
104. First FDA-Approved Vaccine for the Prevention of Dengue Diseases in Endemic Regions. Available online: https://www.fda.gov/news-events/press-announcements/first-fda-approved-vaccine-prevention-dengue-disease-endemic-regions#:~{}:text=The_U.S._Food_and_Drug,who_live_in_endemic_areas (accessed on 31 May 2020).
105. Da Silveira, L.T.C.; Tura, B.; Santos, M. Systematic review of dengue vaccine efficacy. *BMC Infect. Dis.* **2019**, *19*. [CrossRef]
106. Du, S.; Liu, Y.; Liu, J.; Zhao, J.; Champagne, C.; Tong, L.; Zhang, R.; Zhang, F.; Qin, C.F.; Ma, P.; et al. Aedes mosquitoes acquire and transmit Zika virus by breeding in contaminated aquatic environments. *Nat. Commun.* **2019**, *10*. [CrossRef]
107. Monteiro, V.V.S.; Navegantes-Lima, K.C.; De Lemos, A.B.; Da Silva, G.L.; De Souza Gomes, R.; Reis, J.F.; Junior, L.C.R.; Da Silva, O.S.; Romão, P.R.T.; Monteiro, M.C. Aedes-chikungunya virus interaction: Key role of vector midguts microbiota and its saliva in the host infection. *Front. Microbiol.* **2019**, *10*. [CrossRef]
108. Soleimani-Ahmadi, M.; Vatandoost, H.; Zare, M. Characterization of larval habitats for anopheline mosquitoes in a malarious area under elimination program in the southeast of Iran. *Asian Pac. J. Trop. Biomed.* **2014**, *4*, 73–80. [CrossRef] [PubMed]
109. Ziraba, A.K.; Haregu, T.N.; Mberu, B. A review and framework for understanding the potential impact of poor solid waste management on health in developing countries. *Arch. Public Health* **2016**, *74*. [CrossRef] [PubMed]
110. Hori, M.; Shibuya, K.; Sato, M.; Saito, Y. Lethal effects of short-wavelength visible light on insects. *Sci. Rep.* **2014**, *4*. [CrossRef] [PubMed]
111. Puri, A.; Kumar, M.; Johal, E. Solid-waste management in Jalandhar city and its impact on community health. *Indian J. Occup. Environ. Med.* **2008**, *12*, 76–81. [CrossRef]
112. Achudume, A.C.; Olawale, J.T. Microbial pathogens of public health significance in waste dumps and common sites. *J. Environ. Biol.* **2007**, *28*, 151–154.
113. Bell, J.L.; Collins, J.W.; Wolf, L.; Gronqvist, R.; Chiou, S.; Chang, W.R.; Sorock, G.; Courtney, T.; Lombardi, D.; Evanoff, B. Evaluation of a comprehensive slip, trip and fall prevention programme for hospital employees. *Ergonomics* **2009**, *51*, 1905–1925. [CrossRef]
114. Weinhold, B. A spreading concern: Inhalational health effects of mold. *Environ. Health Perspect.* **2007**, *115*, 300–305. [CrossRef]
115. Mattiello, A.; Chiodini, P.; Bianco, E.; Forgione, N.; Flammia, I.; Gallo, C.; Pizzuti, R.; Panico, S. Health effects associated with the disposal of solid waste in landfills and incinerators in populations living in surrounding areas: A systematic review. *Int. J. Public Health* **2013**, *58*, 725–735. [CrossRef]
116. Ferronato, N.; Torretta, V. Waste mismanagement in developing countries: A review of global issues. *Int. J. Environ. Res. Public Health* **2019**, *16*, 1060. [CrossRef]
117. Abeyewickreme, W.; Wickremasinghe, A.R.; Karunatilake, K.; Sommerfeld, J.; Axel, K. Community mobilization and household level waste management for dengue vector control in Gampaha district of Sri Lanka; an intervention study. *Pathog. Glob. Health* **2012**, *106*, 479–487. [CrossRef]
118. SDG7: Data and Projections. Available online: https://www.iea.org/reports/sdg7-data-and-projections/access-to-electricity (accessed on 31 May 2020).
119. Ritchie, S.A.; Cortis, G.; Paton, C.; Townsend, M.; Shroyer, D.; Zborowski, P.; Hall-Mendelin, S.; Van Den Hurk, A.F. A Simple Non-Powered Passive Trap for the Collection of Mosquitoes for Arbovirus Surveillance. *J. Med. Entomol.* **2013**, *50*, 185–194. [CrossRef] [PubMed]

120. Lu, Y.; Bei, Y.; Zhang, J. Are Yellow Sticky Traps an Effective Method for Control of Sweetpotato Whitefly, Bemisia tabaci, in the Greenhouse or Field? *J. Insect Sci.* **2012**, *12*. [CrossRef]
121. García-Betancourt, T.; Higuera-Mendieta, D.R.; González-Uribe, C.; Cortés, S.; Quintero, J. Understanding water storage practices of urban residents of an endemic dengue area in Colombia: Perceptions, rationale and socio-demographic characteristics. *PLoS ONE* **2015**, *10*, e0129054. [CrossRef] [PubMed]
122. Dambach, P.; Jorge, M.M.; Traoré, I.; Phalkey, R.; Sawadogo, H.; Zabré, P.; Kagoné, M.; Sié, A.; Sauerborn, R.; Becker, N.; et al. A qualitative study of community perception and acceptance of biological larviciding for malaria mosquito control in rural Burkina Faso. *BMC Public Health* **2018**, *18*. [CrossRef] [PubMed]
123. Yukalang, N.; Clarke, B.; Ross, K. Barriers to effective municipal solid waste management in a rapidly urbanizing area in Thailand. *Int. J. Environ. Res. Public Health* **2017**, *14*, 1013. [CrossRef]
124. Shockley Cruz, M.; Lindner, R.; Cruz, M.S.; Lindner, R. Insect Vision: Ultraviolet, Color, and LED Light. Ph.D. Thesis, University of Georgia Department of Entomology, Athens, GA, USA, 2011.
125. Van Loon, J.J.A.; Smallegange, R.C.; Bukovinszkiné-Kiss, G.; Jacobs, F.; De Rijk, M.; Mukabana, W.R.; Verhulst, N.O.; Menger, D.J.; Takken, W. Mosquito Attraction: Crucial Role of Carbon Dioxide in Formulation of a Five-Component Blend of Human-Derived Volatiles. *J. Chem. Ecol.* **2015**, *41*, 567–573. [CrossRef] [PubMed]
126. O'Hara, J.E.; UsUpensky, I.; Bostanian, N.J.; Capinera, J.L.; Chapman, R.; Barfield, C.S.; Swisher, M.E.; Barfield, C.S.; Heppner, J.; Fitzgerald, T.D.; et al. Traps for Capturing Insects. In *Encyclopedia of Entomology*; Springer Science & Business Media: Berlin, Germany, 2008; pp. 3675–4007.
127. Zhou, Y.H.; Zhang, Z.W.; Fu, Y.F.; Zhang, G.C.; Yuan, S. Carbon dioxide, odorants, heat and visible cues affect wild mosquito landing in open spaces. *Front. Behav. Neurosci.* **2018**, *12*. [CrossRef] [PubMed]
128. Lorenzi, O.D.; Major, C.; Acevedo, V.; Perez-Padilla, J.; Rivera, A.; Biggerstaff, B.J.; Munoz-Jordan, J.; Waterman, S.; Barrera, R.; Sharp, T.M. Reduced incidence of Chikungunya virus infection in communities with ongoing aedes aegypti mosquito trap intervention studies—Salinas and Guayama, Puerto Rico, November 2015–february 2016. *Morb. Mortal. Wkly. Rep.* **2016**, *65*, 479–480. [CrossRef]
129. Junnila, A.; Kline, D.L.; Müller, G.C. Comparative efficacy of small commercial traps for the capture of adult Phlebotomus papatasi. *J. Vector Ecol.* **2011**, *36*, 172–178. [CrossRef]
130. Sliney, D.H.; Gilbert, D.W.; Lyon, T. Ultraviolet safety assessments of insect light traps. *J. Occup. Environ. Hyg.* **2016**, *13*, 413–424. [CrossRef]
131. Urban, J.E.; Broce, A. Killing of flies in electrocuting insect traps releases bacteria and viruses. *Curr. Microbiol.* **2000**, *41*, 267–270. [CrossRef] [PubMed]
132. Getachew, D.; Tekie, H.; Gebre-Michael, T.; Balkew, M.; Mesfin, A. Breeding sites of aedes aegypti: Potential dengue vectors in dire Dawa, east Ethiopia. *Interdiscip. Perspect. Infect. Dis.* **2015**, *2015*. [CrossRef] [PubMed]
133. UNICEF. *Djibouti Humanitarian Situation Report No. 2 Flood Response*; UNICEF: New York, NY, USA, 2019; pp. 1–5.
134. Krystosik, A.; Njoroge, G.; Odhiambo, L.; Forsyth, J.E.; Mutuku, F.; LaBeaud, A.D. Solid Wastes Provide Breeding Sites, Burrows, and Food for Biological Disease Vectors, and Urban Zoonotic Reservoirs: A Call to Action for Solutions-Based Research. *Front. Public Health* **2020**, *7*. [CrossRef] [PubMed]
135. Banerjee, S.; Aditya, G.; Saha, G.K. Household wastes as larval habitats of dengue vectors: Comparison between urban and rural areas of Kolkata, India. *PLoS ONE* **2015**, *10*, e0138082. [CrossRef]
136. Becher, P.G.; Hagman, A.; Verschut, V.; Chakraborty, A.; Rozpędowska, E.; Lebreton, S.; Bengtsson, M.; Flick, G.; Witzgall, P.; Piškur, J. Chemical signaling and insect attraction is a conserved trait in yeasts. *Ecol. Evol.* **2018**, *8*, 2962–2974. [CrossRef]
137. Billeter, J.C.; Wolfner, M.F. Chemical Cues that Guide Female Reproduction in Drosophila melanogaster. *J. Chem. Ecol.* **2018**, *44*, 750–769. [CrossRef]
138. Boadi, K.O.; Kuitunen, M. Environmental and health impacts of household solid waste handling and disposal practices in Third World cities: The case of the Accra Metropolitan Area, Ghana. *J. Environ. Health* **2005**, *68*, 32–36.
139. Barreiro, C.; Albano, H.; Silva, J.; Teixeira, P. Role of Flies as Vectors of Foodborne Pathogens in Rural Areas. *ISRN Microbiol.* **2013**, *2013*. [CrossRef]
140. Zamora, D.M.B.; Hernández, M.M.; Torres, N.; Zúniga, C.; Sosa, W.; De Abrego, V.; Escobar, M.C.M. Information to act: Household characteristics are predictors of domestic infestation with the Chagas vector Triatoma dimidiata in central America. *Am. J. Trop. Med. Hyg.* **2015**, *93*. [CrossRef]

141. Jawara, M.; Jatta, E.; Bell, D.; Burkot, T.R.; Bradley, J.; Hunt, V.; Kandeh, B.; Jones, C.; Manjang, A.M.; Pinder, M.; et al. New prototype screened doors and windows for excluding mosquitoes from houses: A pilot study in rural Gambia. *Am. J. Trop. Med. Hyg.* **2018**, *99*, 1475–1484. [CrossRef]
142. Che-Mendoza, A.; Medina-Barreiro, A.; Koyoc-Cardeña, E.; Uc-Puc, V.; Contreras-Perera, Y.; Herrera-Bojórquez, J.; Dzul-Manzanilla, F.; Correa-Morales, F.; Ranson, H.; Lenhart, A.; et al. House screening with insecticide-treated netting provides sustained reductions in domestic populations of Aedes aegypti in Merida, Mexico. *PLoS Negl. Trop. Dis.* **2018**, *12*. [CrossRef] [PubMed]
143. Tusting, L.S.; Ippolito, M.M.; Willey, B.A.; Kleinschmidt, I.; Dorsey, G.; Gosling, R.D.; Lindsay, S.W. The evidence for improving housing to reduce malaria: A systematic review and meta-analysis. *Malar. J.* **2015**, *14*. [CrossRef] [PubMed]
144. Massebo, F.; Lindtjørn, B. The effect of screening doors and windows on indoor density of Anopheles arabiensis in south-west Ethiopia: A randomized trial. *Malar. J.* **2013**, *12*. [CrossRef] [PubMed]
145. Musoke, D.; Karani, G.; Ssempebwa, J.C.; Musoke, M.B. Integrated approach to malaria prevention at household level in rural communities in Uganda: Experiences from a pilot project. *Malar. J.* **2018**, *18*, 1144–1156. [CrossRef]
146. Matsui, E.C. Management of rodent exposure and allergy in the pediatric population. *Curr. Allergy Asthma Rep.* **2013**, *13*. [CrossRef]
147. Hopkins, A.S.; Whitetail-Eagle, J.; Corneli, A.L.; Person, B.; Ettestad, P.J.; DiMenna, M.; Norstog, J.; Creswell, J.; Khan, A.S.; Olson, J.G.; et al. Experimental evaluation of rodent exclusion methods to reduce hantavirus transmission to residents in a Native American community in New Mexico. *Vector Borne Zoonotic Dis.* **2002**, *2*, 61–68. [CrossRef]
148. Jones, C.H.; Benítez-Valladares, D.; Guillermo-May, G.; Dzul-Manzanilla, F.; Che-Mendoza, A.; Barrera-Pérez, M.; Selem-Salas, C.; Chablé-Santos, J.; Sommerfeld, J.; Kroeger, A.; et al. Use and acceptance of long lasting insecticidal net screens for dengue prevention in Acapulco, Guerrero, Mexico. *BMC Public Health* **2014**, *14*. [CrossRef]
149. Bonner, P.C.; Schmidt, W.P.; Belmain, S.R.; Oshin, B.; Baglole, D.; Borchert, M. Poor housing quality increases risk of rodent infestation and lassa fever in refugee camps of sierra leone. *Am. J. Trop. Med. Hyg.* **2007**, *77*, 169–175. [CrossRef]
150. Safan, M.A.; Etman, Z.A.; Konswa, A. Evaluation of polyurethane resin injection for concrete leak repair. *Case Stud. Constr. Mater.* **2019**, *11*. [CrossRef]
151. Tseloni, A.; Farrell, G.; Thompson, R.; Evans, E.; Tilley, N. Domestic burglary drop and the security hypothesis. *Crime Sci.* **2017**, *6*. [CrossRef]
152. Carter, A.D. Are Housing Improvements an Effective Supplemental Vector Control Strategy to Reduce Malaria Transmission? A Systematic Review. Ph.D. Thesis, Georgia State University, Atlanta, GA, USA, 2014.
153. Bublitz, D.A.C.; Poché, R.M.; Garlapati, R. Measures to control Phlebotomus argentipes and visceral leishmaniasis in India. *J. Arthropod. Borne. Dis.* **2016**, *10*, 113–126. [PubMed]
154. Kaindoa, E.W.; Finda, M.; Kiplagat, J.; Mkandawile, G.; Nyoni, A.; Coetzee, M.; Okumu, F.O. Housing gaps, mosquitoes and public viewpoints: A mixed methods assessment of relationships between house characteristics, malaria vector biting risk and community perspectives in rural Tanzania. *Malar. J.* **2018**, *17*. [CrossRef] [PubMed]
155. Ogoma, S.B.; Kannady, K.; Sikulu, M.; Chaki, P.P.; Govella, N.J.; Mukabana, W.R.; Killeen, G.F. Window screening, ceilings and closed eaves as sustainable ways to control malaria in Dar es Salaam, Tanzania. *Malar. J.* **2009**, *8*. [CrossRef] [PubMed]
156. Ranjan, A.; Sur, D.; Singh, V.P.; Siddique, N.A.; Manna, B.; Lal, C.S.; Sinha, P.K.; Kishore, K.; Bhattacharya, S.K. Risk factors for Indian kala-azar. *Am. J. Trop. Med. Hyg.* **2005**, *73*, 74–78. [CrossRef] [PubMed]
157. Chan, E.Y.Y.; Shaw, R. *Public Health Humanitarian Responses to Natural Disasters*; Springer: Berlin/Heidelberg, Germany, 2017; ISBN 9781317357445.
158. Ryan, J. Environmental Health in Emergencies and Disasters: A Practical Guide. *Emerg. Med. J.* **2002**, *22*, 610. [CrossRef]
159. Laaser, U.; Dorey, S.; Nurse, J. A plea for global health action bottom-up. *Front. Public Health* **2016**, *4*. [CrossRef] [PubMed]
160. Hou, S.I. *Health Education: Theoretical Concepts, Effective Strategies and Core Competencies*; World Health Organization: Geneva, Switzerland, 2012; Volume 15, ISBN 9789290218289.

161. Naranjo, D.P.; Qualls, W.A.; Jurado, H.; Perez, J.C.; De Xue, R.; Gomez, E.; Beier, J.C. Vector control programs in Saint Johns County, Florida and Guayas, Ecuador: Successes and barriers to integrated vector management. *BMC Public Health* **2014**, *14*. [CrossRef]
162. Demanou, M.; Pouillot, R.; Grandadam, M.; Boisier, P.; Kamgang, B.; Hervé, J.P.; Rogier, C.; Rousset, D.; Paupy, C. Evidence of Dengue Virus Transmission and Factors Associated with the Presence of Anti-Dengue Virus Antibodies in Humans in Three Major Towns in Cameroon. *PLoS Negl. Trop. Dis.* **2014**, *8*. [CrossRef]
163. Poinsignon, A.; Boulanger, D.; Binetruy, F.; Elguero, E.; Darriet, F.; Gallian, P.; De Lamballerie, X.; Charrel, R.N.; Remoue, F. Risk factors of exposure to Aedes albopictus bites in mainland France using an immunological biomarker. *Epidemiol. Infect.* **2019**, *147*. [CrossRef]
164. Reiter, P.; Lathrop, S.; Bunning, M.; Biggerstaff, B.; Singer, D.; Tiwari, T.; Baber, L.; Amador, M.; Thirion, J.; Hayes, J.; et al. Texas lifestyle limits transmission of dengue virus. *Emerg. Infect. Dis.* **2003**, *9*, 86–89. [CrossRef]
165. Bloch, D.; Roth, N.M.; Caraballo, E.V.; Muñoz-Jordan, J.; Hunsperger, E.; Rivera, A.; Pérez-Padilla, J.; Rivera Garcia, B.; Sharp, T.M. Use of Household Cluster Investigations to Identify Factors Associated with Chikungunya Virus Infection and Frequency of Case Reporting in Puerto Rico. *PLoS Negl. Trop. Dis.* **2016**, *10*. [CrossRef]
166. Mathanga, D.P.; Mwandama, D.A.; Bauleni, A.; Chisaka, J.; Shah, M.P.; Landman, K.Z.; Lindblade, K.A.; Steinhardt, L.C. The effectiveness of long-lasting, insecticide-treated nets in a setting of pyrethroid resistance: A case-control study among febrile children 6 to 59 months of age in Machinga District, Malawi. *Malar. J.* **2015**, *14*. [CrossRef] [PubMed]
167. Pryce, J.; Richardson, M.; Lengeler, C. Insecticide-treated nets for preventing malaria. *Cochrane Database Syst. Rev.* **2019**, *11*. [CrossRef] [PubMed]
168. Deletre, E.; Martin, T.; Duménil, C.; Chandre, F. Insecticide resistance modifies mosquito response to DEET and natural repellents. *Parasites Vectors* **2019**, *12*. [CrossRef] [PubMed]
169. WHO. *Handbook for Integrated Vector Management*; World Health Organization: Geneva, Switzerland, 2013; ISBN 9789241502801.
170. Wilson, A.L.; Boelaert, M.; Kleinschmidt, I.; Pinder, M.; Scott, T.W.; Tusting, L.S.; Lindsay, S.W. Evidence-based vector control? Improving the quality of vector control trials. *Trends Parasitol.* **2015**, *31*, 380–390. [CrossRef]
171. Corrin, T.; Waddell, L.; Greig, J.; Young, I.; Hierlihy, C.; Mascarenhas, M. Risk perceptions, attitudes, and knowledge of chikungunya among the public and health professionals: A systematic review. *Trop. Med. Health* **2017**, *45*. [CrossRef]
172. Degroote, S.; Zinszer, K.; Ridde, V. Interventions for vector-borne diseases focused on housing and hygiene in urban areas: A scoping review. *Infect. Dis. Poverty* **2018**, *7*. [CrossRef]
173. Giantsis, I.A.; Chaskopoulou, A. Broadening the tools for studying sand fly breeding habitats: A novel molecular approach for the detection of phlebotomine larval DNA in soil substrates. *Acta Trop.* **2019**, *190*, 123–128. [CrossRef]
174. Moncaz, A.; Faiman, R.; Kirstein, O.; Warburg, A. Breeding sites of Phlebotomus sergenti, the sand fly vector of cutaneous leishmaniasis in the Judean desert. *PLoS Negl. Trop. Dis.* **2012**, *6*. [CrossRef]
175. Vivero, R.J.; Torres-Gutierrez, C.; Bejarano, E.E.; Peña, H.C.; Estrada, L.G.; Florez, F.; Ortega, E.; Aparicio, Y.; Muskus, C.E. Study on natural breeding sites of sand flies (Diptera: Phlebotominae) in areas of Leishmania transmission in Colombia. *Parasites Vectors* **2015**, *8*. [CrossRef]
176. World Health Organization. *Dengue Guidelines for Diagnosis, Treatment, Prevention and Control*; World Health Organization: Geneva, Switzerland, 2009.
177. Iwamura, T.; Guzman-Holst, A.; Murray, K.A. Accelerating invasion potential of disease vector Aedes aegypti under climate change. *Nat. Commun.* **2020**, *1*. [CrossRef] [PubMed]
178. Campbell-Lendrum, D.; Manga, L.; Bagayoko, M.; Sommerfeld, J. Climate change and vector-borne diseases: What are the implications for public health research and policy? *Philos. Trans. R. Soc. B Biol. Sci.* **2015**, *370*. [CrossRef] [PubMed]

Permissions

All chapters in this book were first published by MDPI; hereby published with permission under the Creative Commons Attribution License or equivalent. Every chapter published in this book has been scrutinized by our experts. Their significance has been extensively debated. The topics covered herein carry significant findings which will fuel the growth of the discipline. They may even be implemented as practical applications or may be referred to as a beginning point for another development.

The contributors of this book come from diverse backgrounds, making this book a truly international effort. This book will bring forth new frontiers with its revolutionizing research information and detailed analysis of the nascent developments around the world.

We would like to thank all the contributing authors for lending their expertise to make the book truly unique. They have played a crucial role in the development of this book. Without their invaluable contributions this book wouldn't have been possible. They have made vital efforts to compile up to date information on the varied aspects of this subject to make this book a valuable addition to the collection of many professionals and students.

This book was conceptualized with the vision of imparting up-to-date information and advanced data in this field. To ensure the same, a matchless editorial board was set up. Every individual on the board went through rigorous rounds of assessment to prove their worth. After which they invested a large part of their time researching and compiling the most relevant data for our readers.

The editorial board has been involved in producing this book since its inception. They have spent rigorous hours researching and exploring the diverse topics which have resulted in the successful publishing of this book. They have passed on their knowledge of decades through this book. To expedite this challenging task, the publisher supported the team at every step. A small team of assistant editors was also appointed to further simplify the editing procedure and attain best results for the readers.

Apart from the editorial board, the designing team has also invested a significant amount of their time in understanding the subject and creating the most relevant covers. They scrutinized every image to scout for the most suitable representation of the subject and create an appropriate cover for the book.

The publishing team has been an ardent support to the editorial, designing and production team. Their endless efforts to recruit the best for this project, has resulted in the accomplishment of this book. They are a veteran in the field of academics and their pool of knowledge is as vast as their experience in printing. Their expertise and guidance has proved useful at every step. Their uncompromising quality standards have made this book an exceptional effort. Their encouragement from time to time has been an inspiration for everyone.

The publisher and the editorial board hope that this book will prove to be a valuable piece of knowledge for researchers, students, practitioners and scholars across the globe.

List of Contributors

Eugene Siu Kai Lo
Collaborating Centre for Oxford University and CUHK for Disaster and Medical Humanitarian Response (CCOUC), The Chinese University of Hong Kong, Hong Kong, China

Emily Ying Yang Chan
Collaborating Centre for Oxford University and CUHK for Disaster and Medical Humanitarian Response (CCOUC), The Chinese University of Hong Kong, Hong Kong, China
Nuffield Department of Medicine, University of Oxford, Oxford OX37BN, UK
JC School of Public Health and Primary Care, The Chinese University of Hong Kong, Hong Kong, China

Eliza Lai Yi Wong and Samuel Yeung Shan Wong
JC School of Public Health and Primary Care, The Chinese University of Hong Kong, Hong Kong, China

Kevin Kei Ching Hung
Collaborating Centre for Oxford University and CUHK for Disaster and Medical Humanitarian Response (CCOUC), The Chinese University of Hong Kong, Hong Kong, China
Accident & Emergency Medicine Academic Unit, The Chinese University of Hong Kong, Prince of Wales Hospital, Hong Kong, China

Leif Inge Magnussen, Elsa Kristiansen and Jarle Løwe Sørensen
USN School of Business, University of South-Eastern Norway, 3603 Kongsberg, Norway

Johan Berlin
Department of Social and Behavioural Studies, University West, SE-461 86 Trollhättan, Sweden

Sho Takahashi and Hirokazu Tachikawa
Department of Disaster and Community Psychiatry, Faculty of Medicine, University of Tsukuba; Tsukuba, Ibaraki 305-8577, Japan
Department of Community and Disaster Assistance, Ibaraki Prefectural Medical Center of Psychiatry, Asahi-machi, Kasama, Ibaraki 309-1717, Japan

Yoshifumi Takagi
Nihon Fukushi University, Okuda, Mihama-cho, Chita-gun, Aichi 470-3295, Japan

Michiko Watari
DPAT secretariat, commissioned by the Ministry of Health, Labor and Welfare, Kasumigaseki Chiyoda-ku, Tokyo 100-8916, Japan

Yasuhisa Fukuo
DPAT secretariat, commissioned by the Ministry of Health, Labor and Welfare, Kasumigaseki Chiyoda-ku, Tokyo 100-8916, Japan
Kanagawa Psychiatric Center, Serigaya, Konan Ward, Yokohama, Kanagawa 233-0006, Japan

Tetsuaki Arai
Department of Psychiatry, Division of Clinical Medicine, Faculty of Medicine, University of Tsukuba, Tsukuba, Ibaraki 305-8577, Japan

Tatsuhiko Kubo
Department of Environmental Epidemiology, Institute of Industrial Ecological Sciences, University of Occupational and Environmental Health, Kitakyushu 807-8555, Japan

Alisa Yanasan
Ministry of Public Health, Nonthaburi 11000, Thailand

Teodoro Herbosa
UP College of Medicine, University of the Philippines Manila, Manila 1000, Philippines

Nilesh Buddh
WHO Regional Office for South-East Asia, New Delhi 110002, India

Ferdinal Fernando
The ASEAN Secretariat, Jakarta 12110, Indonesia

Elżbieta Posłuszna
Faculty of Aviation Safety, Military University of Aviation, 08-521 Dęblin, Poland

Krzysztof Goniewicz
Department of Aviation Security, Military University of Aviation, 08-521 Dęblin, Poland

Mariusz Goniewicz
Department of Emergency Medicine, Medical University of Lublin, 20-059 Lublin, Poland

Genevieve Belleville, Marie-Christine Ouellet and Charles M. Morin
School of Psychology, Laval University, Quebec, QC G1V 0A6, Canada

Junwei Ma, Xiao Liu, Xiaoxu Niu and Zongxing Zou
Three Gorges Research Center for Geo-Hazards of the Ministry of Education, China University of Geosciences, Wuhan 430074, China

Yankun Wang and Junrong Zhang
Faculty of Engineering, China University of Geosciences, Wuhan 430074, China

Tao Wen
School of Geosciences, Yangtze University, Wuhan 430100, China

Philip J. Schluter
School of Health Sciences, University of Canterbury—Te Whare Wānanga o Waitaha, Christchurch 8140, New Zealand
Primary Care Clinical Unit, School of Clinical Medicine, The University of Queensland, Brisbane QLD 4006, Australia

Shiori Usami
Department of Mental Health and Psychiatric Nursing, Faculty of Life Sciences, Kumamoto University, Kumamoto 860-8555, Japan

Sonoe Mashino
Research Institute of Nursing Care for People and Community, University of Hyōgo, Akashi 673-8588, Japan

Yoshiharu Kim
National Institute of Mental Health, National Center for Neurology and Psychiatry, Kodaira 187-0031, Japan

Lennart Reifels
Centre for Mental Health, Melbourne School of Population and Global Health, The University of Melbourne, Melbourne, VIC 3010, Australia
Disaster Research Unit, Department of Political and Social Sciences, Free University of Berlin, 12165 Berlin, Germany

Ryoma Kayano and Sarah Louise Barber
World Health Organization Centre for Health Development, Kobe 651-0073, Japan

Emily YY Chan
Collaborating Centre for Oxford University and Chinese University of Hong Kong for Disaster and Medical Humanitarian Response (CCOUC), School of Public Health and Primary Care, The Chinese University of Hong Kong, HongKong, China

Jonathan Abrahams
Country Health Emergency Preparedness and International Regulations Department, WHO Health Emergencies Programme, World Health Organization, CH-1211 Geneva, Switzerland

Virginia Murray
Public Health England, London SE1 8UG, UK

Annelie Raidla and Katrin Darro
Emergency Department at Östra Hospital, Sahlgrenska University Hospital, 413 90 Gothenburg, Sweden

Tobias Carlson
Gothenburg Emergency Research Group (GEMREG), Sahlgrenska University Hospital, 413 90 Gothenburg, Sweden
Center of Emergency Department Development, Sahlgrenska University Hospital, 413 90 Gothenburg, Sweden

Amir Khorram-Manesh
Gothenburg Emergency Research Group (GEMREG), Sahlgrenska University Hospital, 413 90 Gothenburg, Sweden
Institute of Clinical Sciences, Department of Surgery, Sahlgrenska Academy, Gothenburg University, 40530 Gothenburg, Sweden
Department of Research and Development, the Swedish Armed Forces Center for Defense Medicine, Västra Frölunda, 42676 Gothenburg, Sweden

Eric Carlström
Gothenburg Emergency Research Group (GEMREG), Sahlgrenska University Hospital, 413 90 Gothenburg, Sweden
Institute of Health and Care Sciences, Sahlgrenska Academy, University of Gothenburg, 405 30 Gothenburg, Sweden
USN School of Business, Campus Vestfold, University of South-Eastern Norway, 3603 Kongsberg, Norway
Institute of Healthcare Sciences, Sahlgrenska Academy, Gothenburg University, 40100 Gothenburg, Sweden

Hsin-I Shih
Department of Emergency Medicine, National Cheng Kung University Hospital, College of Medicine, National Cheng Kung University, Tainan 70403, Taiwan
School of Medicine, College of Medicine, National Cheng Kung University, Tainan 70101, Taiwan
Department of Public Health, College of Medicine, National Cheng Kung University, Tainan 70101, Taiwan

Yi-Ting Huang
School of Medicine, College of Medicine, National Cheng Kung University, Tainan 70101, Taiwan

Jung-Der Wang
Department of Public Health, College of Medicine, National Cheng Kung University, Tainan 70101, Taiwan

Tzu-Yuan Chao
Department of Urban Planning, National Cheng Kung University, Tainan 70101, Taiwan

Yi-Fang Tu
School of Medicine, College of Medicine, National Cheng Kung University, Tainan 70101, Taiwan
Department of Paediatrics, National Cheng Kung University Hospital, College of Medicine, National Cheng Kung University, Tainan 70403, Taiwan

Tzu-Ching Sung
School of Medicine for International Students, I-Shou University, Kaohsiung 82445, Taiwan

Chia-Ming Chang
School of Medicine, College of Medicine, National Cheng Kung University, Tainan 70101, Taiwan
Division of Geriatrics & Gerontology, Department of Internal Medicine, National Cheng Kung University Hospital, Tainan 70403, Taiwan

Oliver Gruebner
Department of Geography, Humboldt-Universität zu Berlin, Berlin 10099, Germany
Epidemiology, Biostatistics, and Prevention Institute (EBPI), University of Zurich, 8001 Zurich, Switzerland

Sarah R. Lowe
Department of Psychology, Montclair State University, Montclair, NJ 07043, USA

Martin Sykora
Centre for Information Management (CIM), School of Business and Economics (SBE), Loughborough University, Loughborough LE11 3TU, UK

Ketan Shankardass
Department of Health Sciences, Wilfrid Laurier University, Waterloo, ON M5B 1W8, Canada

SV Subramanian
Department of Social and Behavioral Sciences, Harvard T.H. Chan School of Public Health, Boston, MA 02115, USA

Sandro Galea
School of Public Health, Boston University, Boston, MA 02118, USA

Mélissa Généreux
Eastern Townships Integrated University Centre in Health and Social Services—Sherbrooke Hospital University Centre, Sherbrooke, QC J1G 1B1, Canada
Department of Community Health Sciences, Faculty of Medicine and Health Sciences, Université de Sherbrooke, Sherbrooke, QC J1H 5N4, Canada
Sherbrooke Hospital University Centre, Eastern Townships Integrated University Centre in Health and Social Services, Sherbrooke, QC J1J 3H5, Canada

Angela Eykelbosh
National Collaborating Centre for Environmental Health, Vancouver, BC V5Z 4C2, Canada

Viktor Glantz
Institute of Clinical Sciences, Department of Surgery, Sahlgrenska Academy, Gothenburg University, 40530 Gothenburg, Sweden

Phatthranit Phattharapornjaroen
Institute of Clinical Sciences, Department of Surgery, Sahlgrenska Academy, Gothenburg University, 40530 Gothenburg, Sweden
Department of Emergency Medicine, Center of Excellence, Ramathibodi Hospital, Mahidol University, Bangkok 10400, Thailand

Lina Dahlén Holmqvist
Institute of Medicine, Department of Molecular and Clinical Medicine, Sahlgrenska University Hospital, 40530 Gothenburg, Sweden

Emily Ying Yang Chan
Nuffield Department of Medicine, University of Oxford, Oxford OX37BN, UK
Collaborating Centre for Oxford University and CUHK for Disaster and Medical Humanitarian Response (CCOUC), The Chinese University of Hong Kong, Hong Kong SAR, China
JC School of Public Health and Primary Care, Faculty of Medicine, The Chinese University of Hong Kong, Hong Kong SAR, China
GX Foundation, Hong Kong SAR, China
Accident & Emergency Medicine Academic Unit, The Chinese University of Hong Kong, Prince of Wales Hospital, Hong Kong SAR, China

Zhe Huang
JC School of Public Health and Primary Care, Faculty of Medicine, The Chinese University of Hong Kong, Hong Kong SAR, China
Collaborating Centre for Oxford University and CUHK for Disaster and Medical Humanitarian Response (CCOUC), The Chinese University of Hong Kong, Hong Kong SAR, China

Sida Liu
Collaborating Centre for Oxford University and CUHK for Disaster and Medical Humanitarian Response (CCOUC), The Chinese University of Hong Kong, Hong Kong SAR, China
GX Foundation, Hong Kong SAR, China

Tiffany Sze Tung Sham and Tayyab Salim Shahzada
JC School of Public Health and Primary Care, Faculty of Medicine, The Chinese University of Hong Kong, Hong Kong SAR, China
GX Foundation, Hong Kong SAR, China

Kevin K.C. Hung
Collaborating Centre for Oxford University and CUHK for Disaster and Medical Humanitarian Response (CCOUC), The Chinese University of Hong Kong, Hong Kong SAR, China
JC School of Public Health and Primary Care, Faculty of Medicine, The Chinese University of Hong Kong, Hong Kong SAR, China
Accident & Emergency Medicine Academic Unit, The Chinese University of Hong Kong, Prince of Wales Hospital, Hong Kong SAR, China

Shelly L.A. Tse, Kin On Kwok and Pui-Hong Chung
JC School of Public Health and Primary Care, Faculty of Medicine, The Chinese University of Hong Kong, Hong Kong SAR, China

Caroline Dubois
GX Foundation, Hong Kong SAR, China

Rajib Shaw
Graduate School of Media and Governance, Keio University, Fujisawa 252-0882, Japan

Index

www.ingramcontent.com/pod-product-compliance
Lightning Source LLC
LaVergne TN
LVHW082153200926
848484LV00008B/2153

* 9 7 9 8 8 8 7 4 0 1 6 9 0 *